Effective Behavior and Human Development

Fred McKinney
University of Missouri, Columbia
Raymond P. Lorion
Temple University
Melvin Zax
The University of Rochester

Effective Behavior and Human Development

Macmillan Publishing Co., Inc.
NEW YORK

Collier Macmillan Publishers
LONDON

To: Margery Mulkern McKinney

Printed in the United States of America

Macmillan Publishing Co., Inc.
866 Third Avenue, New York, New York 10022

Collier Macmillan Canada, Ltd.

Library of Congress Cataloging in Publication Data
McKinney, Fred, (date)
Effective behavior and human development.

Bibliography: p.
Includes index.
1. Adjustment (Psychology). 2. Developmental psychology. 3. Psychiatry. I. Lorion, Raymond P., joint author. II. Zax, Melvin, joint author.
III. Title.
BF335.M18 155.2'4 75-9582
ISBN 0-02-379340-6

Printing: 1 2 3 4 5 6 7 8 Year: 6 7 8 9 0 1 2

Preface

Some time ago the senior author published *The Psychology of Personal Adjustment*. The book was timely and reflected the concerns of an earlier generation of students. It attempted to present the basic principles of psychology and mental health in a readable and personally relevant form in order to aid students in understanding human behavior. Since the appearance of the third edition of that book, wide-ranging changes have occurred in American society and hence in the needs and interests of students. *Effective Behavior* is a new book by an expanded authorship that seeks to present principles of mental health in a way that is helpful to understanding current behavior patterns.

Two goals have guided the preparation of this text. First and foremost, the concepts presented must "make sense" to the student. If students cannot relate what is presented in the text with what is happening to them and those around them, genuine education cannot occur. Thus, wherever appropriate we have included case material reflecting "real life" manifestations of the concepts presented. Naturally the names and other identifying characteristics of the persons described have been carefully screened out in order to protect their right to privacy. Each case, however, has been selected because of the generalizability of the experience described therein. Hopefully, the reader will approach each case with interest and with the intellectual curiosity needed for understanding human behavior.

Second, the student should be provided the basic tool with which to analyze and understand adjustment. We have therefore begun with a general overview of the psychological variables involved in behavior. In addition to consideration of motivational, coping, and learning processes, we have also included the sociopsychological roles each of us experiences as a member of a given sex, racial, socioeconomic, and cultural group, as background variables necessary to understand human adjustment.

Living involves growing and adapting to new situations. Thus we cannot speak of behavior as effective and ineffective without specifying more accurately the nature of the demands to which it responds. In doing so, we have chosen to discuss adjustment within a developmental framework that provides the reader with a more accurate representation of how people adapt to their changing realities.

Any discussion of adjustment must provide as contrast and reference point those forms of behavior and adaptation commonly referred to as "emotional problems." Here we have given an overview of the major diagnostic categories of mental illness. Additionally, we have considered resources that are available to help individuals deal with their emotional difficulties as well as to maximize their sense of accomplishment and fulfillment.

To aid students in organizing the range of topics presented, we have included study objectives at the opening of each chapter. Since the "technical" jargon of mental health professionals is often confusing, key terms pertinent to the theme of each chapter are given at the end of the chapter and a glossary is given at the end of the book. Hopefully, these aids will make the reader's movement through the text as efficient and informative as possible.

We are indebted to many individuals for their contributions to this text. As in such efforts, the questions and comments of students played an important role in shaping our thoughts about the material considered. The contributions of Judy Rabe Erfling, Janice L. Neumann, Charles Clairborne and John Kersting, Antoinette Pickering, Thomas L. Sexton, and Peggy Thompson were particularly helpful. Additionally, a number of colleagues reviewed and critically commented upon earlier drafts of the material, including Lance Baugh, Kenneth Brown, Robert Dolliver, Joseph Doster, Jerry Fryrear, Mark Thelen, William McReynolds, and especially, A. W. Hillix. To our families, who lived with us during the development of the manuscript, and to our secretaries, who silently bore the brunt of our obsessions, we express sincere appreciation.

F. McK.
R. P. L.
M. Z.

Contents

Part I
General Factors in Adjustment

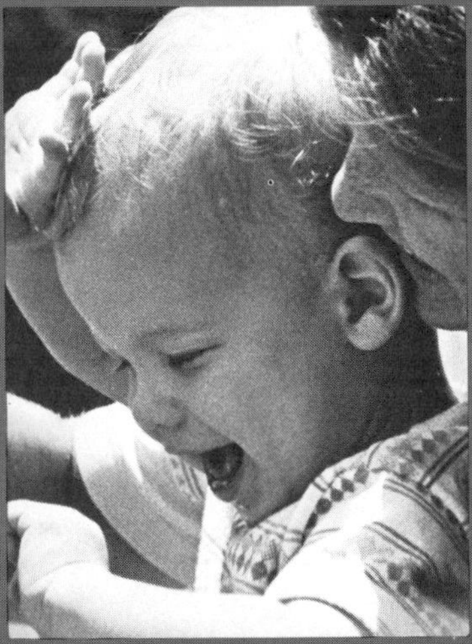

1. Aspects of Adjustment

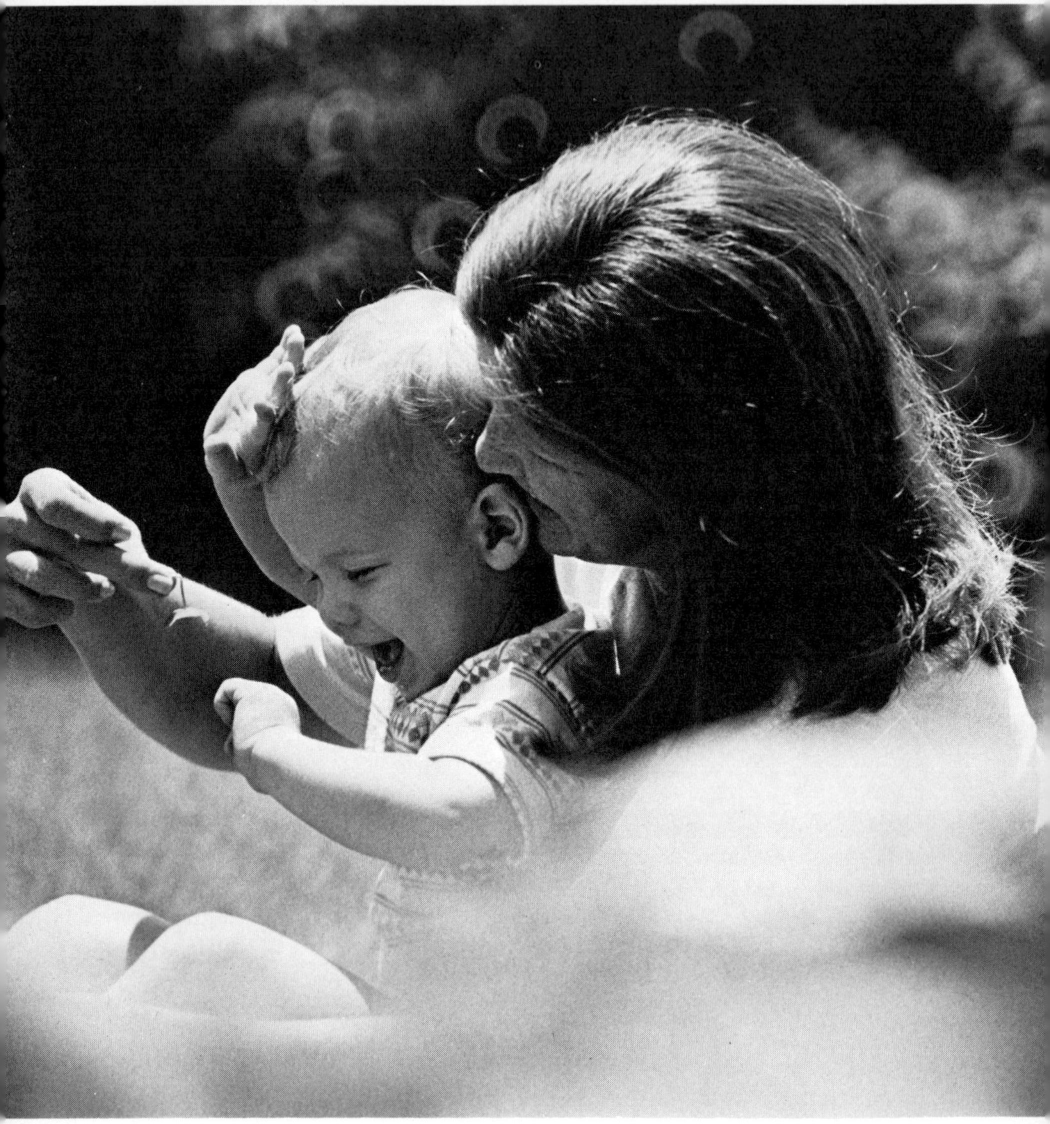

Photo by J. Brian King

Objectives

After studying this chapter the reader should be able to:

1. Describe the general relationships between stimulus and response in explaining human behavior.
2. List the five components in the motivation-adjustment sequence.
3. Identify each of these components in the two case descriptions provided.

In line with our notion that a case study brings alive the abstract concepts that underlie behavior, we introduce Larry and Katherine, some of whose characteristics may resemble those of someone the reader may know. From the information provided in the case studies, we will attempt to understand their patterns of behavior in terms of certain psychological concepts.

Examples of Behavior Problems

The Case of Larry

Larry was a nineteen-year-old sophomore student in an introductory course in psychology when we met him. There was nothing notable about him when he strolled into the classroom with other students. He was somewhat below average in height, smiling, and sociable in manner. If we might say anything about him, he seemed to have more initiative and to be more alert than the average student. At his fraternity house, he was one of the first to come up and greet visitors, and his open, friendly manner in a social situation made him an ideal host. Only on closer, individual contact did Larry's open, outgoing behavior seem somewhat overactive and tense and his social manner forced.

Academically, Larry fared well. He was bright and earned superior grades. He had time and energy to participate in a number of campus activities—including dramatics—and served as an officer in his church's student group. He enjoyed a variety of activities: classical music, tennis, swimming, and golf, and—to the point of provoking his fellow students—controversial discussions.

Larry seemed to be well accepted by his peers. He was more individualistic than most of the other members of his fraternity. He didn't feel compelled to adopt the exact style of clothes that was in vogue on the campus or to mimic the behavior that was accepted in his conformity-oriented fraternity. He did not limit his friendships or activities to his fraternity brothers. He dated regularly, but was never seriously linked with any coed. In general, he seemed self-contained and self-assured.

In discussing himself, Larry rated his standards as very high. Although philosophical about his failure to measure up to these ideals, he kept trying to achieve them. His standards evolved in the context of a close and affectionate family life. He was an only child. Both parents demonstrated their love for him and concern for his growth, encouraging the development of his talents and interests. Larry was well liked by his contemporaries—a fact that he knew pleased his parents—and he was chosen for positions of leadership both in grade school and in high school, although he was always one of the smallest boys in his class. Larry always regarded himself as less mature than most of his classmates, but apparently he experienced no difficulty in being the superior person he thought his parents expected him to be.

From what we already know, Larry seems to be a model of good adjustment. He is rather good-looking, superior in his course work, active in extracurricular activities, quite popular with his fellow students, among the upper 3 or 4 percent of the student "leaders" in the university, and a person of character and conviction.

In spite of these favorable external factors, less than ten years out of college, Larry suffered an emotional episode that required hospitalization. The only previous clue to this possibility was his score on a personality adjustment inventory, which described him as "emotionally maladjusted." (This score means that he checked more statements reflecting anxiety and psychoneurotic symptoms than about 85 percent of the persons who had taken the test.) His answers revealed many subjective attitudes that not many of his friends and acquaintances would have suspected—moodiness, self-depreciation, and feelings of inferiority. Although he knew the implications of his inventory scores and had an opportunity to discuss them with the psychologist (a friend) who administered the inventory, he did not take advantage of this opportunity. Like many people, he sought professional help only after his emotional episode forced him to do so.

After college, Larry had joined the army for four years. Once he left the service, he accepted a job teaching in a small college where his students were predominantly male. He failed miserably in his lectures, despite a long history of successful performances before audiences. He experienced such extreme stage fright, with heart palpitations, heavy breathing, and general discomfort, that he finally had to discontinue lecturing and ask for a leave of absence. He entered a veteran's psychiatric hospital *only* after his dean insisted that he seek professional attention.

Our information about Larry in the period after hospitalization and psychotherapy is meager. What little information is available suggests that he had become more frank and realistic. Also, the gap between what he wanted to be and what he perceived himself to be had narrowed. He returned to his original vocation (accounting) and to his many human contacts and seemed to be functioning efficiently. He had a lifetime of effective habits and relationships that could be used in dealing with events and himself.

Hypothetical Analysis of the Case of Larry

What did Larry's symptoms of extreme stage fright and aversiveness in talking to his predominantly male class indicate? Since Larry had always evaded knowledge of his inner life, it is doubtful that he clearly perceived or sought to analyze the conflict that underlay his panic. In his earlier college days, he apparently could quiet these anxieties by busying himself in study or some extracurricular activity. Now, the classroom, his major source of achievement, required him to prove himself before men younger than himself, which provoked such intense anxiety that he could not function as a lecturer. He had previously developed the skills of dealing with audiences, but no audience aroused such anxiety as this class of young male students. This audience was different; it held a threat for him, a threat he did not want to analyze and that had no objective, realistic basis.

Can we hypothesize that Larry feared that his students would perceive the source of his inner anxieties? Was he concerned over the fact that he had not married, at an age when many of his associates and contemporaries had? Did he worry that his attitudes toward women were different from theirs—a difference that was evident to his students in his lectures? Did he fear that they might reject him and derogate him as their teacher? Larry may have felt a deep-seated conflict between his ideal for himself and his partial perception of his real character. If this conflict existed, it generated anxiety; and much of his behavior—even his achievements—may have been a defense against this disturbing anxiety. We might hypothesize that what he really wanted was self-acceptance, love, warmth, and acceptance by others. He could best obtain these responses by open, nonanxious, self-accepting behavior, which he seemed more capable of exhibiting after hospitalization, psychotherapy, and a lapse of time. Prior to this, his behavior was more defensive—an avoidance of his conflict that also prevented his achieving the kind of acceptance he deeply needed.

Our information about Larry is too limited for a thorough understanding of his emotional difficulties. His early history and later emotional problems illustrate, however, that an individual may display a surface appearance of good adjustment and yet not reveal his actual quality of inner maladjustment, which may be severe. Larry's case demonstrates a belief commonly shared by psychologists that how a person perceives himself plays a vital role in his adjustment. Larry learned rather early to ignore the problems of his inner life and, despite his apparent rejection of conformity, to emphasize the achievement of social and academic skills. Whereas Larry appeared frank and open, there were many aspects of his inner life that he evaded, not only in discussion, but—more important, we hypothesize—in his thoughts. These evasions centered particularly on his assessment of himself as a physically forceful man and on his own impression of his ability to give and receive love from women.

What can an understanding of Larry tell us about personal adjustment and the capacity to control one's behavior? The concepts that help us to understand Larry—*conflict, anxiety, repression,* and *defensiveness*—are a part of the general theme of this book. Understanding these concepts will help in explaining problems in adjustment, whether you perceive them in yourself and others or in the discussions that develop in this book.

Before moving to questions and explanations, let us examine another case—that of a girl who is extremely attractive, somewhat moody, an enigma to her friends, and a problem to her parents.

The Case of Katherine

Katherine is a twenty-year-old junior with sophomore status. She is tall, slender, and when she is well groomed, one of the most attractive girls on campus. Yet she has had relatively few dates in her college years. When she came to the counselor she was a member of a small sorority, but had spent two years on the campus as an independent. (At this university, at the time Katherine was enrolled, status as an independent was socially limiting.)

Katherine has superior ability, but her grades and study habits ranged erratically from the lowest to the highest level. She had a number of acquaintances, and at times she was rather close to them, but most of her associates had difficulty understanding her as a person. She was somewhat aloof when meeting new people. In her discussions with a counselor, she reported that she knew people did not like her when they first met her and that she was scared, tense, shaky, and unable to say the right things. It seemed that she felt socially unsure because of her lower-middle-class background.

She admitted freely to the counselor that she was aware of a number of problems besides that of self-consciousness. She described her work habits as "fitful"; that is, she would work hard for a time and then for a longer time could not bring herself to study. Another problem was a basic uncertainty, which affected every area of her life. She had changed her vocational aims several times since she entered the university. She also left the campus in the middle of the year at one time, to the bewilderment of her parents and her few acquaintances on campus.

During the course of one conference she realized that the source of many of her difficulties was that she did not want to grow up. In recalling her childhood, she could not name many playmates. Apparently, she did not get along well with contemporaries even then. She had an older sister whom she tried to imitate in every detail, even though she felt they were basically different. She described her sister as popular, outgoing, and well integrated and herself as a "willful individual." She was, she said, spoiled by her family in childhood. They tolerated her childish temper tantrums and insubordination, and made excuses for her immature behavior at school when the school authorities reported it to them.

She attended a parochial school during high school, and there she formed two warm friendships. With time, her associates disillusioned her by violating the ideals she had formed with the sisters. In college, she deviated somewhat from the rigorous pattern she wove for herself when younger. She had recently broken away from the Catholic church—an action that deeply disturbed her devout family. In her counseling sessions she reported nightmares, some consisting of dreams in which her mother and sister were horribly mutilated—so shockingly that she wakened.

Katherine's parents both worked so she could have a superior education. They are capable people who have taken advantage of their opportunities to improve their social status. They seem to be competitive, highly conscious of social standards, wish to conform, and place great emphasis on an upper-middle-class appearance. Undoubtedly their plans for Katherine would have enhanced not only her own status but theirs as well. Apparently, she rebelled against them.

In the conferences that followed Katherine's failure to take her degree, the conflict between her attitudes and those of her parents emerged as a long-standing, usually unexpressed, struggle. At times her parents had been very impatient with her, did not understand her, and scolded her for what they termed her shiftless, moody, and dreamy nature. They could not tolerate her unwillingness to strive for the good grades she might have earned with her aptitudes. Although she freely admitted that all they said was true, she did not realize that her problems resulted from her poor social and emotional adjustment. She defended herself with the statement that she does not understand herself. She perceives herself as egocentric, easily hurt, and quick-tempered. It was apparent that she often retreated into daydreams to live in an idealized world where, she said, life proceeds according to some order. She admitted that she was much happier when she was away from home.

Katherine did not graduate because, despite her high ability, she failed a course in her senior year. This failure, along with her uneven record throughout the preceding years, destroyed her chance to earn a degree. When they learned of Katherine's failure, her parents were outraged. Unable to go to college themselves, they had invested their hopes and money to provide their daughter with advantages they had been denied. They came to the campus for the commencement exercises, although they knew that the ceremonies would not include their daughter. They had interviews with her instructor and the dean in hopes of influencing them. Their plea was that this graduation meant so much to them. In view of their many sacrifices, the university officials ought to allow Katherine to get a passing grade in the crucial course so as to graduate with her classmates.

They showed great distress, even to the point of weeping, which deeply embarrassed Katherine. She knew she did not deserve to graduate; she told the instructor that there was nothing she could have done to bring herself to study the material in the course (child psychology!). She seemed to want to destroy her chances to graduate, even though she knew her failure would hurt her parents profoundly. She too was in tears during the conference, and somewhat hysterical. She did not blame herself or her instructor, as her parents did, but she now blamed her parents for not understanding her and not accepting the situation objectively and coolly.

In retrospect, Katherine's life was woven of paradoxes and conflicts. She was strongly attracted to boys, but had very few dates. She was bright, but made poor grades. She had much advice and encouragement (which she called "prodding") from her parents, but behaved contrary to all their urgings and wishes. She refused to openly recognize her strong hostility toward her family, but in her dreams, was actively aggressive toward them. She apparently had difficulty integrating the subculture in which she had developed and the subculture in which she now lived.

Hypothetical Analysis of the Case of Katherine

Again, many questions are raised by Katherine's crisis, the answers to which require more facts than are available to us. We should know her parents' attitudes and behavior during her development, the coercion she felt, and the conditions that produced her low self-esteem. What was the source of the attitudes and behavior by which she opposed the standards of her parents' subculture? This opposition was not conscious and deliberate, but it was effectively obstructive. Her whole personality fought and subverted the goals her parents held up before her and urged her to attain. Torn by these severe conflicts, she was unable to do what she thought she wanted to do. She said, finally, that she hardly knew who she was as a person.

Let us hypothesize about Katherine's unhappiness. Similar to Larry, she was a victim of inner conflict and external pressures. She retained habits that had served her well in childhood but were self-defeating in young adulthood. She perceived herself as not fulfilling her ideals or her parents' expectations. Not understanding these differences and their bases, and unable to behave in a way that would satisfy her ill-defined motives, she became anxious. She defended herself against anxiety by retreating into daydreams and by her obstinancy. The aggressiveness against her family, as reflected in her dreams, was possibly an expression of her frustration and anger, caused by the pressures her parents brought to bear upon her to live the kind of life they had planned.

We have no information on Katherine after the commencement episode. We can, however, on the basis of available facts discuss her strengths and weaknesses for future coping. Much of her problems stemmed from her parents' possessive attitudes and her financial dependence upon them. She seemed to adjust well with her female peers and had the potential for developing in her relationship with men. She still had attitudinal problems which events could help her change. Since she now has an opportunity to become independent of her parents financially, she is in a better position to cope effectively with her problems.

Understanding Behavior

Does contemporary psychology help us to understand behavior like Larry's and Katherine's? It does so only partially. In their present stage of development, psychology and other behavioral sciences do not have—nor do they claim to have—answers to all the problems that can be raised in considering an individual's adjustment to life. Even if all the laws of human behavior were known, we would seldom be able to amass all the information necessary to apply them to an individual case. True, many people now understand more about human behavior and—more important—their own behavior and how to direct it, because they have been aided by psychologists and other behavioral scientists. These workers are continually trying to explain human behavior and to test these hypotheses in the clinic and in the laboratory. Through their efforts, we now have available a body of knowledge and techniques to help people understand the sources of their problems and the means to resolve them. We may anticipate many further refinements in methods and concepts. Let us examine a few of the basic ideas and concepts that are now being used to explain behavior.

UNDERSTANDING ANTECEDENT CONDITIONS

One idea strongly supported by psychologists is that *behavior is lawful and determined.* It doesn't just happen; it has antecedents. The antecedents are, to be sure, highly complex, and we do not always recognize or understand all of them. We do know some important facts about the general classes of antecedents. For example, we say with certainty that Larry was the kind of person he was because of his heredity and the environmental influences that *interacted* with that heredity.

Our understanding of the relationship of even such general classes of antecedents (causes) as heredity and environment is still seriously limited. To extend these limits, when a person comes for advice, we try to get from him as much reliable information as possible about his family and social background, his behavior in infancy, his relationship with his immediate family, and the other close relationships he has had throughout his life. We perceive him as an individual with genetic potentials and limitations that have constantly been *interacting* with events in his environment that are both favorable and disturbing to his well-being. The environmental forces with which he interacts can be more readily known than his genetic resources. He is, in all circumstances and events in his life, an individual with a constitution that is genetically (by heredity) and experientially (by environment) determined. These complex factors are the antecedents to—the causes of—his present behavior.

STIMULUS AND RESPONSE

A second fundamental tenet is that, once we understand the reasons for certain responses, we can change or select antecedent conditions that produce the responses we want. Conversely, we assume that undesired behavior can be altered by removing its causes.

One important kind of antecedent event is a *stimulus.* One common definition for a stimulus is: "A situation or event either within or external to the organism that is responsible for the organism's response." This definition is very general and inclusive. The ring of the alarm clock, the sight of a grade on an exam paper, a whiff of a memorable perfume, a twinge of pain are all stimuli, according to this provisional definition. For Larry, his lecture class was a complex stimulus for an extreme anxiety reaction; for Katherine, schoolwork was a complex stimulus for withdrawal and daydreaming.

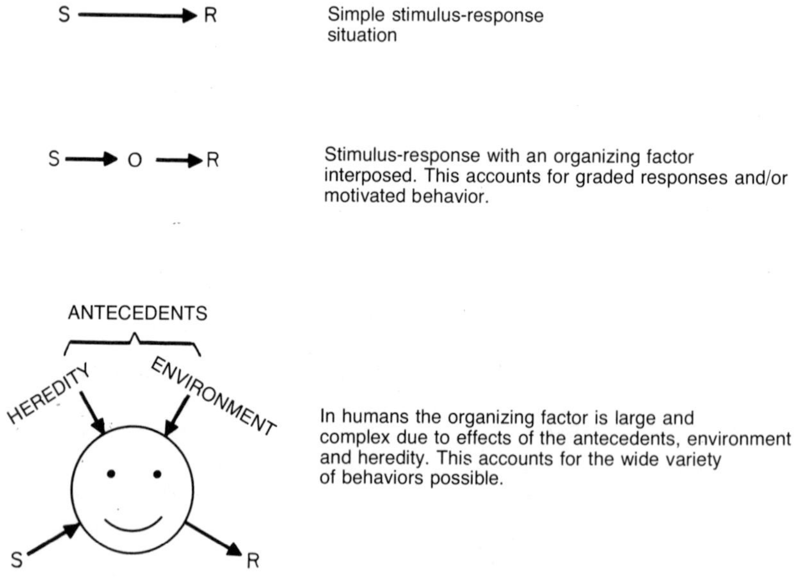

Figure 1–1

Response, the second term to be defined here, may be an activity of the organism, including conscious and unconscious experiences. Some responses are clearly controlled by identifiable stimuli. Although actions are not obviously related to stimuli, we assume that these responses are controlled by unidentified stimuli. (See Figure 1–1.) The increase in heartbeat as one makes love, the relaxation of muscles as one lights his pipe, relief as one awakens from a nightmare, the smile at the approach of a friend—all are examples of direct responses to stimuli. Much of the research and discussion in this area centers on clearly identifiable and measurable responses that are the results of similarly recognized and manipulable stimuli. Other researchers attack more complex internal behavioral patterns (such as thinking, feeling, etc.) that cannot be studied as precisely as simple responses to stimuli.

MOTIVATION AS DIRECTING RESPONSES

The human being, in the thinking of some psychologists, is more than a *reactive* organism. He is also an organism who acts in keeping with his own motivations. This becomes apparent when you reflect that, in your daily activities, you do more than merely react to the many stimulating situations that confront you. You, yourself, initiate some of your actions. Behavior is so complex that many stimuli, some of which cannot be identified even in an experiment, are responsible for what you do. The effects of the unidentifiable stimuli have given rise to the assumption that man is *active* as well as reactive. For example, he displays curiosity and exploration in infancy that are not responses to specific stimuli.

Another factor in understanding behavior is the *meaning* of the stimulus. A student group carrying protest signs means idealism to many activists but disruption to the Dean of Students. Meanings are most significant in the individual's behavior, for they accompany and *regulate* responses to stimuli.

We are trying here to understand complex behavior, to discover the situations that bring it about, and to make careful observations that will lead to valid generalizations about how people adjust. Clinical psychologists speak less often of stimuli and responses and more often of *patterns* of interrelated, well-established behaviors. For example, Katherine's self-consciousness was a pattern of behavior, complex in nature, which occurred as a response to the stimulus-patterns associated with the particular people who elicited that response. Yet Katherine's behavior was far more than a set of *reactions* to stimuli, however patterned and complex. She was an *active* individual with personal traits and dispositions. She actively refused to make (or so it seems to an observer) the expected responses to many situations presented by her parents, family, school, and religion. This behavior was inconsistent with her verbal acceptance of the ideals she expressed. Because of her unique individual traits, her dreams were very difficult to analyze, despite the fact that the dreams seemed to maintain a consistent pattern of responses to stimuli.

In Katherine's behavior the operation of unidentifiable stimuli is apparent. The antecedents of such reactions are often considered in terms of the concept of motivation.

Motivation influences the meaning of behavior and refers to the central *driving and directive* forces of individuals. Chapter 2 is devoted in part to a discussion of motivation, but here we present a skeletal, overall model for behavior that can be used and modified throughout the book.

Motivation-Adjustment Sequence

As a loose but useful framework to help in understanding the behavior of people, we present the "motivation-adjustment sequence," which we have divided into five categories: (1) motivation, (2) frustration and conflict, (3) satisfaction, (4) variable and nonadjustive behavior, and (5) readjustment and satisfaction.

MOTIVATION

When we observe *persistent activity* that ends with some kind of *consummatory sequence,* we usually speak of the person as "highly motivated in that area of behavior." For example, if a young man plans a physical improvement program, uses his summer's earnings to buy weight-lifting equipment, and devotes many regular hours to exercising with bars and weights, he is certainly highly motivated in this area. His improved posture, musculature, and general health are the results of his persistent activity and unflagging motivation.

But when we examine his motivation, we must have certain information that falls into three categories: (1) What were his physical condition and attitudes *before* he undertook his program of self-improvement; did he feel that he lacked good musculature, or did he admire some athlete? (2) Has he *kept up* his program and is he pleased with his progress even though it has been inconvenient to exercise at times and has interfered with more desirable activities? (3) When he discusses his program, is he as enthusiastic about it as when he started, and is his enthusiasm for the activity itself or for the *results* he is getting? If there are discrepancies between these points, we may have difficulty in evaluating his motivation.

Some motives may be extremely short-lived. You are interested in the outcome of yesterday's election; you usually pass by the newsstand near the campus without making a purchase, but today you stop and buy a paper and thus satisfy your curiosity. Others may persist over such a long period of time that we speak of them as "personality characteristics," "traits," or "inner structure." We may say that someone is "ambitious," "shy," or "paranoid," rather than that he is persistently motivated toward a particular goal, that he tends to withdraw from particular persons, or that he inappropriately interprets words and actions as being directed toward him. In these terms, Larry was motivated to retreat from the classroom because of his intense anxiety while lecturing; Katherine was motivated to daydream rather than to study or to engage in social activities.

In the remainder of this chapter we use a broad concept of motive, one that includes highly persistent characteristics along with less long-lived ones. In the next chapter, we will hone our conceptual tools to more sharpness.

FRUSTRATION AND CONFLICT

Physical need and the action it arouses (e.g., hunger in the evening, for example, and eating to satisfy that hunger) may be blocked or frustrated for some reason. To continue our example, there may be no all-night lunch counter in the neighborhood, or you may not have any money. We also have needs that are frustrated by long-term and sometimes remotely related lacks. A young man's desire to make good as a salesman, to appear confident and present convincing arguments when he meets his customers may *conflict* with a long-standing shyness or a fear of rebuff by contemporaries or older people. A collegian who feels a strong need to be popular may find that his tendency to be aggressive in social situations and to be caustically critical of the ideas and behavior of others conflicts with his affiliative need. As these examples show, goal-directed behavior does not always result in satisfaction. Environmental conditions and other motivations that are incompatible with the ongoing motivated behavior may block the motivation. Blocked motivation is called *frustration;* if the blockage is due to other incompatible motivations, it is called *conflict.*

Larry's story suggests that he had a strong need for favorable recognition by his associates and for success in courses and extracurricular activities. On the surface he seemed satisfied with his high grades, his honors, and his extracurricular pursuits. His concept of himself evidently conflicted, however, with the ideal he wished to attain—apparently a primary conflict that undermined his personality with later disastrous results.

Life's realities thwarted Katherine's wishes to reach the ideal she held. The events of everyday life did not fit her ideal pattern. She tried, in an unrealistic, halfhearted way, to win success through excelling in college. She failed, either because her skills were not well applied or for reasons that lay deeply buried in her personality. We have suggested that her behavior was rebellious and covertly aggressive, as though she wanted to hurt her parents or herself.

Motivated behavior, then, may be blocked by environmental situations that prevent the individual from reaching his goals or by other opposing motivation. *Frustration* and *conflict* lead to aggression, anxiety, and other complications.

SATISFACTION

On the other hand, much motivated behavior reaches its goal. A student lives in a dormitory with meal service. He feels hungry at mealtime, so he joins the line in the cafeteria and gets food. Larry, with strong motivation to achieve, had developed good work habits as well as effective ways to deal with people and was satisfying his goals before his deeper conflicts intensified.

The satisfaction that comes through the achievement of goals removes or reduces the motivating condition and relaxes the tensions that are associated with striving toward the goal. The individual might then be said to be adjusting to a given motivation. We are satisfying motives all day long; we eat, sleep, buy what we want, find our way to destinations, see friends, succeeed in tasks we attempt, or watch our favorite programs on television. If the motivations that are primary to a person's life are satisfied periodically through his own striving, he is, very likely, a happy person and is regarded as a well-adjusted and emotionally healthy individual. We shall see later, in greater detail, that the behavior that satisfies motives is usually *learned* and that through such satisfaction effective habits and attitudes become established.

VARIABLE AND NONADJUSTIVE BEHAVIOR

For some goals the behavior is not readily available to reach them. This was true of both Larry and Katherine. Neither achieved the satisfaction they sought. We usually try to achieve our goals, even though they may be blocked or may conflict with each other. This striving behavior may be random or highly variable. *Variable behavior* is valuable in the adjustment of the individual because it may, by chance, result in acts that satisfy a motivation that has been frustrated. On the other hand, it may lead to behavior that satisfies the individual at the moment but arouses other problems. We can say that some of our activities relieve tension and are completely satisfying; others are only partially satisfying. They may produce adjustment temporarily but later create new problems or maladjustments. Larry was quite successful, as measured by his scholastic achievement and social adroitness. However, this partially satisfying behavior did little to reduce the basic unhappiness he experienced over the discrepancy between what he wanted to be and what he was.

Katherine, in modeling her life after the nuns who taught her in her early years, had not built the attitudes and habits her materialistic parents demanded of her. Her failure to meet their goals and their constant dissatisfaction with her resulted in *nonadjustive behavior,* such as daydreams, nightmares, moodiness, and shiftlessness. This variable behavior was nonadjustive because it reduced her self-esteem and caused her associates to perceive her as a disturbed and confused girl.

Under frustration or conflict, then, the individual may employ variable behavior. For Larry, some of this variable behavior was clearly self-defeating, while other behavior disguised his basic and deeper conflicts. Nonadjustive behavior is often the frantic attempt, on the part of the frustrated or conflicted individual to gain relief from anxiety and unpleasantness. Variable behavior may take the form of destruction, daydreaming, apathy, or stereotyped or mechanical responses. The individual may revert to behavior he exhibited in similar situations as a young child. Just as a temper tantrum may make the individual feel better at the moment but worse later, variable behavior may also yield immediate reduction of anxiety but produce undesirable consequences later.

Shaffer and Shoben (1956) point out that this self-defeating behavior, which we have called nonadjustive, is *nonintegrative.* Although it may bring partial and immediate satisfaction, it does not lead to satisfaction of the whole individual. It does not result in a unified personality. On the contrary, it often produces greater problems. Katherine, by daydreaming or sinking into a mood, could fence herself off from people who might, if she were more communicative, have reminded her of her incompatibility with her surroundings. But the daydreams and moodiness, while they defended her from reality, also prevented her from productive activity and social life and thus added to her long-term unhappiness.

Throughout this book we shall examine personal and social problems that are illustrative of nonadjustive or nonintegrative behavior. Alcoholism is a clear example of just such nonadjustive behavior. An individual experiences distress, anxiety, or some other unpleasant state. In his attempts to find relief, he discovers the alcoholic world of blunted perceptions. Drunkenness helps him evade immediate problems, but may create others. He spends money for liquor that he needs for other things, he jeopardizes his reputation and perhaps his employment, and he causes distress to those who are close to him. Other examples of nonadjustive behavior are attempted suicide, drug addiction, withdrawal from society, depression, and prolonged and ineffective hostility. An activity evolving from conflict may, then, be adjustive with respect to the motive at hand, but it may be nonadjustive so far as other motives are concerned. Here we come on a curious but important fact: Much behavior that seems abnormal, incongruous, or socially unsuitable is actually adjustive from one standpoint. It is nonadjustive or nonintegrative in terms of its incompatibility with other motives or in terms of its conflict with prevailing social standards. Yet it does satisfy still other motives that are just as vital to the individual's well-being. Behavior is truly nonadjustive if it leads to subsequent problems and conflicts and prevents the integration of the whole individual. If you reflect on the cases of Larry and Katherine, these points become clear.

READJUSTMENT AND SATISFACTION

If the nonadjustive, nonintegrating behavior leads only to more unhappiness, the individual must seek a new way of adjusting, a more adequate means of satisfying his motives. When Larry finally had to resign from his position and place himself in professional care, he realized the need to change his behavior in some ways. We refer to such a program of change as *readjustment*. Similarly, when Katherine failed to graduate on schedule and precipitated a crisis in her family, she began to recognize that much of her behavior was self-defeating and that it was necessary that she change her habits. In each case, a crisis suggested the need for a change in attitudes and habits, the elimination of self-defeating practices, and an acquisition of habits that would yield more lasting satisfaction. An individual may, through variable behavior, discover these new adjustments himself. But he may need to seek help from someone else—possibly someone in the helping professions, a counselor or psychotherapist. Potential sources of readjustment will be discussed later in the book.

SELF-CONCEPT AND ADJUSTMENT

In discussing Larry and Katherine we have emphasized an *objective* analysis in terms of certain psychological concepts. We have also indicated that they at times took an active part in their adjustment, especially an awareness of their own identity. We will further explore the self-concept in Chapters 2 and 6, particularly one's self-esteem, or how one feels about himself. We shall be interested in one's perception of himself and its closeness to his ideal self. These are important subjective factors in adjustment.

Summary

1. A brief analysis was made of two cases of real persons experiencing difficulties.
2. A frame of reference some psychologists use in understanding behavior—lawfulness of behavior, stimulus, response, and motivation was presented.
3. An initial and very brief outline of the motivational sequence was offered: what happens to the individual when he is motivated in a given direction; how his motives may be satisfied or reduced in intensity; how they may be frustrated or are in conflict with other motives; and finally, how readjustment and satisfaction come about.
4. One's self-concept is an important factor in his adjustment. This is discussed fully later.

Words to Remember

Adjustment
Conflict
Frustration
Motivation
Nonadjustive Behavior
Nonintegrative Behavior
Readjustment
Response
Stimulus
Variable Behavior

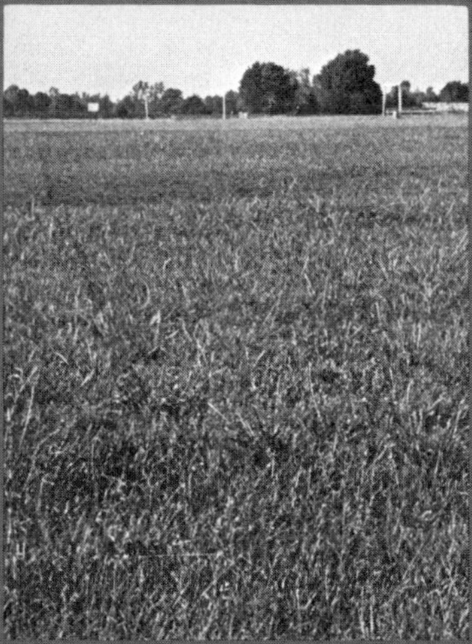

2. Motivation

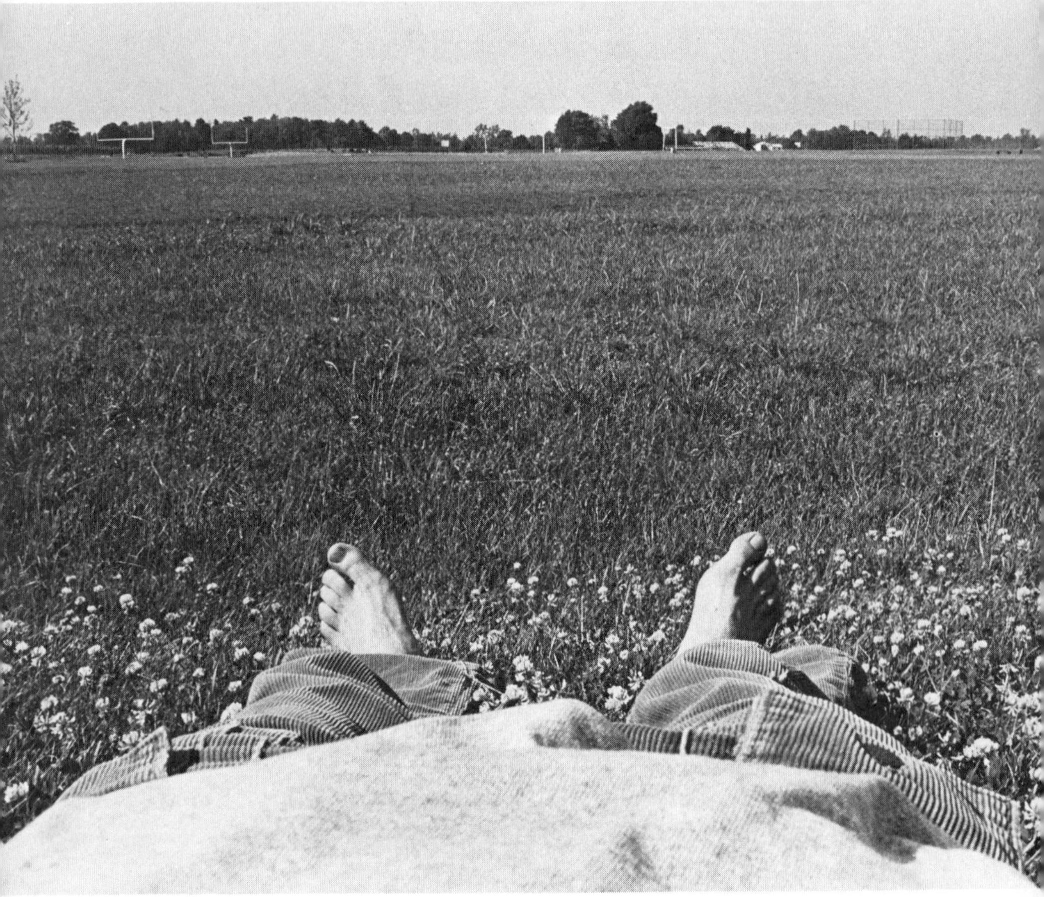

Photo by Andy Franklin

Objectives

After studying this chapter the reader should be able to:

1. Describe motivation in terms of stimulus and response.
2. List several examples of conscious and unconscious motivation along with corresponding examples of motivated behavior.
3. Identify motivation factors in the accompanying case studies.
4. Define "self-actualization."

To introduce our discussion of motivation, brief descriptions will be made of two college men who sought counseling. Their backgrounds and experiences will be drawn on to illustrate many principles of motivation which will be taken up.

CASE STUDIES

The Case of John

John was an 18-year-old sophomore psychology major in a large Midwestern university. Graduating in the middle third of his high school class, he had transferred from a small college, where he majored in physical education. John was the second of three sons in a working-class family. His father, a handicapped retiree, had been unable to complete the eighth grade. His mother, a housewife, finished high school. John came to the University Counseling Bureau because, as he explained, he was uncertain about future career decisions.

The striking aspect of John's appearance was his full beard and the conspicuous protest buttons which he proudly displayed as evidence of his self-proclaimed identification as a "hippie." In discussing his life-style, John explained that he hoped that by adopting the "hippie" subculture and philosophy, he might "find himself." He admitted smoking marijuana since high school and described the "philosophical" awareness and semi-religious experience he had while taking LSD.

John seemed quite comfortable in discussing with his counselor his confusion about his future. A major source of concern for him was his parent's opinion of his life-style. He was strongly attached to them and felt some guilt that the values he had adopted might disappoint or hurt them. Yet John said that he was searching for some meaning to his life and for his place in the world. He felt lonely and alienated from everyone, including those within his adopted group. Since he began using drugs regularly, he had lost all desire for academic achievement. He wanted to establish a close, intimate relationship with someone, yet was unable to give of himself. John explained to the counselor that he felt lost and unsure of how to gain direction in his life.

The Case of Paul

Paul, a 19-year-old sophomore, entered the university as an honors premed student. Both parents had attended college. His father was an engineer; his mother a housewife. He had one sister in high school. Although he graduated in the upper third of his high school class, his university grades were too low to place him in the honors program after his freshman year. He sought counseling because of his apathetic attitude toward school achievement.

The counselor described Paul as a young man of average height and slightly heavy build. In dress, grooming, and general neatness he was below the average male university student. Highly verbal, his speech was, nonetheless, somewhat flat and expressionless. Paul obtained only average grades, cut classes frequently, and was not achieving his academic potential. His vocational aspirations were in medicine, yet he realized that his mediocre college record jeopardized his reaching this goal.

Both Paul's parents and girl friend were disturbed about his apathy. In recent months, he had been in trouble with the police on a serious traffic violation which was complicated by additional charges of drinking and underage possession of alcohol. Paul's relationship with his girl was yet another source of conflict for him. He strongly desired the security and warmth of being with her, but his demanding behavior had caused her to become cool and distant.

Paul described his depression as so intense, at times, that he had considered suicide, but had not attempted it. He was also sleeping more than usual. His relationship with his family was becoming increasingly stressful, with frequent and sometimes violent quarrels. His father's criticism about his grades and lack of religious beliefs ended with name-calling. Paul felt that his parents expected a great deal of him, and were very critical of his behavior. In general, Paul seemed unaffected by opinions others held of him. He showed little realistic planning and had only vague plans for the future.

Aspects of Individual Motivation

We stated in Chapter 1 that the term *motivation* is used for (1) the *arousal,* or *energizing,* aspect of behavior and (2) the *directive* aspect. We also pointed out that motivation is important in understanding behavior. In seeking to understand someone, the following question may be useful: Is he satisfying important motivations (needs), or are they frustrated or in conflict with other motivations? If frustration and conflict obstruct his motivation, he may develop nonadjustive behaviors that lead to increased difficulties. As will be discussed later, when motives are frustrated or blocked, responses like aggression, anxiety, and various defense mechanisms may develop.

In the case histories of John and Paul, it is apparent that each is unable to satisfy his motives. Paul was a high achiever, yet he is no longer in the honors program, and it appears that his grades will bar him from medical school. This is clearly a frustration of his achievement motivation. John has strong interpersonal drives such as succorance (needs aid from others), nurturance (protection of another) and heterosexual needs —but is lonely. He wishes to maintain close ties with his parents, but he has adopted a life-style they cannot accept. He too is in conflict. We may hypothesize that the need frustration of both men is, in part, related to their unhappiness.

Often we notice that people behave much differently under apparently similar circumstances. For example, John and Paul reacted quite differently to the stresses of being college sophomores with highly concerned parents. Their responses differed because the situation evoked differing pressures in each of them—pressures that related to the complex pattern of their motivations. As we begin to understand how individual motives develop and relate to the conflicts that people experience, some of the reasons for their individual reactions will become clearer.

Biological Needs and Learning

In addition to an individual's psychological needs (e.g., aggression, affection, achievement, etc.), he possesses biological needs. The latter are particularly prominent in the first years of life. A baby's early behavior is directed by hunger, thirst, and physical discomforts (e.g., pain, changes in temperature, wetness). These conditions reflect physical deficits—an obvious example is hunger—and the individual, through his activity, attempts to make up for these deficits. In so doing, he learns certain skills and attitudes that may be reflected in later behavior. Biological needs represent primary drives and are the bases for the development of later motive patterns. For example, continued frustration of primary drives may produce a strong need to have any drive responded to immediately. The interaction between inner bodily states and environmental pressures often produces specific adult behaviors that are socially important—friendliness or withdrawal; courage or fear; meekness; concern or indifference. Modern advertisers and merchants clearly recognize the power of these motives and spend vast sums of money to associate a certain product with the primary drives of hunger, thirst, sex, and pain reduction. Behavioral scientists have also recognized the strength of such motives in attempting to describe behavior.

Murray (1938) discusses human motivation in terms of needs. Since behavior may be aroused either by *internal* (hunger, a physiologic need) or *external* events (a sight or sound), a need may follow either kind of antecedent event—internal or external. Activity in response to a need is continued until the internal or external environment is somehow changed to satisfy the need. For example, a gregarious person becomes restless and irritable until he sees an acquaintance and can talk to him. Needs then may be associated with particular emotions or feelings and may serve to elicit specific behaviors that bring about the desired alteration of environment. *This arousal and direction of behavior by a need is what we mean by motivation.*

Murray (1938) defined five criteria that are useful bases for inferring needs. For example, hunger brings about (1) the desire to achieve a certain end result—satiation; (2) a definite behavioral pattern—eating; (3) a selective response to a particular class of stimulation—eating soft food; (4) the expression of a particular emotion or affect—pleasure; (5) the expression of (a) satisfaction when a given effect is achieved or (b) frustration when it is not achieved.

Constitutional Influences on Motivation

In considering the differences between John's and Paul's response to their situation, it may be appropriate to ask: Are there any influences in their basic physical constitutions—in terms of anatomy, physiology, or biochemistry—that, in conjunction with early environmental experiences, may have engendered their early preferences, aversions, enthusiasms, and dreads? It is certainly easier for some people, because of their unique natural equipment, to become (in a favorable environment) interested in art, music, athletics, or other people. It appears that basic temperamental qualities—tendencies to be active or quiet, to respond quickly or slowly, and to differ in mood—observed in infants continue throughout life. As individuals, we are apparently more responsive to certain environmental stimuli than to others. This persistent selective process contributes to our development as the kinds of persons we are in early adulthood.

Murphy (1947), in his attempt to understand personality, begins with a consideration of the individual physical constitution. He observed that:

> Some children turn toward lights, sounds, and touches more actively than others. Color preferences are distinct in early infancy. . . . Small infants differ considerably in the kinds of sounds to which they make positive orientations, and vary strikingly in their interest in sounds in general. . . .

> Individual kinesthetic differences are suggested by comparison of active and passive, rhythmical and non-rhythmical, fine-muscle and large-muscle users, activity-streamers and stop-and-goers (p. 74).

We differ, then, in our early sensory receptiveness, the degree and kind of activity we initially demonstrate, and in levels of arousal. There is some evidence, for example, that individuals characterized by extremely low arousal levels or extremely high levels are more susceptible to breakdowns in adaptive behavior (Sechrest & Wallace, 1967). Thus early predispositions affect the direction our behavior takes. As they interact with various specific environmental influences and experiences, our behavior becomes more selective. We no longer want just food, but ham or gum; no longer do we want mere activity, but soccer or chess.

Nondeficit Motivation

Experiments with basic drives have shown that we are motivated by deficit. If deprived of food, water, or rest, we engage in behavior that might satisfy these needs. We approach those objects or conditions that could relieve us. When we have eliminated the deprivation state we have achieved *homeostasis* (i.e., physiological equilibrium in the organism). When we run, breathing and heart rate increase, thereby keeping within allowable limits the oxygen available to our tissues; when we are cold, we shiver, and thereby keep our body temperature within limits. All such actions help to restore the body physically or chemically to a state of equilibrium, and are thus homeostatic mechanisms.

Are we motivated solely to reduce tensions produced by physiological need states or, in the absence of such needs, may the individual also seek new experiences, explore and manipulate his environment? Maslow (1954) distinguishes between two kinds of motivation: One group of motivations seeks to reduce "deficit" and the other to achieve "growth." Maslow suggests that as one satisfies deficit motivation, he feels more secure, is less self-centered, and is freer to reach out beyond himself. Even early in life the child is motivated by something besides hunger, wet clothing, cold, or thirst. He plays with his fingers and feet; he observes and enjoys toys and rattles. He devotes hours to explorations and manipulations of his world and develops valuable skills as a result (White, 1959). A child less than one year old already approaches stimuli that are colorful or novel (Berlyne, 1966). As soon as he is afoot he is curious and explores much of the household. John adopted a particular life-style to "find himself," since his growth need was apparently not being adequately met.

Much of this nondeficit-related, spontaneous behavior leads to new abilities and to the development of complex needs. One who has enjoyed music all his life will find that when his days are filled with routine activities and he has little opportunity to hear or play music, he has a conscious need for it. Former athletes are glad to get out and throw a ball when they are away from the game for a while. Thus, since early activities shape later needs, the conditions in the family which encourage the child's natural inclinations to explore, manipulate, and exercise his developmental potential are very important. For both John and Paul, family pressures to achieve success became early determinants of behavior and of later adjustment difficulties.

The two forms of motivation, deficit and nondeficit, differ in an important way. While the psychogenic needs can become excessive, they weaken with deprivation. On the other hand, increasing deficit strengthens *biogenic* needs. The longer an animal is without food, the more fiercely (within limits) he tries to get it. (See Figure 2–1.) In the case of a psychogenic need, the probability of satisfaction is an important factor in the effort one puts forth to satisfy it. For example, Stagner (1965) points out that as a black worker realizes that a sense of job security, status, and prestige is unattainable, he may divert his energies to needs more readily satisfied.

Variety of Adult Motives

Walk into a large magazine store and glance over the periodicals on the racks. You will find a publication related to nearly every interest, hobby, amusement, and recreation. Add to these books all habits, attitudes, goals, drives, and physiological states that *arouse* or *direct* behavior, and you begin to see the range of human motivation in our culture.

The wide range of motivation can, in part, be understood in terms of a person's age group. The major interests of the "normal" adolescent differ obviously from those of the first grader. The later adolescent has his interests and directions; the young married person his; the middle-ager his; and the aging citizen differs in some respects from them all. New motivations constantly replace those motives that were previously important.

Behavior has consequences, and the consequences maintain or disrupt that behavior. The sailing enthusiast doesn't have to eat fish (satisfy an innate drive) to maintain his sailing behavior, but he must experience pleasant sensory events associated with wind, sun, and sea in order to maintain it. Adult behaviors are susceptible to change because the reward systems are not usually related to primary biological drives.

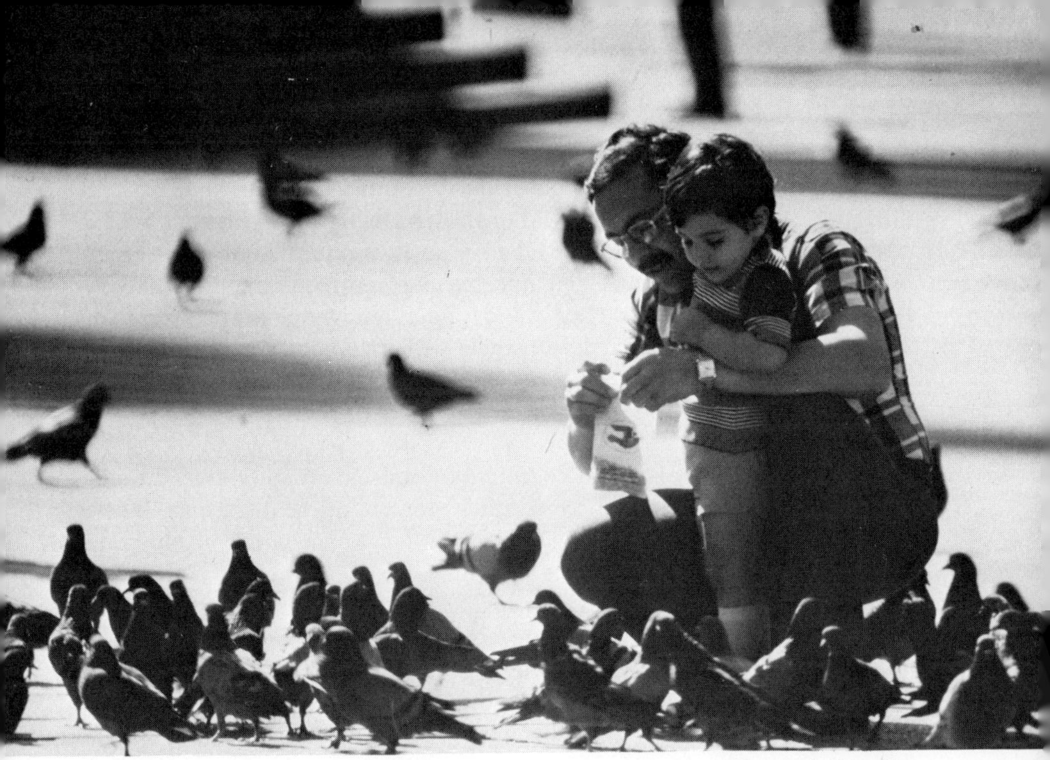

Photo by J. Brian King

Figure 2–1 Feeding the Birds.

Conscious Aspects of Motivation

Great attention has been paid to the drive or motorlike nature of motivation. However, when you ask the average student to name his outstanding motives, he will usually refer to ones that are conscious in nature. He is aware of his hopes, plans, and intentions—to marry the right person, to gain happiness, to find the most suitable vocation, or to gain worldly success. We know we want to "get ahead," to be prepared for a better job, to help other people, to make more money, to improve in amateur sports or some leisure pursuits. We are aware of the fact that we need other people and want to work with others for a cause or, on the other hand, we want to spend little time in social gatherings.

For most of us our awareness of goals, aspirations, intentions, ambitions, fears, and concerns are significant determinants of when, where, and what we do. Simply stated, such awareness is the *why* behind much of our behavior. We think about what we want and set out to achieve satisfaction for such conscious motives. Yet, as will be explained more completely later, more subtle, *unconscious* processes may also influence our behavior patterns. Typically, *unconscious* motives arise from early experiences in which needs are frustrated or, for reasons to be reviewed in later chapters, denied. When behavior is guided by such unconscious motives it often appears maladjusted and leads to further conflict and frustration. For example, Paul consciously wanted to achieve success, yet other motives, related to his relationship with his father, hampered his efforts. Hence, in understanding behavior it is important to pay attention to both the conscious and unconscious motives directing that behavior. Neither John nor Paul could understand why they continually acted in ways that conflicted with their verbalized goals.

LEVEL OF ASPIRATION

Psychologists have studied cognitive or conscious motivation through the experimental examination of the process of goal setting. These studies are concerned with research in the *level of aspiration* that characterizes a person's performance on a task. Simple tasks, such as solving arithmetic problems or throwing rings at pegs, are presented to the subject, who is then asked to estimate how many problems he can solve or how many rings he can get on the pegs. His answer tells us something about his level of aspiration. After he states his estimate, the subject begins the tasks and observes his actual performance level. (See Figure 2–2.)

Such studies have identified a number of variables that are related to the subject's estimate of his performance. Past success or failure is an important factor. Sears (1940) reports that children who have a past history of success tend to set more realistic goals than children who have had little success. The latter group of children, by contrast, tend to set goals that are too low in order to avoid failure or set goals that are so unrealistically high that they could not be expected to succeed. A person's reaction to past experiences plays an important role in his motivation to succeed or avoid failure. Such motivation, in turn, relates to the degree of involvement one has in the task presented. These same variables and tendencies are present in our everyday decisions as we set goals. As will be seen later, our well-being is influenced by our ability to reach these goals.

EXPECTANCY IN MOTIVATED BEHAVIOR

Atkinson (1964) has done extensive research in an attempt to understand more completely what determines a person's level of involvement in a task. His work suggested that motivation to perform on a task relates not only to one's goals but also to the task's particular *incentive* or stimulus and to the individual's *expectation* of achieving success. Atkinson's theory to explain motive arousal states that the person with a motivational disposition to succeed "should work hardest at a task of intermediate difficulty when the outcome has a 50/50 chance of success or failure . . . a task of very high probability of success has low incen-

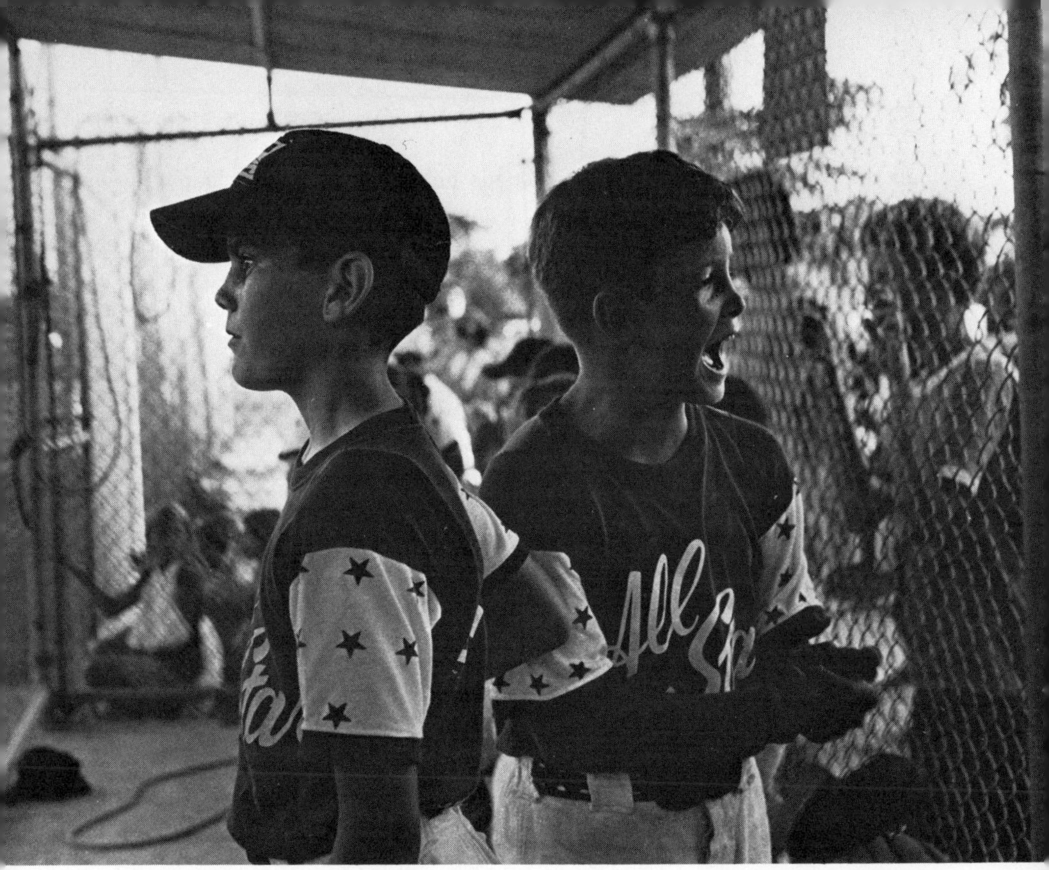

Photo by J. Brian King

Figure 2–2 Aspiring for Success.

tive value, while a task of low probability of success discourages effort even though its incentive value is high" (Hilgard, Atkinson, & Atkinson, 1967, p. 156). We should expect persons who are high in achievement motivation and low in fear of failure (anxiety) to favor tasks of moderate difficulty, to take moderate risks, and to hope thereby for success. On the other hand, those who have low achievement motivation and high anxiety will choose very easy tasks and thereby prevent failure; or they might favor very difficult tasks—a flash of bravado. These ideas, coming from empirical work, should have some significance for everyday decisions such as vocational choices, work styles, and so forth.

Unconscious Motivation

As stressed above, it is important to understand that behavior is influenced not only by conscious decisions but also by aspects of our personality about which we are minimally, or not at all, aware. In a sense, all motivation has an unconscious aspect. No one is completely aware of all the inner forces that help direct his behavior. Nor is it clear why we are sometimes greatly aroused by a given event and at other times not. For example, a friend may make a casual remark that for no apparent reason evokes a hostile response.

Vaguely conscious motives are constantly influencing and being expressed by our behavior. For example, the mild person who rarely gets into arguments may be openly aggressive in his dreams, where he sees people being hurt, but he stands by, unconcerned by their plight. Movie and television programs that express aggression may have special appeal for him. He may be rigidly critical of others' errors and misbehavior and be strongly hostile toward them. This mild person may urge adoption of more severe laws and greater powers for the police and "right-behaving citizens" to enforce these laws and punish violators. These indications of aggression or hostility would astound or shock him if he recognized them as such.

Needs or motives about which our society has a number of taboos (such as aggression or sex) are quite likely to function in an unconscious, or only partly conscious, manner. They may be permitted only indirect, symbolic expression. Clark and Sensibar (1956) conducted an experiment with male college students that dealt with this aspect of our emotional lives. After the subjects had been presented pictures of attractive nude women, they were shown some pictures of neutral content. The experiment was conducted under two conditions: (1) in the classroom, and (2) at a fraternity beer party. In the first condition, the neutral pictures evoked much less expression of overt sexual imagery than they did at the party. The imagery was apparently suppressed in the classroom situation, where, however, indirect or symbolic expressions of sex did occur. At the fraternity party, where there was more evidence of overt sexual imagery, there were fewer indirect or symbolic expressions than in the classroom. There was no need under party conditions to disguise the sex responses and to employ symbolism. Symbolism is accepted as one means of expressing unconscious motivation.

DYNAMIC QUALITIES OF UNCONSCIOUS MOTIVES

Freud dramatized, probably more vividly than anyone else, the *dynamic* qualities of unconscious processes. He argued that the motivation they produce acts as both a guiding influence and an energizing agent in our response to stimuli. We are energetic mainly because we are living beings. This energy, however, varies from time to time, and certain conditions (emotional, for example) intensify behavior because they arouse these unconscious processes. A young man responds far more energetically than usual to the ringing of a phone when he is expecting a girl to return his call. Freud believed that the motivational system is so active that, even when it is apparently dormant, it influences our dreams, errors or slips of the tongue, the forgetting of unpleasant matters, and the specific direction abnormal behavior takes. If this is true, we should expect our self-control and emotional stability to improve if we could give conscious direction to those activities we have brought out of the unconscious.

The idea that directing and energizing factors in our behavior operate without our complete knowledge is disturbing to some people. We have grown up in a culture that teaches us that events happen for logical reasons and that we have "will power" and must be in control of all of our behavior. When we fail to know the reasons behind our own actions, we feel threatened. Freud and his early associate, Jung, have consistently pointed out the seeming irrationality of some behavior (dreams, for example) even in the most rational people. Increasingly, knowledgeable people are accepting the fact that much of human behavior is, in part, guided by unconscious forces. Infatuations, impulsive temper tantrums, and oversights are all examples of behavior with motivational factors of which we are not completely aware.

Knowledge of this unconscious part of our selves, and our attempts to accept and understand it, will lead eventually to sounder self-understanding. The genius of Freud was not his demonstration that behaviors previously thought rational were irrational; rather, it was his demonstration that when we understand the unconscious motives behind them irrational behaviors stand clearly revealed, in all their logic.

Inordinate Motivation

Some motivations are intense and seemingly insatiable states that lack the creative aspect of growth motivation. The person is driven to satisfy such motives but rarely achieves the subjective satisfaction he seeks. No matter what he does, he can never do enough to feel relief. This kind of motivation and striving has the characteristics of self-defeating, nonintegrating behavior discussed earlier.

Horney (1942) observed from her clinical practice that *inordinate motivation* or extremes of normal trends often plague adults and seem to relate to early frustration of basic needs. A few adult examples follow:

1. An extreme need for affection and approval, shown in attempts to please everyone and to be liked and approved by everyone, or in a fear of self-assertion.
2. An intense need for someone, usually a spouse, who will assume all responsibilities; a fear of being on one's own—of having to make independent decisions.

3. A strong tendency to restrict one's behavior and life within narrow borders, as reflected in an urge to save rather then to spend, to remain entirely inconspicuous, or to belittle one's abilities and to overemphasize modesty.
4. A tendency to exploit and to get the better of others, as shown by a great emphasis on power, money, bargaining, or sexuality.
5. A need for perfection, as shown in dread of mistakes or personal flaws.

Among other traits found in personal tendencies in their extreme form are needs for prestige, admiration, personal achievement, and independence.

Inordinate motivation reminds us of defective animals who overeat because their nervous system does not provide the feedback that directs them to stop. This analogous behavior suggests that we may have to examine the *feedback nature* of the behavior that is excessively motivated. Why does not a great deal of affection, power, or the world's goods result in satisfaction and a "turning off" of the need mechanism? Since many of man's motives are learned, it is evidently possible to learn how to begin and engage effectively in a behavior without learning how to turn it off. Special training or psychotherapy might enable individuals with such inordinate motivation to learn when to stop their striving.

The issue of inordinate motivation reminds us that there are problems in motivation besides those of starting behaviors. Motivation to behave is related to the behavior it arouses. This behavior may lead to a goal not easily reached and therefore must be sustained. On the other hand, aroused behavior may bring satisfactions that are short of, and inimical to, reaching the original goal. Social drinking, for some people, leads to inebriation, which makes them no longer sociable.

How often have you heard examples such as the following:

"I wish I really wanted to study."

"I'd like to make good grades, but I just can't get down to the books."

"I usually start the semester with a great head of steam, but it goes down every time."

"I've got to quit eating so much. This blubber I carry around makes me look pudgy."

The first and second students are talking about motivation for *starting* behavior; the third is concerned with *maintaining behavior* after he has started; the fourth is concerned with *stopping* ongoing behavior. Some authors have looked at biological motivations in terms of the analogy of starting, maintaining, and stopping a motor (Dethier, 1964; Premack, 1965). This analogy is also helpful in dealing with more complex psychogenic motivation.

STARTING

Here are some cherished goals: competence in golf or tennis; playing a musical instrument well; having a better functional vocabulary; being successful in amateur dramatics; developing skills that would help to bring about changes in society like the ability to convince people in small or large groups. In many cases the person who desires these goals may subjectively wish to reach them, and know or not know that achieving such goals requires learned skills. The acquisition of these skills requires enthusiasm, emotional arousal, previous success in similar tasks, and appropriate practice. The importance of each of these prerequisites explains why getting started on a complex activity is more difficult than merely wanting to do it.

MAINTAINING MOTIVATION

Sometimes one is fortuitously or spontaneously catapulted into an activity in which he consciously desires to reach some greater competence. The initial enthusiasm for a sport or for some social activity may wane because, at the beginning, competence was at a low level. The beginner may not realize that previously acquired contrary attitudes may inhibit his enthusiasm, or earlier mistakes or fears may discourage him. The disastrous results of his first trials may make him withdraw from the activity, and his initial motivation arousal and enthusiasm may not continue. Can he arrange a more agreeable situation that will help him to maintain his motivation, like working with and being encouraged by a good friend? Positive feedback and reinforcement, success and encouragement are often necessary for the maintenance of ongoing motivated behavior.

STOPPING BEHAVIOR

Some undesired behavior is strongly established—too strongly motivated. Eating fattening foods, smoking or drinking to excess, frequently expressing aggression toward others, and exploiting people are a few examples of behavior a person might want to curtail. How can one check such behaviors? The feedback from these initially satisfying activities may be immediately reinforcing. The later consequences of the behavior is regret or negative social comment.

Recognizing the condition that led to the undesired behavior may help to change it. Introducing negative consequences to follow immediately the undesirable behavior would be effective, but often difficult to arrange. Possibly, the performance of other behaviors incompatible with the undesired behavior can result in the gradual replacement of positive for negative behaviors. In such situations it is best to find professional help, as suggested later in the chapters on learning and behavioral therapies.

Personal Motivation

Recall how an ordinary task can loom large and important when it is somehow associated with your reputation or status as a person or when you become deeply involved in it. A student's study behavior suddenly becomes more intensive and more preoccupying with the announcement of an important quiz, whose results will become part of his permanent record. A student group may have little impact on a member until he becomes an officer with opportunities to initiate plans. Motivations that have a strong self-reference influence behavior much more strongly and more persistently than those that do not.

Another way in which the concepts of motivation and self become intertwined is an individual's discovery of inconsistency between how he regards himself and what he would like to be, which is termed the *self-ideal discrepancy* (see Figure 2–3); the discovery may well motivate him to bring about closer congruence and reduce the discrepancy. A student may find himself carried away by the behavior of a group and do things he could not do as a solitary individual. If the group's behavior is condemned later by his peers or by himself, he is likely to be quite disturbed and think: "I really got out of hand; I was really *not myself.*" This kind of conflict in self-awareness is an example of *cognitive dissonance.* It has motivational power in that it prompts the individual to behave so as to reduce the incongruence. In some way he has to justify his behavior to himself and to others.

Aversions Involving Selfhood

Recall some of your deep dislikes of people, places, and events, as well as the things you hate to do. You may have been embarrassed, shamed, confused, criticized, or frightened by a given situation or person; now this aversion is transferred to similar situations or persons. Many aversive feelings accompanied by avoidance of a stimulus are due to experiences that involved you as a person. In addition to these aversions because of a real experience, there are those that result from a feeling or fear of failure in a certain kind of situation. The youth who avoids athletics may have been kidded about his awkwardness earlier in life. The girl who is terrified by public speaking may never have experienced success on the stage. A boy or girl who has been excluded from a prestigious group may avoid small groups as they gather around the school premises. Any such experience may have induced brooding about one or another aspect of himself. The inclination to withdraw from a complex situation that taps persistently unpleasant memories is an aversive motive, then, and may become associated with one's self as a person. This inclination is especially strong if it is associated with words that are heavily charged with unpleasant emotions, like *nonentity, ineffective, weak.*

Figure 2–3 Self-Ideal Discrepancy.

Photo courtesy of *Columbia Missourian*

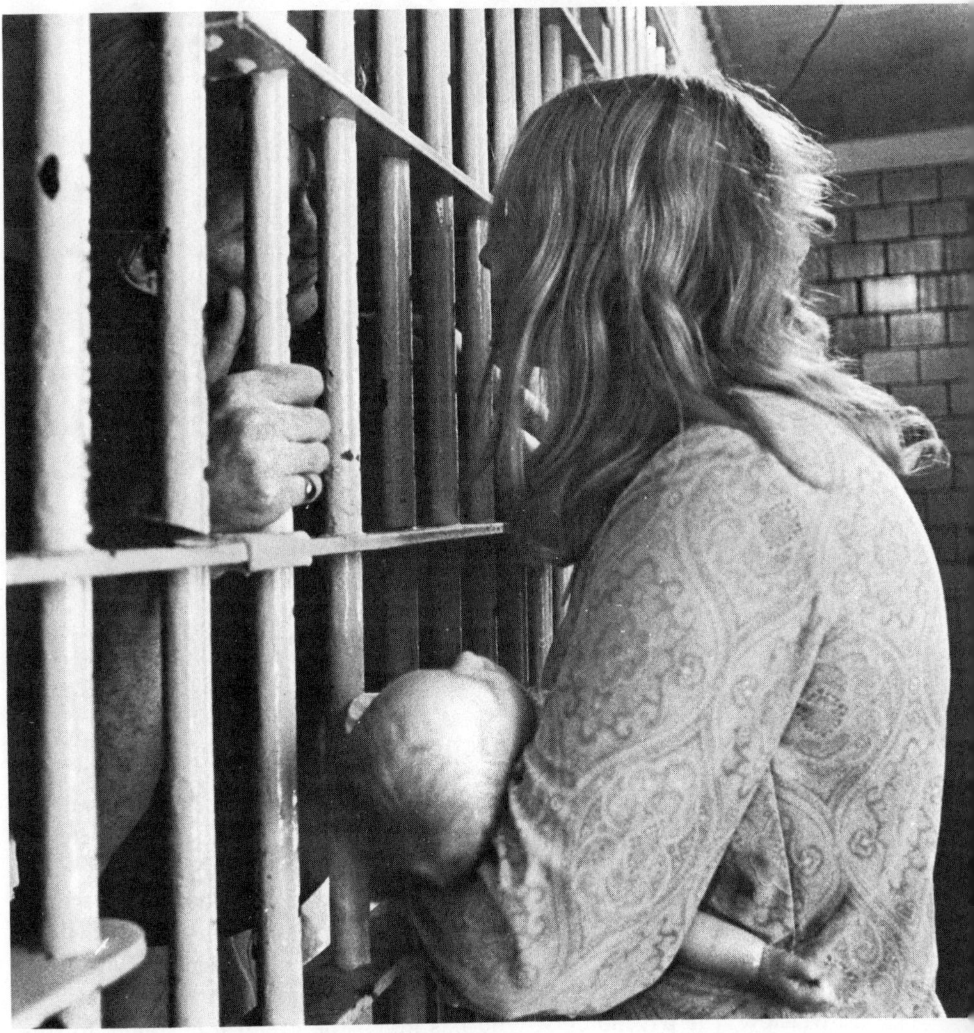

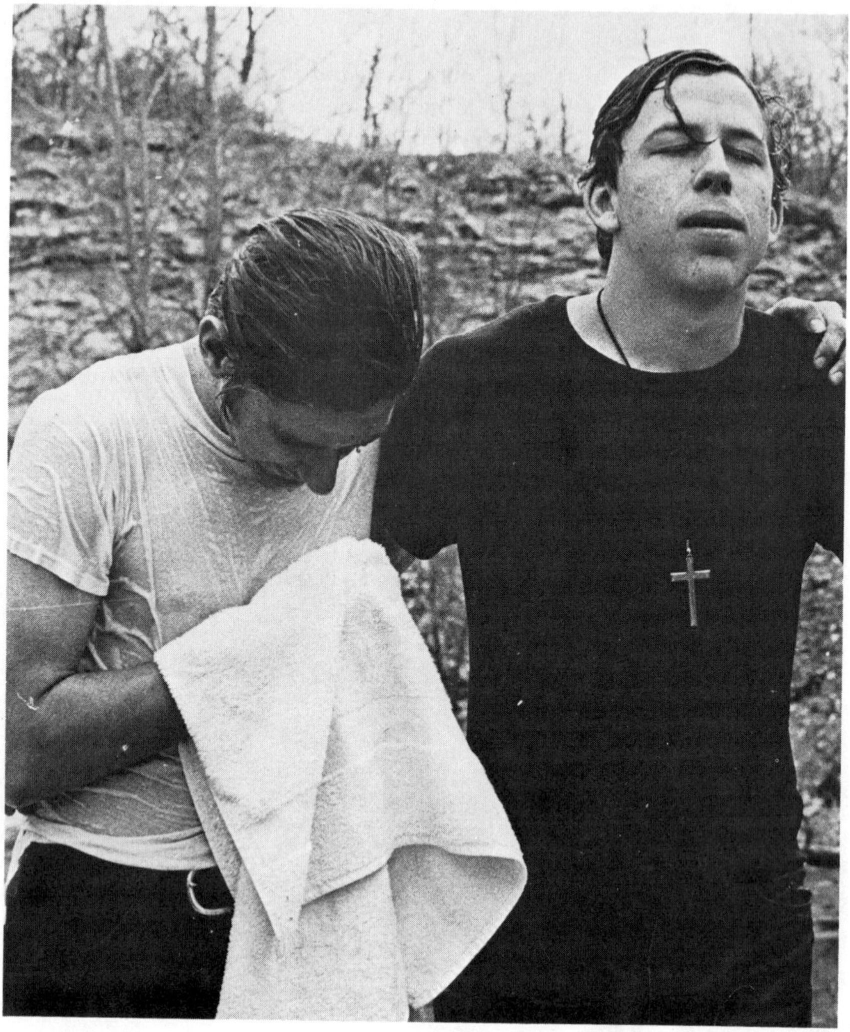

Photo courtesy of *Columbia Missourian*

Figure 2–4 A Peak Experience.

Motivation Toward Self-Actualization

Some motivation is intimately tied up with that which is central to the person as he identifies himself. The hypothesis has been advanced that if physiological and safety needs are satisfied early in life, the individual is able to turn to the satisfaction of other, more creative ventures and develop to his greater potentiality, unity, and individuality (Maslow, 1954, 1962). This development to seek greater fulfillment of one's potential as a person is called *self-actualization.*

Maslow, the psychologist who has given the greatest currency to this concept, has studied individuals who seem to be most self-actualizing and who represent that small part of the population (1 percent) who are emotionally healthiest. They are not only relatively free of symptoms of maladjustment; they also use their talents and potentialities well. Maslow's study of *peak experience* among college students indicated that all of us are self-actualizing some of the time. (See Figures 2–4 and 2–5.) The peak experience is one that stands out in memory as the moment of highest happiness and fulfillment, accompanied by a feeling of wholeness (versus conflict), aliveness, uniqueness, self-sufficiency, and worth. Students have given these examples of peak experiences: warm response from a loved person, listening to music, response to a new place, a gathering with good friends, an accomplishment or recognition, a friend's wedding ceremony. It has been found that the more self-actualizing the person, the more peak experiences he has (Maslow, 1962).

Pause in your reading, and think back over your own peak experiences—those moments when everything was going well, when you felt

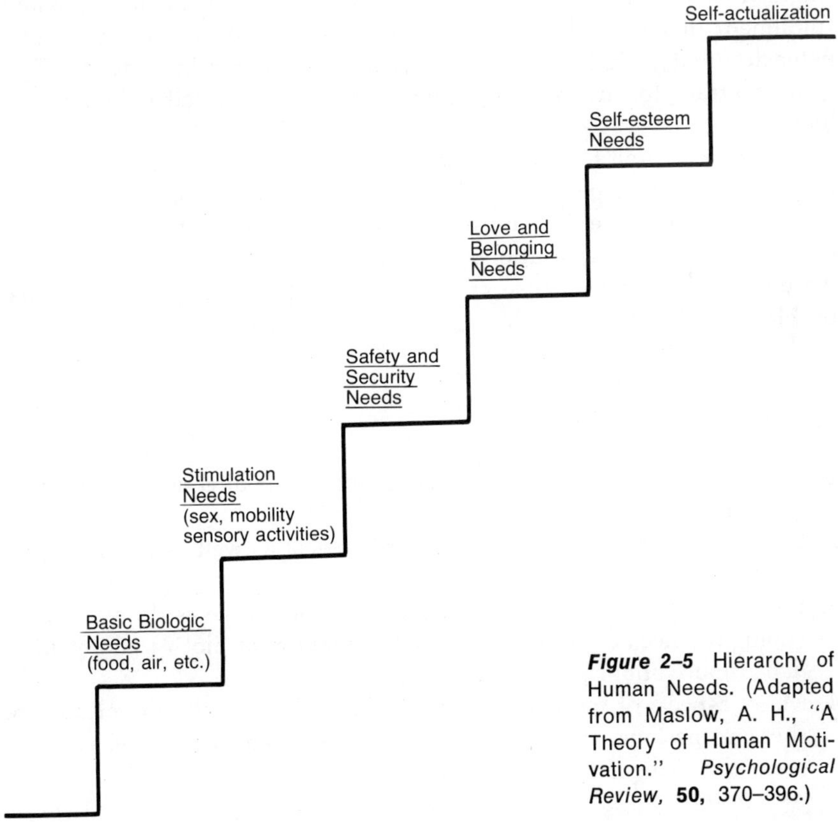

Figure 2–5 Hierarchy of Human Needs. (Adapted from Maslow, A. H., "A Theory of Human Motivation." *Psychological Review,* **50,** 370–396.)

you were a unified person and you were able to accept yourself as a valuable and an integral part of the world around you. Such moments are times of nonstriving and nonself-centeredness.

Several studies indirectly support Maslow's theory. Kaplan and Singer (1963) administered a dogmatism scale, which measures inflexibility, to a group of students and correlated their scores on it with a test of "sensory acuity," in which the subject had to make perceptual judgments. He found a substantial negative relationship between dogmatism and sensory acuity. These data may be related to Maslow's descriptions of the self-actualizer as more efficient in perception of reality.

Another study tends to support the belief that the more self-actualizing individuals have a high degree of emotional stability and better mental health. Knapp (1965) used a personality inventory to measure neurotic tendencies and found negative correlations between a neuroticism scale and characteristics of self-actualization.

Rogers (1951) points out that the individual becomes more differentiated, more expanded, more autonomous, and more socialized as he grows and matures. To actualize one's potentials one must be able to distinguish between progressive and regressive ways of behaving. Obvious fulfillment of potentials is seen in the development of skills and competencies that include social and self-management achievements. This is in contrast to antisocial, egocentric pursuits and self-defeating behavior.

It is time for you to ask what the above discussion of human motivation means to you personally. In what ways do you understand your own motivation better? To be sure, it is early in the project, because we have yet to discuss frustrations or conflicts in motivation. With conflict we find anxiety and defense or, conversely, challenge toward personal problem solving and growth.

Summary

1. Motivation may be defined as the arousal and direction of behavior by a need.
2. Man's motivation can be related to biological as well as psychological needs.
3. Basic biological drives involve *deficits* of some type as do many psychological needs. In addition much behavior is motivated by *non-deficit* motivation.
4. Many aspects of motivation are conscious, but equally important are the unconscious aspects whose presence often causes behavior to seem confusing.

5. Inordinate motivation is reflected in the problems found in stopping behaviors that seem to be maladaptive.
6. When basic needs are adequately satisfied, man seems more likely to seek satisfaction of higher-order needs involving fulfillment of his potential as a person.
7. In considering the motivation of behavior we must attend to its maintenance and cessation as well as its initiation.
8. The destiny of an individual's motivation relates to his attitude toward himself and his fulfillment as a person.

Words to Remember

Biogenic
Cognitive
Cognitive Dissonance
Deficit Motivation
Feedback
Inordinate Motivation
Level of Aspiration
Nondeficit Motivation
Peak Experience
Self-Actualization
Self-Ideal Discrepancy
Unconscious Motivation

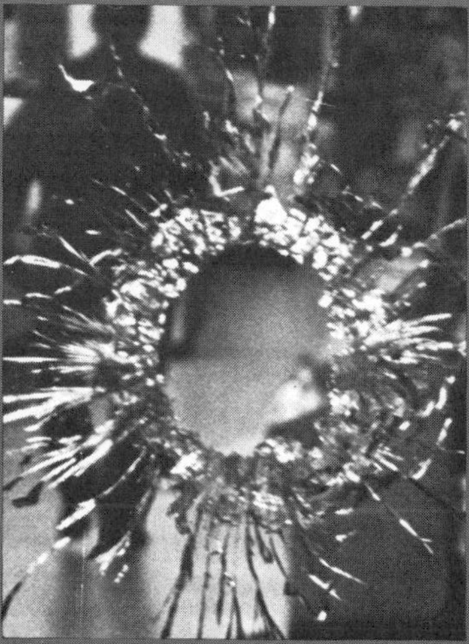

3. Frustration and Conflict

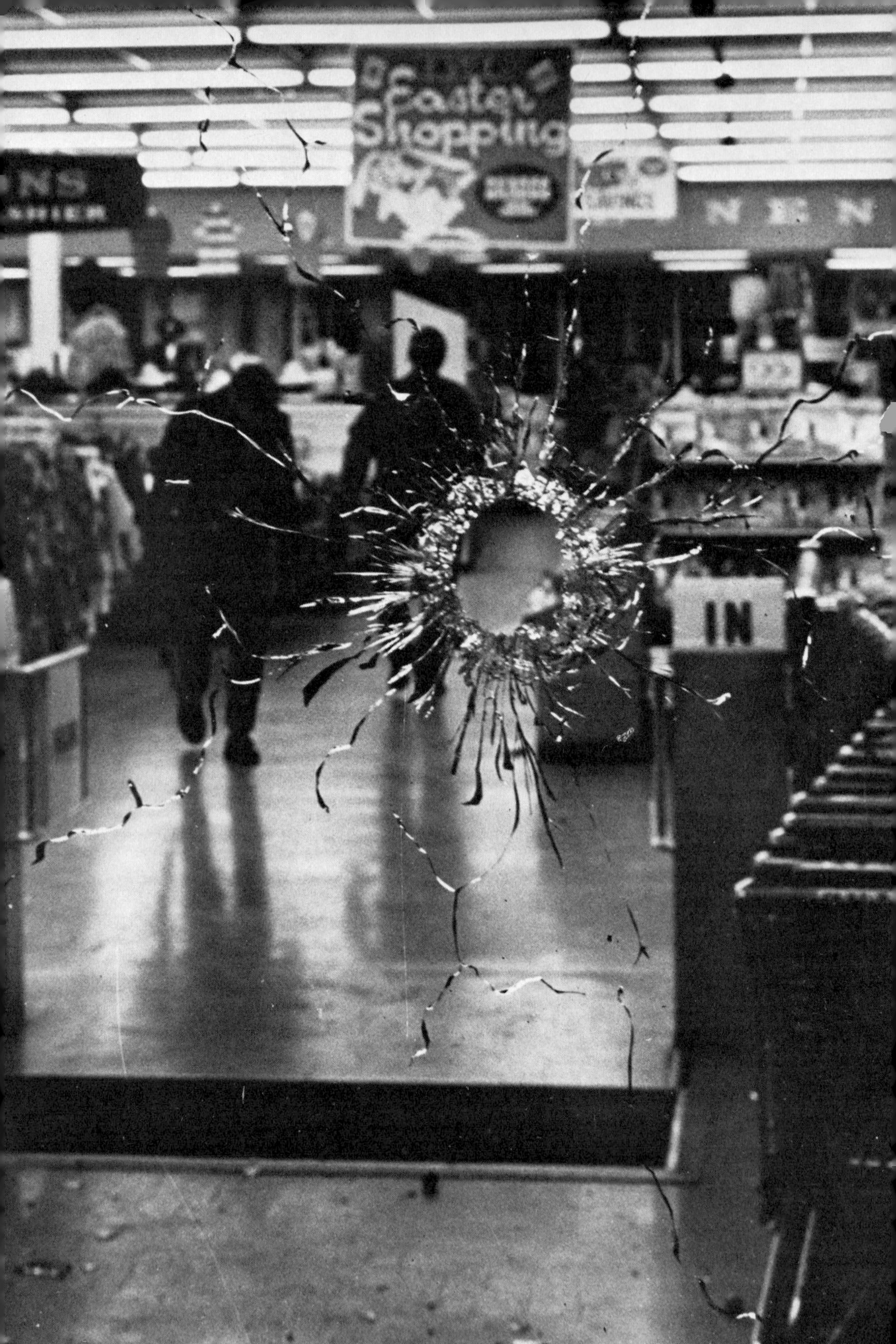

Photo courtesy of *Columbia Missourian*

Objectives

After studying this chapter the reader should be able to:

1. Define *frustration.*
2. Define *conflict* and describe three types of conflict.
3. List some examples of the ways that humans react to frustrations and conflict.
4. List the variables that determine the strength of aggressive response to frustration.
5. Identify the factors of conflict, anxiety, and regression in the accompanying case study.

Frustration and conflict are not difficult to find on the campus. Students' talk amply reflects these feelings:

> "I get C's in German no matter how hard I study."
>
> "I got a nothing part in the play, and I went to every tryout!"
>
> "I like John and we can have fun on a date, but he has these mannerisms and habits that really irritate me."
>
> "I'm no good in anything—looks, sports, the girl department, grades," Marty confides after a few drinks. "And dammit I try. That's the tragedy."
>
> Bill complains, "I like history but that creep that teaches it drives me out."
>
> Jerry thinks human society is in an "awful mess": "We have the bomb hanging over us; we elect congressmen to represent us, but they're more interested in making sure they'll stay on in Washington than in finding the causes of poverty, war and race prejudice and doing something about them. When I join an organization to protest and to attack the stupid establishment, I'm a dangerous radical and my father starts talking about sending me to see a psychiatrist."

Like the above students all of us at times are *frustrated*—blocked in our efforts to get what we want. To be thwarted in certain pursuits either infuriates or crushes us. In addition we are sometimes in *conflict*—an inner frustration—we want what we realize is "bad" for us and we like people who make us uneasy.

We will now look at the frustration and conflict of *motivations*—major and minor—attempt to understand their dynamics, and review how people react to them. We will try to evaluate our responses to frustration and conflict and the role these responses play in the development of personality. Some patterns of response to frustration and conflict, such as escape or defensive behavior, become established ways of behaving and create deeper problems on their own account.

CASE STUDY

The Case of Irwin

Irwin was an 18-year-old freshman when he came for "psychoanalysis," as he called the counseling session. He was expensively dressed and good-looking, but his slight build made him seem no more than 15 years of age. Although he seemed shy and awkward when he entered the office, he talked quite openly. He explained that while he makes a good first impression on people who seem ready to like him, they quickly become cool toward him and seem to prefer others. This pattern has recurred many times—most noticeably at camp and now at college. With considerable emotion, he told how he was elected to a fraternity office soon after he pledged; now he thinks no one in the house respects him.

Irwin, the only child of a large, rich, successful, and prominent family, received much attention and protection from his parents and relatives. Camp and college provided his first opportunities in making his own decisions. Concerned about doing well, he broods constantly over his mistakes. When he learned that he had done poorly in his college entrance ability test, he felt even less capable. In general, he sees himself as inadequate, a self-image that is in *conflict* with the image his parents and relatives have always tried to convey to him.

His self-consciousness makes him think others are critical of him. He finds it difficult to maintain a conversation with his peers. He worries about his reluctance "to look the fellows straight in the eye"; his desire to withdraw to his room alone; and his inability to carry out many of the plans he envisages. For example, he is so sure that a girl would not enjoy his companionship that he backs off from asking for a date.

There is a clear conflict between the *self he perceives* in his group and the *ideal self* he strives for. He does not understand that his social inadequacy is a consequence of a sheltered childhood, which kept him from acquiring social skills.

While he analyzes the motives of others, he rarely evaluates his own behavior in a mature, objective fashion. For instance, Irwin initially tried to explain his interpersonal difficulties as due to anti-Semitic feelings. His experiences at camp and in his all-Jewish fraternity have since convinced him that his difficulties lie within himself.

After a few counseling periods he had a talk with his father, a self-confident, successful man well into his sixties. Irwin's father apparently blocked discussion of Irwin's emotional and subjective symptoms by telling him there was nothing the matter with him, that he was better in every way than most of the boys in the fraternity, and that self-analysis is a poor idea. Yet Irwin continued to feel that he needed counseling and needed it badly. He continually wanted to be told just what to do because he felt that his own efforts were so fruitless. The counselor pointed out how much advice he had already been receiving from others, and that what he needed more than advice was the opportunity to talk out his feelings and act out the behavior of which he was most capable. He asked, "Aren't you expecting to learn new social attitudes and skills at an impossibly fast rate?" This idea impressed Irwin, but the feelings of inadequacy he experienced many times a day were overpowering. He was extremely sensitive to any slight, and sharp comments by any of the more critical fraternity men accentuated this feeling of rejection by the group.

As time wore on and the conferences continued, Irwin became less negative about himself, and tended to be more realistic about his traits and possibilities. When he saw the movie *Doctor Zhivago* he recognized in the central character many of his own qualities, but saw him as much firmer and assured. On the other hand, he felt himself to be cowardly and afraid to face the world. After viewing the movie a second time, Irwin emerged with a number of insights, which he expressed in a letter to the counselor:

"I saw the picture again, and I have come to some definite ideas. I think if you will straighten out these ideas for me I will hit upon something. I believe that I am divided into three parts: *first,* the part that makes me so anxious to make friends that I leave myself open (to criticism). I don't act naturally. I think that everything I do offends someone. I am always afraid that I will do the wrong thing. The *second* part is the bad part—the deep cowardice—the part in which I think that a person is my friend only because of what he can get from me. This is the suspicious part of me—judging things for their money value—the cheap part. This is the part that will not allow me to love anybody, to be true to anybody, because I think that this will lower my status; that people won't like the persons I go with, either boy or girl—the part that looks at people's faults instead of their good qualities and affects my conversation and feelings. Then there is the *third* part—the part that feels that I can't get enough knowledge, the initiative part of me—the part that I hope some day will be natural—the part that wants to do things but is conquered by the other parts, the good intention side of me, the part that judges a man by what he is, the part that is not like the second part, which judges a man by what other people think. The problem then is to determine what I should do to eliminate the first two parts and strengthen the third. The way to do this is to find a cause of the two parts and try to eliminate it. That is where I need your help."

What conflicts was Irwin experiencing? One entailed his strong motivation to be accepted by others (need for affiliation) opposed by anxiety over mistakes that might lead to rejection. Another conflict pitted affiliative needs against hostility bred by suspicion that others were exploiting him. His motivation to develop into a competent person was concealed by *anxiety* that destroyed his openness, objectivity, and confidence. These deep-seated conflicts disturbed Irwin's daily life and prevented the development of more mature and satisfying attitudes.

FRUSTRATION

When any ongoing behavior sequence is blocked, the individual is frustrated. As shown in Figure 3–1, frustration may be caused by three

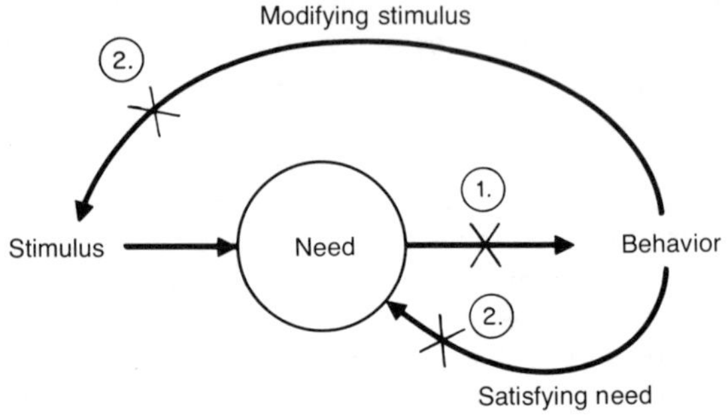

Figure 3–1 Frustration may occur at any one of the three points shown. Frustrations that interfere at point number 1 tend to be of the *loss* or *lack* type, while frustrations that interfere with the resolution of the situation (points 2) tend to be of the *obstruction* or *barrier* type.

factors. Frustration may result from *privation* or *lack,* and we experience it in many situations: insufficient time, knowledge, or intelligence may cause extreme frustration during an exam; lack of money frustrates many people, lack of athletic or social skills frustrates others. Frustration may also result from *loss,* as when one is separated from those he loves, fails in some pursuit, or wrecks a car. The kind of frustration experienced because of a physical handicap due to wounds, illness, accident, or birth defect is constant, and sometimes unendurable. Finally, frustration may be caused by an *obstruction* or *barrier,* such as the frustrating effect of noise during study, of a low grade when working hard, or of being forced to live with an annoying person. Young adolescents see their parents' restrictions as frustrating to their efforts to be popular. Parents' rules about dress, behavior, grooming, and late hours keep them from conforming to the current patterns.

Any of us may be deeply disturbed if a lack, loss, or obstacle thwart strong motivation, such as a desire for love or for status or some ambition that is strongly related to one's self-concept. Not all frustrating situations, then, are external. Some deficiencies are *within the individual.* When the obstruction is within the individual, as in the case of fear or guilt, we speak of *conflict.*

Motivation may be blocked because it conflicts with an opposing motivation. This conflict is traditionally regarded as a more serious maladjustment than frustration, possibly because it occurs so often in the histories of seriously disturbed people. Also, conflict—particularly the more trapping, anxiety-producing kind—is not obvious to the individual who experiences it, since he does not readily perceive the frustrating factor (Symonds, 1946). Mental conflicts are frequently observed by college counselors in students who come to them unhappy, worried, anxious, and disturbed. It was this kind of conflict that Irwin experienced.

Type of Conflicts

Conflicts can be classified into three types: approach-approach conflicts, avoidance-avoidance conflicts, and approach-avoidance conflicts. As will be seen from the discussion that follows (and Figure 3–2) some are more trapping and disturbing than others.

APPROACH—APPROACH CONFLICTS

In these conflicts one is attracted by two equally desirable but incompatible goals. For example, Jack wants to room with an old friend, but also wants to room with a new acquaintance who is stimulating, different, and probably a person with whom he would really enjoy living. Mary wants to marry Frank this semester, but she also has her heart set on finishing her work toward a degree and qualifying as a nurse. Frank is employed in a city where she cannot continue her training.

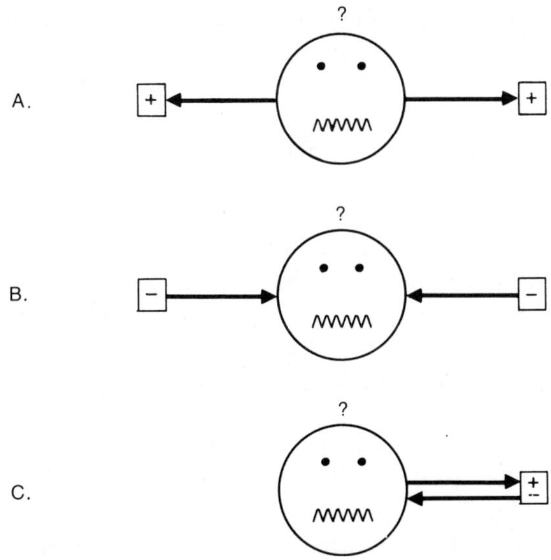

Figure 3–2 Three Types of Conflict. In (A) the individual must choose between two desirable goals. This is called *approach-approach* conflict. In (B) the individual must choose between two undesirable goals. This is called *avoidance-avoidance* conflict. (C) illustrates *approach-avoidance* conflict in which the goal contains both positive and negative features. The individual is both attracted to and repelled from the goal.

It can readily be seen that these are intricate approach-approach conflicts. In their complicated settings there is an aversion to losing one of the alternatives. Each goal has a desirable and undesirable consequence, the undesirable aspect being the loss of the alternative. An example of this sort of conflict is the *perfectionist.* He wants to satisfy all motives, to be highly successful in *all* pursuits, but time, energy, and aptitude permit success in only some of them. He wants everything: perfect grades, student offices with prestige, social life, girls, parties, and rap sessions, and the sleep that will keep him in physical shape to function without irritability. He decides to give up social life, then feels he cannot be without it; relinquishes study time to activities, then is bothered by lower grades; and finally he is unable to make up his mind, so he vacillates between one goal and another. Alice hates to give up her plausible plan for creative writing as a career to go into teaching in order to please her mother and to provide a definite income. She thinks she will "abhor teaching" and will not do well in it. At present she is so undecided that she has become listless because of the conflict.

APPROACH—AVOIDANCE CONFLICTS

In an approach-avoidance conflict one is drawn to a goal having both positive and negative features. For example, John let his hair grow long and began to associate with students who dressed and behaved unconventionally. He found his new identity satisfying; developed some friendships; enjoyed long discussions with his friends about the ills of present-day society; and no longer felt himself a nonentity. His new way of life, however, conflicted strongly with that of his parents—conventional, churchgoing people. They thought he was degenerating, and they objected to his associating with dirty, immoral (in their opinion) characters. Some of his "straight" contemporaries kidded him, but others, when he was walking along the street alone, pushed him off the sidewalk and called him a "queer," or "dirty hippie." During the first few months of his new identification he experienced an approach-avoidance conflict.

A student wants a prominent office, but attaining it will require electioneering, public speaking, back slapping, all of which he thinks is cheap politicking. A girl is strongly attracted to a man who has a car and dresses well, but she is turned off by his loud manner, his efforts at public caresses, and his drinking. These are further examples of approach-avoidance conflicts.

Most inferiority conflicts fall in this category. The individual has strong ambitions to excel in athletics, the social world, or in some enterprise, but he feels inadequate, lacks confidence, and is discouraged by any obstacle or minor failure. Sometimes merely the thought of an obstruction or possible failure discourages him. The motive to compensate for inferiority is strong, but the fear of failure is intense enough to halt any efforts to win his goal.

Sex conflicts are often of this type. The girl who is brought up on conventional middle-class taboos regarding petting and sexual intimacy before marriage is attracted to a boy who induces her to spend hours with him in his apartment. She is struggling with a conflict produced by her physical attraction for him and the pleasure in their hours together and by a strong fear of being detected by her more conventional friends and parents. She not only experiences conflicting pleasure and guilt over the memory of her hours with him but also a disturbing fear of pregnancy and subsequent rejection, since the boy has made it very clear to her that he has no intention of getting married. Most so-called struggles with conscience represent a conflict between a strong impulse and an aversion to the consequences of acting on that impulse.

Many situations in life do not involve choices between clear-cut, "good" and liked alternatives and obvious "bad" and disliked ones. Choosing in such cases would hardly involve a choice! Real situations and real people have both positive and negative associations. We simultaneously like-approve and dislike-disapprove many situations. We are constantly faced with approach-avoidance conflicts. Any of us can reflect on specific events, people, and places and recall positive and negative feelings about them, particularly if we have had many realistic experiences with them. If we accept the reality of many approach-avoidance conflicts and ambivalence, we come to understand ourselves and events more clearly and become less puzzled over our puzzlements. The stalemate of select or reject is broken only as one pole of the approach-avoidance conflict is greatly strengthened as we get closer to the situation.

AVOIDANCE—AVOIDANCE CONFLICTS

Occasionally an individual will feel forced to respond in an undesirable manner to avoid a situation even more undesirable. This is the old dilemna of being "between the devil and the deep blue sea," "damned if you do and damned if you don't." A student feels forced to introduce an acquaintance whom he does not genuinely like into his social group. He knows that he will lose friends by pushing the case, but he will also feel like a "heel" if he does not. A boy feels that he must marry a girl whom he no longer loves because breaking the engagement will hurt her and her parents and embarrass himself and his parents.

Anxiety

THE STATE OF ANXIETY

In many of our conflicts we experience anxiety. We are concerned lest we make the wrong choice and suffer from it. When we feel trapped and unable to respond, anxiety sets in. At such times we are so troubled that we doubt ourselves and our abilities to cope with the simplest problems. Memories of previous failures or shortcomings rise up to threaten our self-assurance and reduce our ability to meet the present crisis. Anxiety is that *generalized state* of uneasiness and fear that characterizes many of the preceding situations and will be described below.

Anxiety is described here in its *normal* everday expression as well as in its function as the basis of *pathological* behavior. In considering anxiety it is important to distinguish between the *state* of anxiety and the *trait* of anxiety. Threatening situations may cause a transitory *state* of anxiety until we adjust to them. This "anxiety state" may occur in anyone, regardless of his trait structure. For some, however, anxiety is a more permanent condition. In the anxiety-prone person a variety of conflicting situations evoke apprehension, nervousness, and concern, and lead to constant feelings of stress. When anxiety is aroused in such individuals, the sense of dread and tension generalizes more broadly and persists longer than in less anxious persons. Such individuals are said to be characterized by *trait* anxiety.

Anxiety as a trait is sometimes described as a result of *insecurity*, possibly originating in infancy, when the child is dependent on adults to protect him. Neglect, loss of affection, or deprivation arouses emotional behavior in the infant which may be labeled anxiety. This kind of anxiety is associated with other people. It includes isolation or loneliness and lack of affectionate responses from other people. Sullivan (1949) suggests that *things* can cause fear, but only *people* can cause insecurity or anxiety.

Another way of looking at anxiety is that suggested by the physiological psychologist Malmo (1957). In a review of studies of anxiety and behavioral arousal, he refers to anxiety as a "disease of over-arousal." Some individuals have been chronically subjected to situations that arouse them physiologically, and thus have difficulty in inhibiting this arousal. We move in the direction of understanding their anxieties when we locate the *situations* that cause abnormally high arousal. Two of these conditions that give rise to strong arousal and in consequence disturb and disorganize behavior are *frustration* of strong, self-centered motivation and *conflict*.

ADJUSTMENTS TO CONFLICT AND ANXIETY

Humans become *anxious* when frustrated, possibly because being blocked in an ongoing activity is punishing in some way. Both animals and humans, when frustrated, *regress* (i.e., return to behavior used earlier in life), or they *fixate* (i.e., continue to rely on behavior that was appropriate at one time in their early life) on some random act that may seem senseless to the observer, and repeat it over and over. Humans find many methods to escape or defend themselves from the disturbing anxiety produced by severe frustration. One escape is to turn impulsively away, physically and mentally, from the disturbing situation. Children seek their source of security, the parent, and adopt the behavior, attitudes, and ideas of the parent model. This *introjection* of their parents' standards becomes their "conscience"; however, other models with different behavior are introjected, and conflict ensues, which produces more anxiety, builds more defenses, and favors escape. In fact, *adjustments to life* for most people *is not always a logically worked-out plan but a pattern of motivation and frustration and a series of defenses and escape from the anxiety produced by the thwarted motives* (Symonds, 1946).

Another frequent response to frustration and conflict (inner frustration) is aggression. Since punishment is a frequent consequence of aggression in our culture, it will be explored following the discussion of aggression.

Aggression

PAIN AND AGGRESSION

Fighting, malicious gossip, verbal attacks, prejudicial deprivation of others of their civil rights are examples of aggression, just as are assault and murder. We have already noted that one of the most primitive reactions to frustration or thwarted behavior is aggression or hostility (see Figure 3–3). Azrin (1967) shows that when pain is administered to an animal, he will attack any other animal that happens to be in the same cage. This tendency of pain to produce aggression or hostile action seems to be widespread among animals, but the pain-provoked attack is not stereotyped. Different animals attack in different ways—with their limbs, their teeth; often humans attack through speech. Suffering individuals may attack inanimate objects that are near at hand. The amount of aggression exhibited depends on how intense the pain is, how long it lasts, and how frequently it occurs. Aggressive responses can be eliminated by providing the individual with some nonaggressive means of escape or avoiding pain. A laboratory animal, for example, can be taught to avoid shock and pain by pressing a lever in the experimental cage.

An interesting finding is that *psychological equivalents* to pain produce aggression. For example, if the reward that the animal has learned to receive is abruptly terminated, he becomes aggressive. This "psychological" pain, produced experimentally in animals, reminds us that humans become aggressive when blocked in efforts to obtain something valuable, including an object of love, or when something goes wrong, such as the car's running out of gasoline on the way to an important appointment.

Any strong motive, then, that is severely frustrated may provoke a person to anger. This reaction to frustration is demonstrated early in life; the very young child shows anger at restrictions to movement and directs his irritability and temper tantrums outward.

Figure 3–3 Learning to Aggress.

Photo courtesy of *Columbia Missourian*

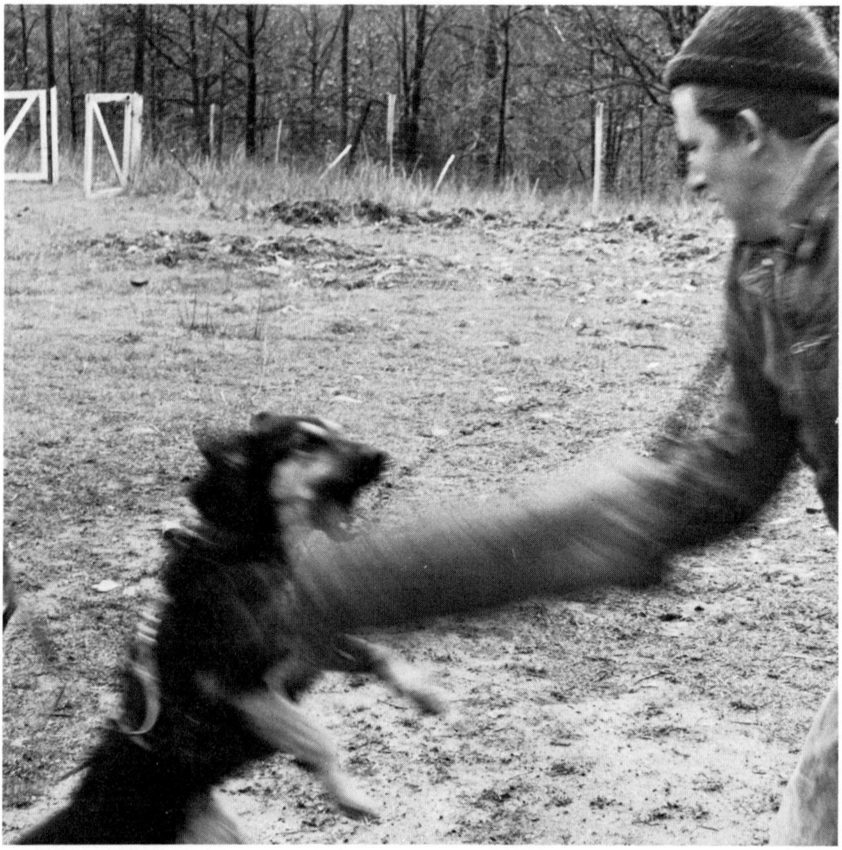

FRUSTRATION—AGGRESSION HYPOTHESIS

"Aggression is due to frustration,"—a simple statement of an important relationship, the classic *frustration-aggression hypothesis.* Frustration may produce other responses, however—crying, withdrawal, anxiety, and passive resistance (see Figure 3–4). Which response occurs as the result of frustration is determined by previous training and experience and by the variables that control the strength of the aggression, and the intensity, duration, and frequency of the frustration.

While teaching at a university in Turkey, an instructor used in his lectures the same examples of accumulated frustration as he had in classes in the United States. These examples were failure to get breakfast one morning, traffic delays in trying to meet an appointment, and walking along a muddy street and dirtying polished shoes. He then asked the students to indicate their reaction to these annoyances. Never was their reaction aggression; rather, it was sadness, disappointment, or withdrawal. The events and annoyances mentioned were not really frustrations to the Turks, but circumstances of daily life. With the many unpredictable privations in the austere Turkish society of the time, the students did not have the hopes and anticipations held by their contemporaries in the nonpoverty sectors of the affluent American society. Aggression could be produced among these students, however. One day when, in accordance with the dean's order, the instructor announced that class would be held instead of a celebration to honor the birthday of the national hero, Ataturk, strong, overt expression of aggression (shouts of anger, leaving their seats) erupted from a previously well-behaved class. On impulse, the instructor recalled his admiration of this great democratically oriented autocrat and said to the angry class, "As a visitor from the United States I feel as you do about Ataturk, and I will join you on your pilgrimage across town to Ataturk's tomb after we settle a few matters here in class." The cheers from the students were loud and reassuring. Here is an example of palpable aggression that resulted from arbitrary frustration of a strong motivation that was rather close to a goal. The situation contained all the elements (if they

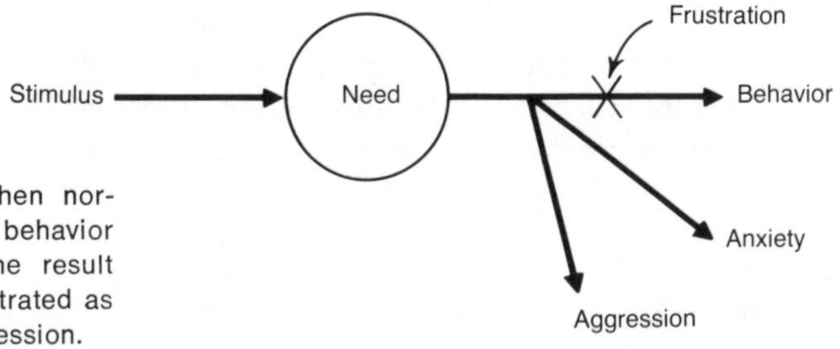

Figure 3–4 When normal motivated behavior is frustrated, the result may be demonstrated as anxiety or aggression.

had been anticipated) by which one could have predicted strong aggression. Removal of the frustration turned the anger to joy and excitement.

Frustration does not invariably lead to aggression. There are situations in which people exist under great deprivation and dire cruelties, but because of tight social control they show responses other than aggression, and these responses include passive resistance.

VARIABLES IN AGGRESSION

The variables that control the strength of aggression include (1) *strength of the motive* that is frustrated; (2) the *point in the ongoing behavior* at which frustration occurs; (3) the *extent of interference with ongoing behavior;* (4) the *number of frustrated response sequences* that have previously occurred; and (5) the *arbitrariness* of the frustration.

To illustrate the effect of the above variables, apply them to the behavior of the Turkish university students. (1) Ataturk was their greatest national hero, and, furthermore, they greatly enjoyed celebrations; their motivation was doubly strong. (2) They had already planned to attend the celebration; therefore, the frustration occurred fairly near the goal of their motivated behavior. (3) The statement from their instructor, backed by the dean's announcement that they had to attend class, was complete interference with their ongoing behavior. (4) Since they lived in an authoritative structure, in which their parents and older people make most of the decisions that govern their lives, they had been frustrated many times in the past. (5) The frustration doubtless seemed arbitrary to them because everyone in Turkey reveres Ataturk.

It may be of interest here to pause and recall the event that preceded your most recent aggressive behavior. The aggression may have been an angry verbal outburst or a real attempt to inflict punishment or to be destructive. To what extent was each of the above factors operating?

DEVELOPMENT OF AGGRESSION

In studies of children a relationship is found between the punitiveness of the child's mother and the degree to which the child expresses aggression toward her doll in play (Sears, Whiting, Nowlis, & Sears 1953). In adults such displaced aggression is often seen in prejudice toward minority groups or toward groups representing a subculture with different attitudes, such as protesting college students. Displaced aggression constitutes a serious social problem in the United States, and its effects are observable in most of our current domestic and international crises.

Parents vary from prohibiting and punishing aggression to permissively allowing a child to shout angrily at them or even hit them. Most highly aggressive children—boys, slightly more often than girls—had mothers who were either very permissive or punished them severely. A smaller percentage of highly aggressive children had mothers who were not permissive about aggression and administered mild punishment. Sears, Maccoby, and Levin (1957), in commenting on these results, suggests that if parents wish to produce a nonaggressive child, they should make it clear that aggression is not approved, should stop aggression when it occurs, but should avoid punishing the child when he is aggressive. Punishment, as we shall see, has complex effects and is likely to generate hostility in the child and lead to aggression at some other time and place, and perhaps against another person or object. Parents who punish also act as a model for aggressiveness which the children imitate. Some parents use and encourage "justified" hostility. They encourage their children to retaliate for any aggression toward them.

Children of authoritarian parents—that is, of parents who are high in conformity, prejudice, and rigidity and who show hostility and are intolerant of ambiguity—build up a great reservoir of aggression. They are more aggressive than children of equalitarian parents—that is, of parents who show normal aggression, no extreme prejudices, independence from conformity, and flexibility in judgment of others' behavior (Siegal, 1956).

IMMEDIATE CUES TO AGGRESSION

The man in the street tends to explain aggression in terms of some event that touches off hostile behavior. In fact, aggression is a complex phenomenon involving a number of variables, some of which have been mentioned above. A person becomes aggressive not merely because someone mentions a word that offends him or because someone interferes with his ongoing behavior. These events may be cues to elicit aggressive behavior in an individual who has *built-up aggressive propensities.*

A recent experiment demonstrated the importance of cues in the outburst of aggression. The subject who participated in the experiment did not know its real purpose. It was interpreted to him as an experiment to measure his partner's (in the experiment) physiological reactions to stress. The subject was to evaluate the partner's report on a previous project. If he approved the report, he was to press a telegraph key, which would presumably give a mild shock to his partner. If the subject did not approve his partner's report, he was to administer as many as ten shocks. Sometimes the table at which the subject sat was clear; at other times, objects such as badminton rackets and shuttlecocks, which had no relation to the experiment, were placed on it. During one condition of the experiment, the table contained a twelve-gauge shotgun and a snub-nosed .38 revolver. The presence of these firearms increased the number of shocks the subjects gave their partners (Berkowitz, 1968).

INHIBITION OF AGGRESSIVE ACTS

There is one well-recognized *inhibitor* to aggression—the threat of punishment for the aggressive behavior. (See Figure 3–5.) Punishment is defined broadly to include scolding, embarrassment, and various forms of disapproval. Most children do not aggress directly against authorita-

Figure 3–5 One of Society's Ways of Inhibiting Aggression.

Photo courtesy of *Columbia Missourian*

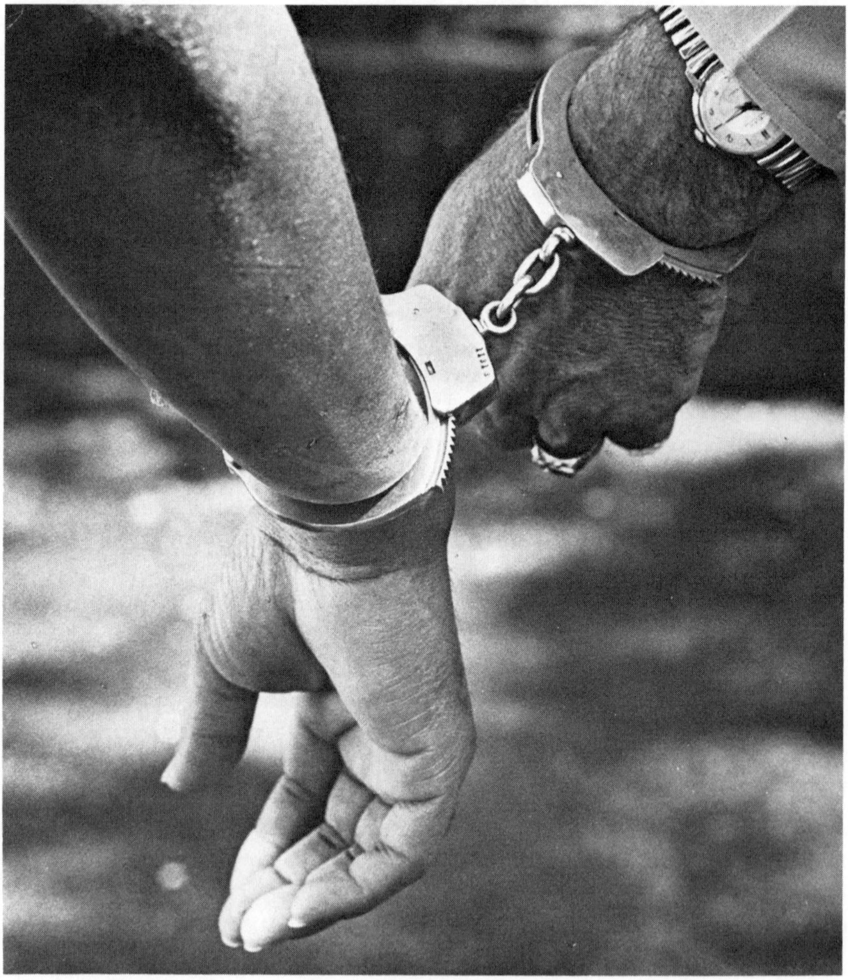

tive parents, teachers, or others in authority; their aggression is only temporarily inhibited. An angry child or adult who does not display aggression toward an individual with powerful retaliatory potential may, however, show *displaced* aggression toward a weaker peer or toward a toy.

In addition to fear of punishment the individual's standards of conduct act to inhibit aggression. These inhibitions vary widely, for they are the product of experiences during growing up. Despite these individual differences, inhibitions inculcated in early life, and some of the attitudes that regulate aggression, are shared by members of a given subculture, such as a social class or ethnic group.

AGGRESSION AND CATHARSIS

One theory concerning aggression has been loosely derived from Aristotle's view of the role of tragedy in plays or literature. It proposes that violence, as experienced vicariously in viewing a play, movie, television program, or in reading fiction, drains off accumulated aggression in the individual. The fictional violence releases tensions and the potentiality of overt expression of violence by the individual. This process is called *catharsis*.

Numerous experiments throw doubt on the theory that the vicarious experience of aggression reduces active aggression in the viewer. In one such experiment college volunteers were made angry with a classmate, following which they viewed a film that included a violent prize fight. The peer with whom they were angry had the same name as the victim of the violence in the film. The reactions of the volunteer group were compared with those of a control group, who saw an exciting but nonviolent horse race. Immediately after the film each subject was provided with a socially sanctioned opportunity to give an electric shock to the person who had angered him before the film. The method used was similar to that described in the experiment that involved firearms. Instead of showing *less* aggression after the violent film, experimental group subjects freely administered shocks, a reaction which was in marked contrast to that of the control subjects who saw the nonaggressive film (Geen and Berkowitz, 1966).

Another study does lend some credence to the doctrine of catharsis. Subjects in this experiment were assigned a task, but the assignment was presented in a very insulting manner in which it was suggested that the subjects' motives were socially valueless and their talents dubious. The experimenter allowed one group of subjects to express their aggression by telling stories after they had viewed a series of pictures. Control group subjects had no means of release. They were immediately given some routine pencil-and-paper tests of clerical and spatial abilities. The control group manifested greater aggression than the one that had an opportunity to vent their aggression in their stories about the pictures. The control group were more irritated with the experimenter and said so openly. They also showed reluctance to volunteer for further experiments. This study suggests that for the first group the storytelling was an *outlet* for their aggression (Feshbach, 1955). Apparently, experiencing aggression vicariously actually *increases* aggression within the individual. On the other hand, if the individual is allowed to somehow express his aggression (real rather than vicarious catharsis), he shows less aggression in later tests. The question arises, however, of whether the individuals who are allowed to aggress through storytelling are inhibiting their aggression on later tests, not because of a reduction of aggressive feelings, but rather because of guilt over their own previous expression of aggression.

AGGRESSION IN CONTEMPORARY SOCIETY

Ever since the violence of the Nazis, psychologists have been attempting to explain violence in a society in terms of previous frustrations. Anyone acquainted with man's history will have no difficulty citing a number of examples of waves of violence in the form of war, cruelty, and atrocities, including people with religious motivations who wage a holy war or engage in systematic persecution. (Figure 3–6 shows an act of aggression committed in contemporary society.) The issue of man's aggression has a current popularity as a subject for debates, and man's behavior has been contrasted with that of infrahuman animals. Infrahuman animals make a show of aggression that causes the weaker animal to withdraw and the more aggressive animal to cease his attack; the fracas does not end in death (Mathews, 1964). This fact has led to the generalization that man seems to be the only animal that routinely kills his own species and makes a career or business of it.

The issue of man's aggressiveness becomes especially serious at this time in our history because of the possibility of large-scale extermination of human life and the means to support the remnants. Doubtless, biological as well as cultural factors intertwine to produce man's aggression (Lazarus, 1969). The previously quoted studies and others indicate that psychologists are discovering some of the variables that are significant in aggression. With the strong motivation of contemporary man to deal with the problem of aggression, we may, hopefully, persuade governments, local and national, to use knowledge gained in the laboratory and to control domestic and international aggression.

A relationship has been found between the annual farm value of cotton in southern states and the number of lynchings of blacks. This suggests that the blacks may have been used as scapegoats in lean years (Gaudet, Caril, & Dennagar, 1950). Another contemporary example of

Figure 3–6 Aggression in Contemporary Society.

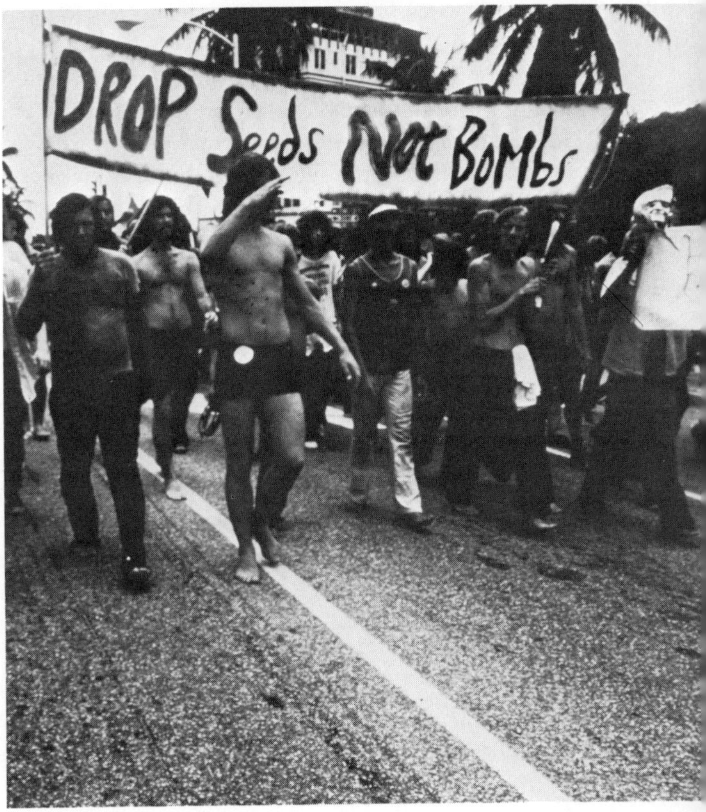

Photo by J. Brian King

aggression in society is the occurrence of riots attending the efforts to implement civil rights legislation and those on the college campuses to protest war and racial inequities. Chronic frustration and conflict are seen in the background of those who riot; more stable and conventional backgrounds showed among peaceful and legal activists. The actual riot is set off by some external event. Once triggered, the violence is self-perpetuating.

These comments suggest that in order to reduce outbursts of violence, it might be well to reduce as far as possible socioeconomic frustrations, strengthen through education the inhibitions toward violent action, and also lessen the immediate cues that can set off aggressive acts. Admittedly, this is a big order, but violence and destruction are serious enough problems to merit such efforts.

Conflicts and Mental Health

Conflicts are, of course, inevitable in our daily lives. We often both like and dislike people, events, or activities.

Personality maladjustment, as we shall see, has many expressions, ranging from the psychoses or insanities to transient personal maladjustment in the essentially normal person. It has been demonstrated that severe conflicts and the way the individual responds to them are basic to neurotic behavior. On the other hand, a recognized and potentially resolvable conflict can be motivating, especially if the individual mobilizes his resources and attacks the problem in a coping way. He may actually develop skills and attitudes like venturesomeness in this effort. The individual differences in reaction to conflicts are circumstances of the individual's development, his present environment, and his various learned capacities to cope effectively with situations. It is also possible that some individuals have particularly intense drives (i.e., sex and aggression) that lead to socially undesirable behavior despite opposition or punishment. On the other hand, some individuals have stronger capacities to inhibit and suppress unwanted behavior. The various ways in which we adjust to conflicts are discussed in detail in the next chapter.

Summary

1. *Frustration* is defined as the blocking of an ongoing sequence of behavior. These frustrations may be privations, deprivations, or obstructions.
2. *Conflict* is the term for inner frustrations or obstructions *within* the individual. Conflicts are classified as (1) approach-approach; (2) approach-avoidance (ambivalences); (3) avoidance-avoidance.

   This classification helps us to understand how conflicts differ. Most disturbing personal problems are basically conflicts.
3. Associated with conflict is the phenomenon of *anxiety*. This is a vague generalized fear state. It may become a trait, a more permanent reaction to threat. Anxiety may be viewed as a state of *insecurity* or, from the physiological point of view, as a condition of *overarousal.*
4. One common important reaction to frustration is aggression. Pain has been found to produce aggression in animals, but even in animals there are *psychological equivalents* of pain produced by terminating the reward the animal has learned to receive. An important hypothesis relating to much human aggression is the *frustration-aggression hypothesis,* which relates to aggression and frustration.
5. Some of the variables related to aggression are (1) the strength of the motive that is frustrated; (2) the point in the ongoing behavior at which frustration occurs; (3) the extent of interference with the ongoing behavior; (4) the number of frustrated response sequences that have previously occurred; and (5) the arbitrariness of the frustration.
6. The degree of *aggression* shown in an individual is related to his ex-

periences in development. To rear children to be nonaggressive adults, it is suggested that they learn that aggression is not favored but checked and that aggression not be rewarded but also not be punished when it occurs. Aggressive tendencies can be evoked by such cues as the sight of a gun.

7. Aggression can be *inhibited* by a person who has retaliatory powers or by individual standards of conduct. Seeing a movie on aggression does not act as vicarious *catharsis* or a purging of aggressive tendencies. Rather, it tends to increase aggressive tendencies. Man has a long history of aggression, and more than ever today, with the destructive potentials available to him, it is necessary to reduce it. Work in this area suggests that aggression can be diminished by reducing frustration as far as possible and by strengthening inhibitions against violent action.
8. Aggressions are sometimes displaced to some other object or person rather than toward the person who instigates it. If aggression is displaced to a less threatening person, this is known as scapegoating. Among the forms aggression may take is intropunitive behavior, by which the individual blames himself or is self-punishing.

Words to Remember

Aggression
Anxiety
Approach-Approach Conflict
Approach-Avoidance Conflict
Avoidance-Avoidance Conflict
Catharsis
Frustration-Aggression Hypothesis
Ideal Self

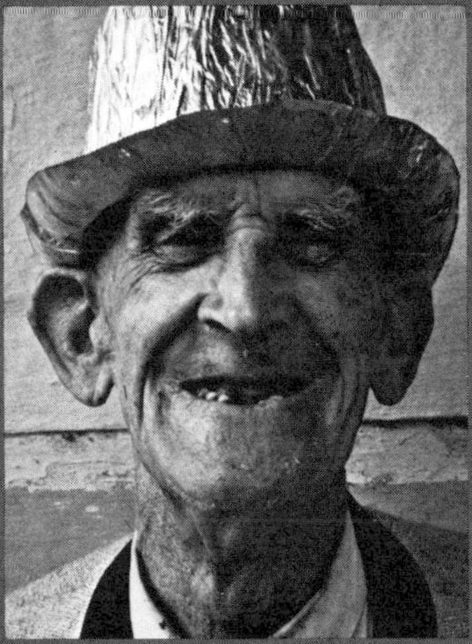

4. Defenses and Coping

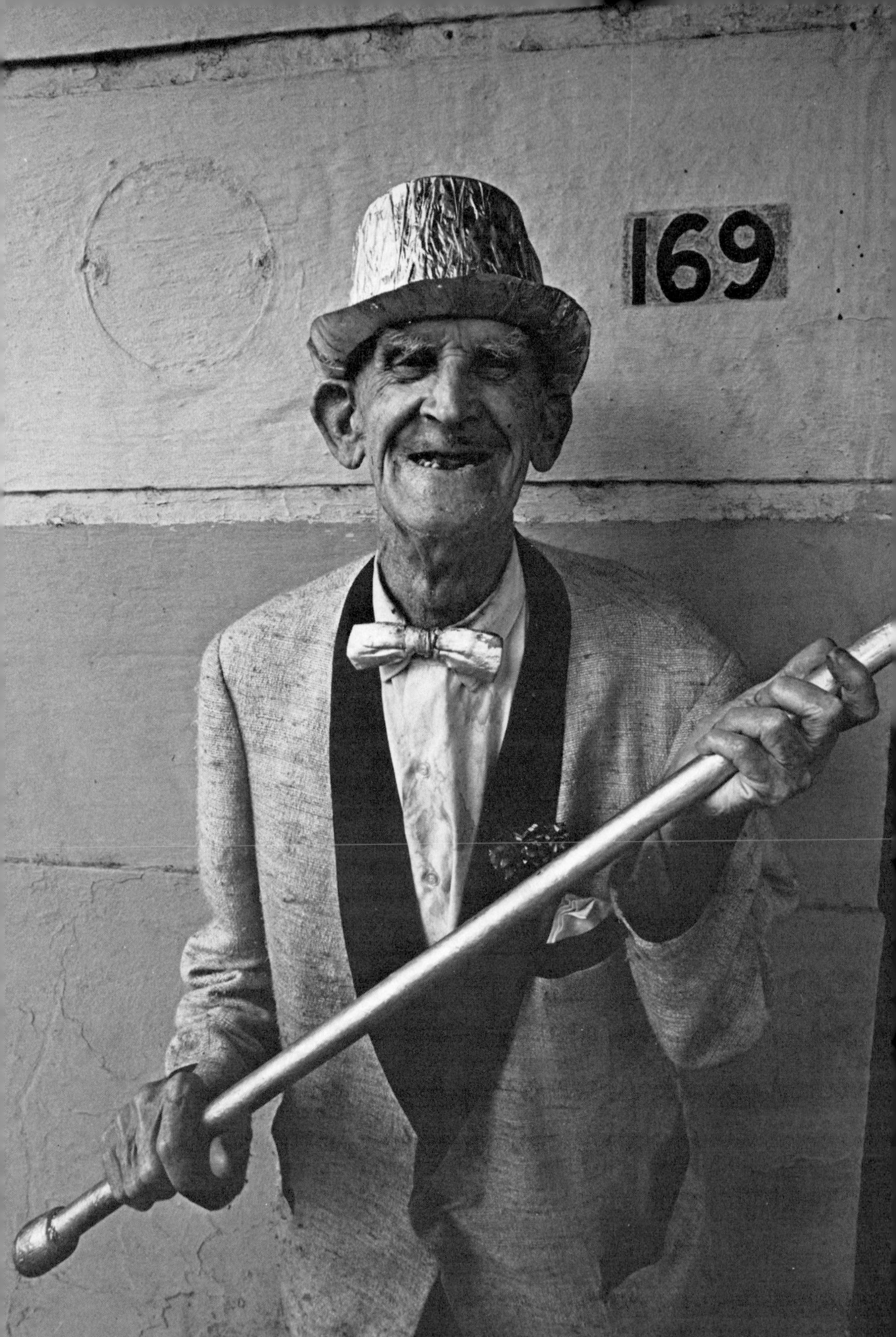

Photo by J. Brian King

Objectives

After studying this chapter the reader should be able to:

1. Define *defense mechanisms.*
2. Describe the two classes of defense mechanisms and list examples of each.
3. Identify the positive and negative aspects in the use of defense mechanisms.
4. Contrast defenses with effective coping behavior.
5. List factors required in developing effective coping behavior.
6. Describe abnormal behavior in terms of ineffective coping and faulty defenses.

Let us begin our discussion of reaction to frustration and conflict, considered in the previous chapter, by presenting a case. Sam, the subject of this case, experienced severe conflicts and anxiety. He used defenses and, later, coping responses to deal with them.

A CASE STUDY EXEMPLIFYING CONFLICT AND DEFENSE

When Sam came to the counselor, he was an 18-year-old recent high school graduate. Below average in height, Sam makes a good general appearance, dressing neatly and conventionally. He was referred to the counselor by his stepfather because, although he wanted to enter a large state university, he did not have the necessary high school grades.

Sam's appointment with the counselor was made by his stepfather, who telephoned and outlined exactly what he wanted accomplished in the counseling session; the counselor was to get Sam registered in the university by any means and despite any rules that might stand in the way. The counselor agreed to see Sam but made no promises except that he would judge the boy's abilities and make recommendations for action in Sam's best interests. The meaning of this statement seemed lost on Mr. M., who replied, "I have full confidence that you will clear the way for my son to enter the University." He did have enough insight into his own personality to say that Sam had none of his own tendency to talk loudly and behave aggressively—clearly, characteristics he did not regard as faults in himself.

Mr. M. made the startling revelation to the counselor in their conversation that although Sam did not bear the M. family name, he was actually his son. Mr. M. had not married Sam's mother until the boy was twelve years old. On the positive side, Mr. M. described Sam as a "fine boy," a plugger who usually achieved what he wanted. The counselor sensed that although Sam's father wanted to dominate the boy's life, his motivations were basically good and affectionate.

In the conference with the counselor, Sam was quite open about his concerns. He wanted very much to enter the university, and was confident that he could make respectable to superior grades. He had been informed several months previously that if he came to summer school, took several basic courses, and earned passing grades, he would be admitted to the university in the fall semester. Instead of registering for summer school, however, Sam had taken a job, working with underprivileged youth in the inner city as a playground supervisor, a job he had succeeded in during the previous summer. He realized that it was a mistake not to have gone to summer school, and he was disappointed that now he would have to enter a small state college for his freshman year instead of the university.

This failure to attend summer school was only one of several examples of negativism toward his parents and persons in authority that emerged during the interview. Sam knew that his behavior was rebellious and in the end self-defeating, but apparently, at the moment of action, his impulse to defy authority overpowered discretion.

Sam's school records had not always been poor; he had made good grades in elementary school, junior high, and even in high school until he was shocked to discover that he was really the son of Mr. M., his present "stepfather," conceived while his mother was married to "his real father." The discovery was shattering to the boy; he felt confused and lost. People whom he loved and considered as blood relatives were not, in fact, relatives at all. He hated his mother, both for her involvement with Mr. M. and for her marrying him. He lost all feeling for anything or anyone. He felt alienated and alone. He hated himself and had no wish to continue living. He retired to his room, refused to talk to anyone or to attend school, and buried himself in comics and other time-wasting activities.

His father reacted violently to this withdrawal. He told Sam to go back to school and to "take hold of himself," and during one heated confrontation, even struck Sam. Instead of fighting back, the boy hit himself in the head with a blunt instrument, knocking himself unconscious. He later wrote a suicide note before taking some pills that merely made him sick, but thinks his parents are unaware of this attempt at suicide.

For several months Sam refused to go anywhere and initiated no contact with his parents. In retrospect, he thinks that he was "mentally sick" at the time, and his mother took him to a psychiatrist. He was beginning to make some progress toward acceptance of himself and his situation when his parents, who did not perceive his improvement, terminated the conferences with the psychiatrist just when Sam felt he was gaining control over his emotional life.

He angrily decided one day that he would take charge of his life and make something of himself. He volunteered for work in the ghetto, and found that being able to help people worse off than he improved his attitude. He discovered that he was especially good as a counselor, and this success prompted him to choose volunteer work again instead of summer school.

During the later stages of his own illness, Sam came home one day to find his mother unconscious from an overdose of sleeping pills. He immediately called for professional help. For some time, the physician was not sure she would recover. What puzzled Sam most about this incident was his lack of concern for his mother. Almost at the same time, the dog he had had all during his childhood died. Despite the fact that he had loved the dog dearly, he felt no loss; indeed, the night the dog died, he went to the movies.

Sam hates everything his father represents, especially his father's Catholic background, since Mr. M. forced him to attend Catholic rather than Jewish services. His antipathy extends toward his father's successful business. He has refused to accept his father as a father and has made his lack of respect clear. He told his father that he would accept his support only until he could become independent. He wants to change his name, leave home after college, and never see either of his parents again. He regards his birth certificate as a lie; he feels he doesn't belong to the family or any other place. Altogether, Sam exhibited throughout the interview an honesty and integrity that doubtless was one of his great strengths.

At the end of the interview he stated his plans to enter a small state college that would accept him and to make a good record there, so the university will eventually allow him to enter. He presented these plans with conviction and with apparently some anticipation of pleasure in this decision.

Sam's treatment by his father did not result in a completely cowed and submissive son. Sam's self-concept is low, but his strong distaste for his father and everything he represents has given unity to Sam's choices. He consistently acts in opposition to his father's wishes, as when his father objected to his volunteer social work, thought he should get out and earn money instead, and opposed the selection of teaching as a vocation because of its low earning prospects. Sam's strongly negative feelings toward his father have been a reliable source of motivation to become independent and to achieve. He has no hopes of being understood by his father and, in fact, does not care to be.

PERSPECTIVES ON SAM T.'S CASE

Sam's crisis illustrates details of psychological stress that were discussed in the preceding chapter. He suffered severe frustrations and conflicts and also showed the complex of defense mechanisms that may be used under stress to protect the individual from psychological pain, which may appear to others as abnormal behavior. The reader will find it helpful, as we review defense mechanisms, to recognize those used by Sam.

What are some of the frustrations and conflicts Sam experienced? He had a history of six years of domination and derogation by an aggressive, dominant "stepfather," years of felt personal failure, produced by Mr. M.'s constant comparison of Sam to his brother, to Sam's disadvantage. His "stepfather" constantly forced him to do what was foreign to him in his religious life and in his relationships with his former relatives. He was subjected to a series of frustrations, which he reacted to with negativism and by surreptitiously going his own way. When he discovered that his despised stepfather was actually his real father, the conflict was almost too great to endure. He defended, then, by denying all feeling and withdrawing from his parents and all social life. He *couldn't accept himself* as a product of adultery between his mother and a man he hated. The aggression resulting from this frustration was too great to be expressed directly against his parents, who had caused it; he therefore turned it upon himself by seeking self-destruction physically as well as psychologically. The report of his condition when he was taken to the psychiatrist suggested that he was seriously disturbed psychologically. His withdrawal and his leveling of feeling were symptoms as well as defenses.

The psychiatrist helped to give him a verbal and emotional outlet for his feelings, some perspective on his life, and help in integrating his resources. Although he did not appreciate his teacher's help at the time, his success and recognition through his violin recital brought much-needed ego satisfaction. Later, finding a need-satisfying outlet for his energy by helping others was therapeutic, as he himself recognized. Sam's father served as a negative model, and since many of his inclinations were antithetical to his father's to begin with, he had motivation for rebuilding an inner structure that had added value to him because it was so different from his father's.

In summary, Sam's *defenses* included denial of feelings and withdrawal. Luckily, part of his defense was plunging, against his father's will, into a job that helped him to satisfy needs, build self-respect, and feel valuable to society. Early in life he had personal resources that stood him in good stead when he sought a way to build a new life. He was not completely trapped by the situation; he could get out of his home situation, attend school, and develop plans for the future. In Sam's case we see how defenses operate in a stressful crisis and how one moves toward coping reactions and recovers from the possibility of a serious abnormality. We will refer again to Sam's behavior to illustrate the various defense mechanisms as well as coping behavior.

Definition of Defense Mechanisms

Defense mechanisms are patterns of behavior designed to protect the person from the anxiety of facing his own unacceptable feelings. People who feel intense anger toward a parent, or sexually attracted to a person of the same sex, or jealous of their own children's relationship with the other parent are hard put to admit what they feel, even to themselves. It is far more acceptable, and even necessary, to become a doting son to the hated parent, to condemn the homosexual heatedly, or to over-indulge the resented child. The problem posed by such defenses is that they fail to permit expression of the true feelings that must continually be controlled, thereby draining the energy that might be devoted to more productive pursuits. The advantage of the defense mechanism is that it makes it unnecessary for the person to acknowledge negative aspects of himself. All of us exhibit defense mechanisms. In fact, we need the more harmless defenses in order to carry on our essential daily activities. Our culture often furnishes us with ready-made defenses and reinforces our use of them. After we have examined the various forms that defense mechanisms take, we will evaluate various kinds of defenses. Incidentally, although our definition of defense mechanisms seems to imply that the diversions that are practiced are conscious, actually, defense mechanisms are virtually always unconscious.

Classification of Defense Mechanisms

Any division of defensive behavior into separate mechanisms is arbitrary, and the borderlines between these mechanisms are not always clear. Classification of the mechanisms into major groups is also arbitrary, but often helpful in relating those that are somewhat similar. We will use the following broad classification: (1) *withdrawal reactions,* which include behavior such as repression, denial, and so forth; and (2) *compromise reactions,* which include more subtle responses such as compensation, rationalization, and projection.

WITHDRAWAL REACTIONS

Repression. Repression is one of the most basic of defense mechanisms. It develops as an early and easy adjustment to frustrations and taboo situations. Repression is defined as the banning from consciousness of dangerous or embarrassing thoughts or impulses, and exemplified clearly by the failure to recognize or recall impulses, memories, or actions, any of which may cause anxiety. This defense simply blocks from consciousness any *ideas* related to negative experiences. Sam T.'s story illustrated repression of feeling; also Katherine, described in Chapter 1, repressed her negative feelings for her sister. Consider for a moment how many unpleasant events you have pushed out of mind—the embarrassing moments when you felt foolish or ignorant; the times you

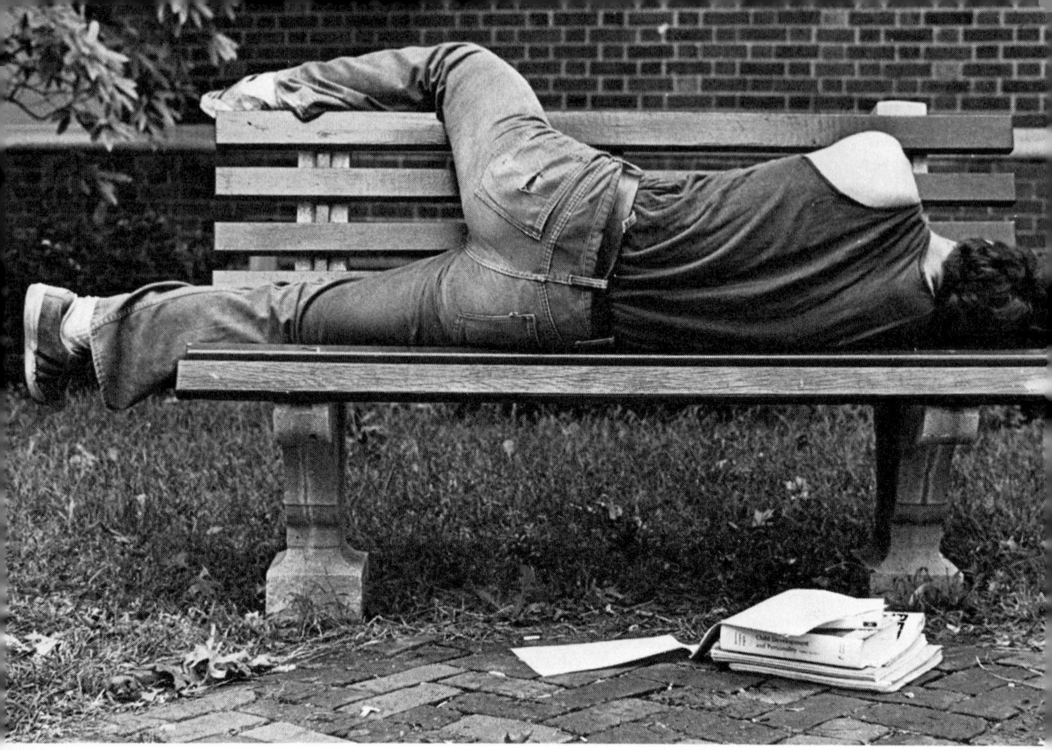

Photo courtesy of *Columbia Missourian*

Figure 4–1 Turning Off a Difficult Problem—Withdrawal.

have taken advantage of someone; the horrifying sights like accidents or cruelty. Those who have been in combat, in prison, or in concentration camps have lived through experiences they wish never to recall and that recur only in dreams. Often these memories are too heavily laden with anxiety and guilt to be reviewed voluntarily by the individual.

Although repression can make life more pleasant, it can also complicate our adjustment to problems. It prevents us from understanding the forces of conflict within us. Rather than accept, discuss, and settle our inner feelings either temporarily or permanently, we flee from them.

SUPPRESSION AND DENIAL

A distinction is usually made between *repression, suppression,* and *denial.* Repression is entirely unconscious, so the person is neither aware of the impulse or thought nor of the process by which these ideas are blocked. In *suppression* (Figure 4–1), there is a conscious and volitional inhibition of the unwanted. The person banishes irrelevant and annoying impulses so that he can carry on his activities. It is as though he says to himself, "This is a matter I cannot accept at present, and I must turn my attention to other, more satisfying activities." Sam, described in the beginning of this chapter, *suppressed* his reactions to his "father," but after he learned that this man whom he hated so intensely was not his stepfather but his real father, he *repressed* his feelings about events that would earlier have moved him deeply.

Through denial, a person attempts to avoid recognizing and dealing with negative feelings he may have toward another. Denial also is employed to reduce or remove the anxiety and stress that might accompany complete awareness of one's situation. Thus the traveler who is lost refuses to admit that fact for to do so would in itself increase his fear. Similarly the family of a dying patient ignores the significance of the medical reports, for to accept it would bring on a very painful feeling of sadness. How often have you seen and heard people say that they simply don't want to hear bad news because if they know about it they will feel worse? Sam's father, for example, refused to admit his son's inability to enter the university.

Denial, when used extensively as a defense mechanism, is seen most frequently in children and severely disturbed adults. It is considered a more primitive form of defense than repression, since it does involve unconscious mechanisms that enable a person to establish greater distance between himself and the source of unpleasant feelings. Denial is often reflected in our wish-fulfilling fantasies and dreams, as will be seen later in the chapter.

APATHY

Several studies give evidence that apathy develops when individuals are trapped in situations such as concentration or prisoner-of-war camps. Prisoners held in the Nazi concentration camps at Dachau and Buchenwald under conditions of continual deprivation, torture, and threat of death, without hope of escape, developed attitudes of detachment and inattentiveness (Bettelheim, 1943). Americans in prisoner-of-war camps in Korea were reported to behave in a similarly listless and indifferent manner to their frustrating and stressful situation. As prisoners the Americans were observed to lack emotional expression and to be completely absorbed in themselves. These men were not psychotic, as they showed in their speech and behavior when approached by their compatriots. In fact, the attention and support of a friend were a powerful factor in helping them to come out of their state of apathy (Stressman, Thaler, & Schein, 1956).

FANTASY

Another reaction to disturbing frustrations and conflicts in the real world is to turn to the world of dreams or fantasy—a world of our own making. A study that involved college men and women from different universities in two different decades of time and representative of a wide

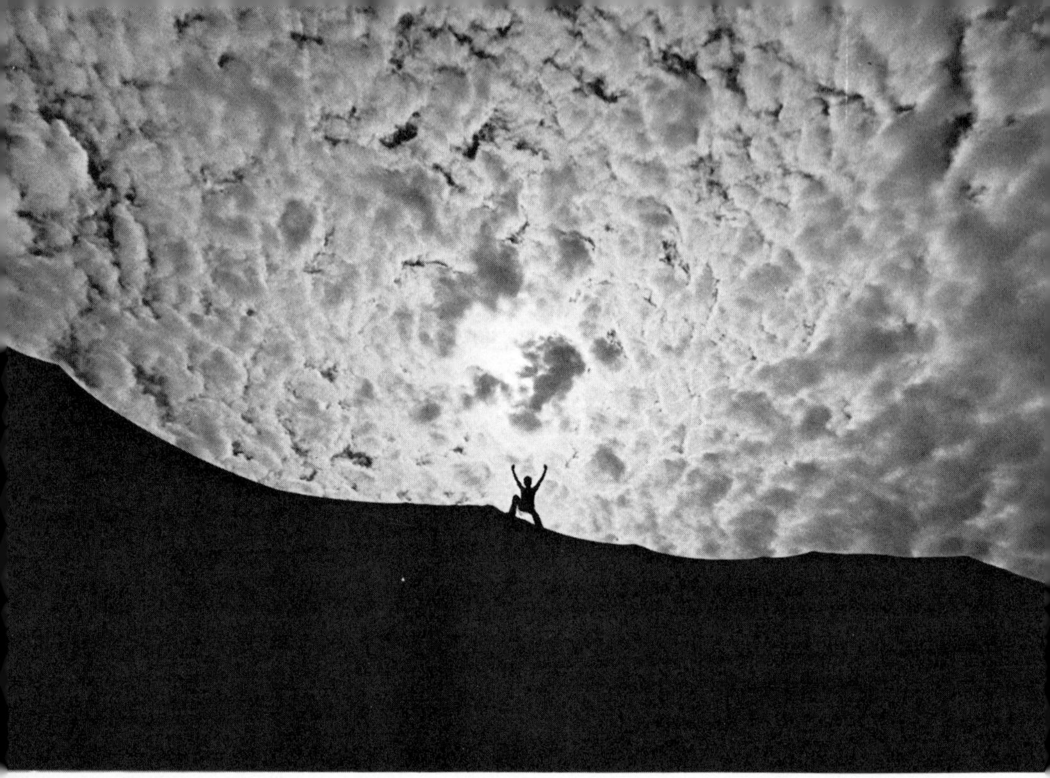

Photo by J. Brian King

Figure 4–2 A World Mastery Fantasy.

age group—from 18 to 50—revealed that only 3 percent of the entire group reported no *recent* daydreams (Shaffer & Shoben, 1956).

Some fantasies are the results of frustration, and as such, may be classified as *defense mechanisms.* The motivation for fantasy is dimly conscious or unconscious. Daydreams may involve a preoccupation with traumatic situations. The individual who has been embarrassed or hurt might engage in a fantasy of retaliation against the person who has injured him. Fantasy permits one to withdraw from painful or upsetting circumstances, as evidenced by the lonely nature of fantasy. When an individual impulsively builds an elaborate fantasy life as a substitute for real events that produce anxiety, the fantasy becomes a *defense mechanism.* The fantasy world of some psychotics is richer and sometimes more meaningful to them than reality.

Some of the *themes* found in both normal and abnormal fantasies have been characterized as the "conquering hero" and the "suffering hero." In fantasies of grandeur the dreamer pictures himself as a great person, winning successes and applause—a conquering hero. (Figure 4–2 depicts a fantasy of mastering the world.) The central character of James Thurber's short story (later a motion picture), *The Secret Life of Walter Mitty,* is a man who indulges in daydreams in which he accomplishes amazing feats. "Walter Mitty" was, for a time, a widely recognized term for the man who is in reality a mouse but in his dreams a roaring lion. The suffering-hero fantasy is represented by the dreams of the child who has been sent to his room for punishment and who fantasizes the mourning of his family and friends when he runs away and meets a tragic end. Another kind of fantasy is of the death of an enemy or the death of a friend who wills the dreamer a small fortune. The death or destruction dream, although one of the less frequent, is reported as occurring in 39 percent of the men and 44 percent of the women in the study made by Shaffer and Shoben (1956).

DISSOCIATION

When we are successfully pursuing desirable goals and satisfying needs, we tend to behave as unified organisms. Our thoughts, feelings, and actions are integrated and represent a coherent whole. But when strong conflict and anxiety enter the scene, we tend to vacillate, and the unity may become disrupted. This disunity due to anxiety is referred to as dissociation. Certain aspects of the total activity or experience are inhibited or excluded totally. At times irrelevant acts are added making our behavior a less appropriate response to a situation.

Some psychoneuroses, particularly hysteria, are examples of dissociated behavior. In World War I a number of individuals developed hysterical paralysis or blindness. The disability was not the result of any lesion in the nervous system but a psychological mechanism to deny the horrors of warfare and to defend the individual from observing combat activity that he abhorred. Some psychoneurotic patients have compulsions. They repeatedly engage in certain ritualistic actions, especially when they are under tension. They show tics and twitches, such as eye blinking or ritualistic finger movements that have little relationship to their coping behavior.

Many lecturers have irrelevant speech and behavioral mannerisms that probably developed early in their careers when they had to grope anxiously to find the right words to communicate ideas effectively. It has been hypothesized that some individual ritualistic activity stands for something that is not recognized by the person; it is an act that reduces the anxiety and tension of the moment and becomes learned. Any of us may show awkward mannerisms, nervous actions such as eye blinking, facial twitches, and hand gestures, or, conversely, we may fail to inhibit certain spontaneous gestures under strong anxiety or conflict.

COMPROMISE OR SUBSTITUTE REACTION

Compromise and substitute behaviors reduce anxiety by at least partially resolving a conflict. Instead of repressing or withdrawing, the person who expresses compromise or substitute reactions does not entirely relinquish the goal he is seeking. Rather, he seeks a similar substitute or symbolic goal. Sam, in the case with which we began the chapter, used withdrawal to his room and dissociation of feelings from actions as his defenses. Later, however, he plunged into a volunteer job to help other people who were "worse off than" himself—behavior that was a compromise. He could not face his own state of conflict and anxiety and could not work through its difficulties. He was overcome by the anxiety involved in his sense of loss of identity, and being cut off from meaningful, early relationships that had provided him with much affection and support as a child. His solution was neither to surrender to his impulse, to withdraw, nor to face and resolve his conflict. Rather, his defense was to enter a lower economic neighborhood and help others to work out their problems.

Let us look at some of the various kinds of compromise or substitute adjustments that attempt to reduce the clash of motives and the intensity of the accompanying anxiety.

RATIONALIZATION

The compromise that requires finding "reasons" for our failures to reach goals and evade the real causes and consequences of our difficulties can take many forms. Most of us at times use *rationalization* or false reasons to explain an event that would cause anxiety and loss of self-esteem if faced frankly. When the mother gives the "reason" for her child's apparent misbehavior, she is rationalizing for him and providing a model for the child's own rationalizing. Most prejudices are supported by rationalization rather than by examination through reasoning.

Sometimes whole areas of thinking are in such *logic-tight compartments,* which the individual cannot expose to open thinking. Religion, for some people, remains in a logic-tight compartment. Selfishness, when exposed, is bulwarked by statements like "The Lord helps those who help themselves," "You have to protect your family," or it is bolstered with statements like "Our country was built on *individual* initiative." Such statements are used to defend all kinds of exploitation. The traditional churchgoer who finds that his affiliations with institutional religion conflict with his weekday hostilities and shrewd practices belittles the "wild-eyed idealist" and says, "You got to be practical."

When all the effort that we can muster fails to achieve a goal, we decide it wasn't worth having anyhow. In addition to this "sour grapes" rationalization, there is the "sweet lemon" approach. When legislation to improve the housing and civil rights of minorities remains unimplemented, this "sweet lemon" rationalization can be heard: "Look how far we have come in helping minorities in the last ten years." The *status quo,* no matter how undesirable, assumes new value when changing it requires more talent or courage than we possess, or means that we lose cherished perquisites. It is shocking sometimes to see how good, moral adages are quoted out of context as rationalizations to justify some basically immoral practice. Elaborate expenditures on a church building, when the man for whom the religion was named emphasized good works instead, is often justified by the statement, "Nothing is too good for the House of God."

The line between reasons and rationalizations is sometimes thin. Rationalizations, if they are defense mechanisms, are not conscious means of resolving the conflict, in the sense that the individual wholly realizes what he is doing; he fails to see his false premises clearly, so he thinks his position is valid. In reasoning, the issue is stated unmistakably and arguments pro and con are evaluated objectively. Some of the same arguments may appear in rationalization, but the personal motivation and method of dealing with them are different.

The reader should consider some of his "reasons" for selecting courses, dating a certain person, or accepting or rejecting associates, particularly whose behavior differs from his. There will be some "reasons" that are justifications for behavior for which the true motivation is not readily stated. These are not reasons: they are rationalizations. Curiously, listing the rationalizations our acquaintances use is less difficult!

PROJECTION

This defense mechanism is the process by which a person protects himself from recognition of his undesirable traits by attributing them to others. An interesting study of college fraternity men indicated empirically the existence of projection (Sears, 1936). Members of the group rated themselves on a number of traits that could be observed, such as disorderliness, obstinancy, and stinginess. They also rated their housemates and were rated by them on the same characteristics. With these data, a student's self-rating may be compared with his fraternity brothers' ratings. Students who did not recognize in themselves traits observed by those who lived with them were the very students who used projection. Students who lacked insight tended to attribute socially undesirable traits, such as stinginess, to other students. It is interesting that these other students were not generally rated by their other fraternity brothers as stingy. It seems, then, that when we fail to recognize in ourselves traits that are regarded as negative, presumably because of the unpleasantness involved in this recognition, we may attribute these traits to others.

Each of us has certain aspects of personality that we have learned to dislike through discipline or taboos. We learn to deny some of them as being part of ourselves, or we attribute them to someone else and thereby gain relief. This process—"misery loves company"—takes many forms. Pointing to guilt in others is satisfying when one is troubled with impulses that make one feel guilty. Seeing characteristics like greed, dishonesty, immorality, and ruthless, self-seeking behavior in others may possibly be projection. "She knew all about me long before I ever saw her, so she can't blame me," argues the fellow who feels guilty for treating a girl shabbily. In this way he places the blame for his behavior on her.

COMPENSATION

A real or imagined obstacle or defect engenders substitute behavior or attempts to overcome it. Response to deficiencies is an established biological phenomenon. A defective thyroid gland, by compensation, grows larger; breathing and heartbeat increase in speed to accommodate the greater needs of the body during exercise. Stories of individuals who have attained greatness despite physical or social handicaps are legion. They have been discussed at length in connection with the inferiority complex. Oddly enough, the greatest asset a high school or university student can have is a vague feeling of inadequacy, if it motivates him to productive compensation or personal problem solving.

Compensation as a defense mechanism is an impulsive attempt to cover up or balance failure by strenuous effort. Several kinds of compensation may be distinguished: (1) *Direct, or compensation in kind.* Here, the individual vigorously attacks his deficiency and attempts to overcome it. The youth who is underdeveloped in size or musculature spends hours in systematic exercise; the plain girl uses a variety of cosmetics. These ways to compensate differ from *rational coping* behavior in which the difficulty is faced openly, the cause or remedy for the felt failure is recognized, a program for improvement is planned, and its effectiveness is checked. (2) *Indirect or substitute compensation.* The individual with physical or social handicaps in a given area turns impulsively to other areas for accomplishment. The bright, slight boy who becomes a public defender and the tall, heavy girl who develops social charm, competence, and leadership ability illustrate this kind of compensation. A Vietnam amputee became active in needed but neglected public services and spent many hours a day with it. A youth from a black ghetto with a boyhood record of stealing became a successful college football player and later an outstanding youth worker.

The process of turning a handicap into an outstanding asset is called overcompensation. The comedian with an oversize nose or mouth or other asymmetrical physical feature who calls attention to the feature and makes it his standard joke is well known to the entertainment world. Similarly, the highly successful man who began in poverty and obscurity and struggled upward is an example of this process; the champion athlete who overcomes, through unrelenting exercise, a physical disability, is another.

It is pointed out that compensation may lead to socially approved or socially disapproved behavior. The borderline student becomes outstanding in extracurricular activities, in athletics, or as a campus entrepreneur. The freshman who arrives on campus feeling lost in the crowd excels as an upperclassman in music, art, or scholarship. On the negative side, an individual who has suffered rejection or has felt socially or physically inferior may act arrogantly, talk loudly, or behave in unconventional or destructive ways. Compensation accounts, too, for the rise of some world leaders. They compensated for their provincial origins by identifying themselves so vigorously with the causes of the mother country that they forced their way to her rule. Napoleon, a Corsican, ruled France and, through it, much of Europe; Hitler, an Austrian, became Feuhrer of Germany and its conquered countries; and Ataturk, a Macedonian, led Turkey to its modern status as an independent Western country.

Lord Byron's career reflected many of the various kinds of compensation. His basic insecurity was generated by an unstable childhood. Furthermore, his crippling by infantile paralysis was a defect he could not face. Byron's greatness as a poet, his cynical acceptance of adulation, his swimming skill (he swam the treacherous Hellespont), and the scandals he created—all can be hypothesized as compensations. Compensation fails, sometimes, to meet the deep personal need that is central to self-esteem and acceptance by the individual himself. It is as though he becomes a prisoner of his frantic efforts to gain simple acceptance of himself. As Murphy (1947) remarks about Byron's notorious free love—it was neither free nor love.

SUBLIMATION

The greatest conflict seems to occur, not between basic motives, but between *methods of satisfying* these motives. Therefore, it is quite possible to substitute socially accepted means of satisfying impulses that push toward antisocial satisfaction. That is *sublimation*. For example, aggression and hate result from an accumulation of frustrated motives. Any socially acceptable means through which these motives can be satisfied, thus preventing the more violent types of aggression or hate, represent sublimation. (See Figure 4–3.)

Most of the forms of play and sports, social gatherings and parties, service to others, art and creative work, outings and travel are socially approved methods of satisfying complex motives. The whole process of readjusting when we are emotionally disturbed consists in finding avenues through which our basic motives may be satisfied in a manner that will merit our approval and self-respect as well as the approval and respect of society. Motives differ with the individual; they represent his personal history. The creative means of satisfaction will therefore vary from person to person. As each one succeeds in a special interest or in a recreational or social activity, he feels more secure and is better able to accept and redirect those of his traits that have been producing anxiety.

REACTION FORMATION

Reaction formation is the defense mechanism in which the behavior that is expressed is the *opposite* of that which the individual actually feels; the unexpressed behavior is disapproved. The overly pleasant individual may be using pleasantness as a façade for inner tendencies to be aggressive. Reaction formation is compensation for socially taboo

Figure 4–3 Sublimation.

Photo by J. Brian King

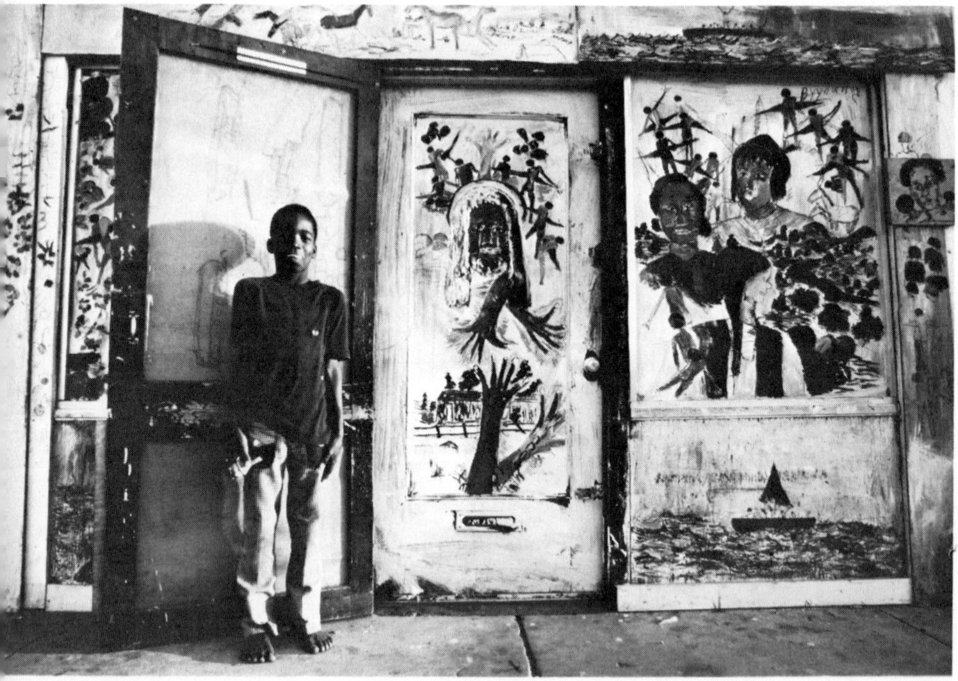

impulses by substituting behavior that will mask these impulses. The individual who is unable to face his tendencies toward aggression or lust feels that he must go to the opposite extreme to prevent this behavior. Many idiosyncracies that differentiate an individual from others fall in this group. The person who must be meticulously neat, inordinately careful, or overly honest may be fighting the opposite impulses he dare not express, even in their mildest forms. Reaction formation may motivate some censors; their work requires them to read all the questionable books, see all the films and plays that are suspected of being pornographic so that they can protect the morals of the general public.

Defense Mechanisms in Perspective

On the positive side, defense mechanisms (which we all use to some extent) allow us to maintain self-esteem and reduce strong anxiety (Figure 4–4). This positive aspect is balanced, however, by the negative fact that they are a form of self-deception and deprive us of a rationality

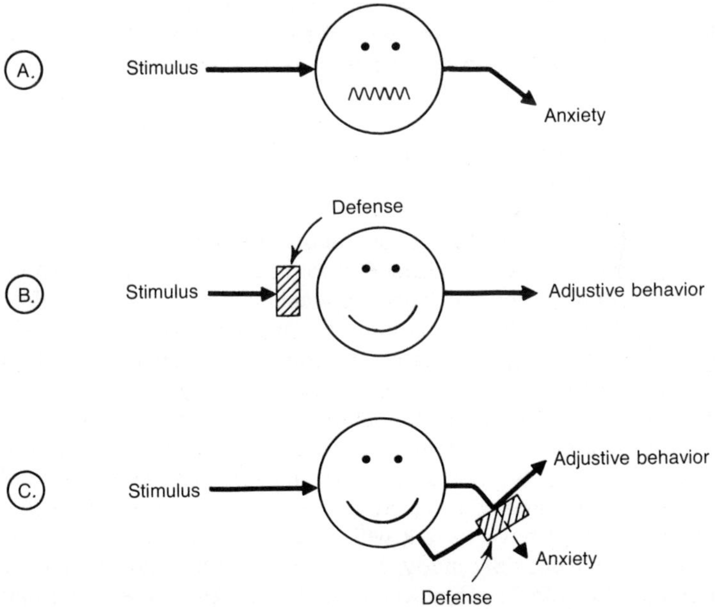

Figure 4–4 (A) illustrates a normal anxiety reaction to stimulus condition or frustrated behavior. (B) and (C) illustrate the erection of defense mechanisms that serve to modify the negative aspects of the stimulus or head off the anxiety. Defenses of the type shown in (B) are withdrawal types; those of the type shown in (C) tend to be compromise reactions.

that could lead to problem solving. They persist despite their detrimental effects, and the negative pattern continues because they are valued for reducing anxiety.

The defense mechanism is a form of adjustment, but usually not the most effective form over a long period of time, as shown by the case of Joe T., which follows. It does adjust the individual to the unbearable anxiety, but it is likely to produce even more severe problems than the anxiety itself. Individuals who are armed with previous successes in coping with their problems come to respond to anxiety with behavior of a more rational or coping nature.

THE CASE OF JOE T.

Joe T. decided he wanted to be a lawyer after he had worked in a law office during the summer break. He had become closely and successfully involved in the office's activities, and he came to admire and use as a model one member of the firm—a relatively young lawyer. He told his psychologist adviser, with great enthusiasm, when he returned to the campus in the fall, "Things will be different now. I've never felt so excited about a vocation. I'm going to improve my rotten grades, and I'm sure I'll be accepted into law school. I've got to be! I have some lawyer friends practicing in the city. I've talked with them, and I think I can get them to write letters of recommendation to the Dean of the Law School." (Joe's grades were just high enough for him to remain in the university, but not high enough for him to be considered for a professional school.)

Joe's grades did improve—but not enough. Although his abilities were adequate for entering Law School, his prelaw grades were damagingly low, and his work habits were too poor to produce the high grades he needed to balance his previously low record. His adviser, viewing the probabilities of Joe's candidacy in Law School realistically, suggested that Joe consider alternate options, in case he washed out. Joe *denied* the possibility of rejection by the law committee and defensively referred to his strong motivation, his good intentions, and the influence of his friends in the profession to bring him special consideration by the Dean.

The night before the last examination of the semester in which he had been trying to make grades to qualify for Law School, Joe phoned his psychologist adviser. He was so panicky his voice quavered. His defenses were weakened; at times during the conversation he seemed on the verge of tears. He said, "I have to talk with you. I'm in the worst mental shape of my life. I can't possibly study. I don't remember anything I've learned in the course. My mind's a blank. I know I'll just sit in the exam tomorrow and shake. I've never been so scared. I've done my best this semester. I've studied regularly, but it's all gone now."

His adviser encouraged him to keep talking, and in the pauses he reflected some of Joe's feelings with remarks like, "You feel that, despite your hard work all semester, you won't know *anything* tomorrow. . . .

You believe you've failed already and that's why you can't study. . . . How do the other students feel—have you talked with them? Aren't they having difficulties and panicky feelings too?" As Joe talked, he began to sound calmer. His adviser suggested that he focus on the actions necessary to prepare for the exam. He also suggested that when Joe began those preparations for the next day's ordeal, his anxiety would subside. The adviser said, "You can't do anything about the past now. Quiz yourself on major topics, see that you do remember the correct answers, and tomorrow begin the exam by answering the questions you know. That's all you can do, but do that! Put your full attention on preparation for the exam; that's all that is in your control now. All the consequences of the exam are out of your hands."

The cathartic effect of talking out his panic, together with a plan for action, calmed Joe greatly. He later reported that his anxiety was initially so great that merely bringing it under control gave him confidence, and he became less concerned about the results of the exam.

Joe didn't make it into Law School, but the crisis experience brought him to view his abilities more realistically. He settled for a less demanding vocation—one that was within the scope of his abilities—and was able, by continuing his hard work and application, to finish the required course work and find a job.

Joe's story illustrates the immediate reason for defenses. It also shows the quasi-adjustive but unrealistic role of defenses, for Joe's defenses were finally broken down by the reality of the exams. His anxieties intensified when he perceived that failure in this exam threatened his prospects of entering the Law School and, later, the profession of law. After several hours of panic, Joe turned to a person whom he trusted and to whom he could express his anxiety. The complete venting of his feelings exposed how unreal his thinking was. The suggestion of action that would yield concrete results produced some self-control and a return of enough confidence for him to go to the exam the next day and try to answer the questions. Later, Joe said that this experience—the initial panic and confusion and later control and action to cope with the reality of the exam—was a salutary experience that he would use in the future, and it may indeed have been of some permanent value for him.

Abnormality and Defense Mechanisms

Much that we call abnormal, neurotic, or psychotic can be seen as consisting of defense mechanisms that result in exaggerated and disorganized behavior. In attempts to defend one's self from persistent and intense anxiety, the individual engages in behavior that may become strongly self-defeating and that results in a serious problem in its own right.

A difference between the "normal" and the pathological individual is that in the normal individual the quasi-adjustive or defensive reaction does not absorb so much of his energy that he cannot carry on the adjustive functions of everyday life; whereas in the abnormal person, disruption of everyday activities usually ensues. Chronic procrastination, alcoholism, and habitual lying are examples of such destructive defenses. The goals of the development of personality, often mentioned by laymen and mental health personnel, are toward a more mature, sociable, adaptive, integrated, and zestful person living in the present real world.

An important aspect of a course in personal adjustment involves self-understanding. An ingredient of such insight is recognition of defense mechanisms, particularly as they keep us from facing and trying to cope with problems. The reader may ask: What recurring defense mechanisms do I find in my life pattern? What specific anxieties do they defend me from? How can I reduce the anxieties and thereby eliminate some defenses?

Factors That Affect the Presence of Defense

There is some evidence that we show a certain degree of consistency in the use of our defense mechanisms. A study of children, made over a period of years, has shown that they tend to use the same kind of defenses at various stages in their lives. A young child who turns away from stimulation uses withdrawal as a frequent defense later in childhood. Variations occur, of course, but the consistency is remarkable (Murphy, 1962).

Presumably, as differing events in early life interact with differing basic constitutions, some individuals develop *ego strength,* a term for strong tolerance of frustration and anxiety and greater coping capacities. Stated another way, some people have, through previous successes, gained confidence or resistance to overpowering anxiety. Others have learned well to evaluate and react to stress, such as criticism. Still others suffer intense anxiety, which requires various kinds of defensiveness rather than efforts toward problem solving.

What conditions give defense mechanisms a preemptive role over coping activities? First, the degree of threat or the *intensity* of the anxiety is a factor. A threat that is perceived as devastating might well arouse more primitive behavior, which may lead to deterioration of the normal problem-solving behavior or the usual effective personal functions. A second factor is the *location* of the frustrating or threatening force. Can the individual perceive and react to that which is frustrating him, or is it too vague or hidden? If the location of the frustration is too vague or hidden for him to perceive its source, his anxiety and defensiveness increase. A rumor circulated about one's competence or one's character is more vague and threatening than the truths that emerge during a quiet, objective evaluation in a friendly professional office.

Rational Coping—Problem Solving

DEFENSE VS. RATIONAL COPING BEHAVIOR

We remark offhandedly and in a joking manner that life is filled with frustrations and conflicts, but we are, in fact, constantly striving earnestly to adjust to them. Defenses thus are universal and accepted as inevitable, and they are a kind of adjustment to anxiety at various points in personal growth. From one viewpoint, defenses indicate that the person has strength and is in the process of adjusting to an overwhelming situation; instead of being panicked, he defends himself. On the other hand, the temporary defense may be detrimental to adjustment at a higher level.

Symonds (1945) asked a class of teachers at Columbia University to write on the ways they deal with personal problems. They described frustrations and situations that were obviously related to anxiety. In analyzing these papers Symonds found that the adjustments were primarily reactions to frustration and defensive attempts to avoid anxiety. Few of the larger problems of their lives were solved through reasoning. He concluded that *rational coping* requires great maturity, which is reached by slow accretion of experience.

When do defenses become self-defeating and create problems for the individual? When they are adopted impulsively and without thought of the effects they may have on the individual's development of effective behavior for dealing with life. The defense must also be evaluated in terms of cultural goals or daily satisfactions. A student may be effective in extracurricular activities, which absorb most of his study time, so he earns poor grades. Is his extracurricular activity a defense from his aversion to reading texts? Possibly. But he does develop social skills that may be useful in his vocation after graduation.

A graduate student whose work is borderline in quality perceives the academic hurdles (comprehensive exams and dissertation) as insurmountable. He defends himself from this agony by taking a temporary job; eventually he settles into the job permanently and forgets the graduate degree. This solution, arrived at indirectly and as a defense, may be a more realistic adjustment for him than to continue his struggle toward a doctoral degree and mediocre performance later.

Psychological abnormalities (psychoses and neuroses), as mentioned above, are often cited as examples of defense mechanisms of an extreme kind, which dominate the individual. A psychotic person may be

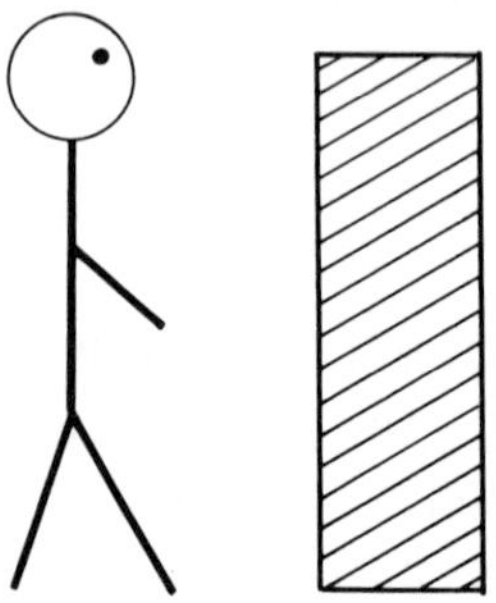

Figure 4–5 Defenses often prevent us from clearly seeing a problem, finding the antecedents to it, and changing them, thereby preventing effective coping.

preoccupied by a repetitive fantasy life or may withdraw from responsibility to adjustment in a perceived hostile world. He may refuse to leave his room or to talk to anyone, as Sam did. Because the defense mechanism in such cases takes so much of the individual's time and energy, yet does not permanently reduce the anxiety, the individual is hampered in dealing with his environment (Figure 4–5). Effective coping requires *clearly seeing a problem, finding the antecedents to it, and changing them.* Therefore, we can assume that the detection and redirection of defense mechanisms is a worthy goal. Those mechanisms that distort our perception of reality and also distort our personality as judged by our culture make adjustment most difficult.

DEFENSE MECHANISMS AS INDIRECT PROBLEM SOLVING

A person may be so emotionally involved with a personal problem that he is at least temporarily incapable of solving it directly. Furthermore, the problem itself may be so complex or emotionally weighted that rational solution is difficult. In such instances defense mechanisms may increase the individual's sense of well-being and serve to protect him until he can move toward a more rational solution or, eventually, to a more satisfactory adjustment. On the other hand, if the defense mechanism itself is too satisfying, it may become a long-term behavior, entrenched in the personality.

In one sense, defense mechanisms represent an *indirect* kind of problem solving. For example, rationalization *may* start a search for reasons that might be productive. Defense mechanisms may be viewed as distorted adaptations of effective ways of coping with conflicts, and as such they are potential adaptive processes that have gone astray (Kroeber, 1963). It should be noted here that many mechanisms have a productive or coping aspect as well as a defensive aspect. Denial, for example, or the refusal to face unwanted thoughts or unpleasant feelings, is, in a sense, a kind of selective awareness. From a positive standpoint it is *concentration.* It is the ability to ignore painful thought for the time being, in order to attend to the business of the moment. Projection, in a sense, is a sensitivity to another person's feelings or thoughts, although, to be sure, it may be erroneous and exaggerated. In its positive form this sensitivity is known as identification or the ability to feel and think as another does. Here again is the suggestion that defense mechanism, under the proper conditions, may move into effective coping responses.

A good example of a borderline process is *identification.* The child emulates his parents and ideal persons, and he identifies himself with them. A related process is *introjection.* In this process the child makes the ideal person's behavior and attitudes his own. Some of this introjection is attributable to admiration of a person or the association of motive-satisfaction or pleasantness with him. This process has been called *modeling* or learning to emulate admired models. At other times the child follows the direction of the parents to avoid punishment or the withdrawal of love. He behaves as though he has taken into himself the regulating commands of his parents, and this behavior has the quality of a defense mechanism. Previously, we termed this regulation as the superego; it is loosely equated to the popular concept of conscience. The parents inculcate their standards, with the belief that their admonitions and examples will keep the child out of trouble and help him, as an adult, to avoid serious problems. Introjection has a problem-solving or coping flavor if the child's attitude toward his parents is positive. If the parents' standards are not valid or consistent or if the child's attitude toward his parents is negative, the introjection may lead to conflict instead of to relief of anxiety. Another negative result is that the continual identification with parents (defense) may not allow the child, in adolescence, to adjust to his peers and thus impedes his development.

GOAL-DIRECTED AND COPING BEHAVIOR

We have already emphasized the point that defense mechanisms, which become established rigid forms of behavior, can disrupt essential goal-directed behavior. In a sense they are often digressive means of adjusting to the environment. Allport (1961) uses the phrase *rational coping* to contrast broadly satisfying goal-directed behavior with defense mechanisms. Coping involves reality testing, effective repression, attempts at reaching self-insight, progressive organization or integration of behavior, the development of frustration tolerance, and personal autonomy. This kind of behavior is in contrast to the uncontrolled self-centeredness, automatic, dissociative, compulsive, and self-defeating characteristics of the pathological individual.

The concept of *ego strength* is used to describe the characteristics of individuals whose adjustment involves much rational coping rather than defensiveness. Barron (1968), in his study of patients who improve in therapy as compared with those who do not improve, finds some empirically established characteristics that validate the importance of rational coping as a factor in total personal adjustment. The improved patients exhibited, among other characteristics, good physical functioning, spontaneity, ability to share emotional experiences, undogmatic religious beliefs, permissive morality, good contact with reality, feelings of personal adequacy and vitality, physical courage, and the related lack of fear. Important questions concern the extent to which positive characteristics can be acquired and facilitated in the adult, and what the best program for teaching these characteristics might be.

The implication of Barron's study and previous comments point to previous successes as important in allowing the individual to engage in problem solving. Some studies suggest that children who are rewarded for active problem-solving behavior and in whom an attitude of confidence is fostered, tend to show the effects of such treatment later (Sears, Maccoby, & Levin, 1957). Jack (1934) and Page (1935) showed some success in modifying dominance levels of young children by providing timid children with certain "confidence-building experiences." Keister (1937) showed that reactions to frustration can be altered to produce more persistent and constructive actions by indicating to small children that frustration can be overcome. Davitz (1952) found that "prior training" can affect the occurrence of responses to frustration. Children were encouraged to play aggressive games and later responded to frustration with more responses involving initiative.

Summary

1. Adjustment can be generally classified into two categories: defenses and rational coping. To see these processes realistically, we take the case of a young man who is on the verge of serious emotional disturbance, observe his defenses, and note that some of his adjustments represent coping with a difficult life situation and that others are ego defenses.
2. The defense mechanisms have the characteristic of *denial* or disguising the impulses that are in conflict with other aspects of the individual's personality. They protect the individual from anxiety resulting from threat to his integrity as a person. Defenses are unconscious, to varying degrees. It is sometimes difficult to discern the extent to which a given response has been learned as a means of satisfying motives and to what extent it is an attempt to avoid or reduce anxiety.
3. Some defenses continue to function for years. We have classified these activities into general categories: (a) *withdrawal reactions,* and (b) *compromise reactions.*

4. The withdrawal reactions include *repression,* which is a clear denial of impulses. *Denial* involves the conscious avoidance of negative feelings and situations. Also included is *suppression,* which is conscious and voluntary inhibition of unwanted behavior. *Apathy* is still another withdrawal defense mechanism.
5. A different class of defense mechanisms is seen in compromise reactions. The individual substitutes some partially need-satisfying activity rather than face and deal with the source of the anxiety. *Rationalization* or "finding reasons" for failures or inconsistencies and evading the real causes of the difficulty is classified under this rubric. *Projection,* similar to rationalization, in that the individual defends his anxiety-laden experiences by pointing to similar behavior in others is also classified here as are *compensation, reaction-formation,* and *sublimation.*
6. Defense mechanisms are inevitable and universal and represent one kind of adjustment to anxiety. They sometimes temporarily quiet anxiety until the individual can engage in rational coping or until the complex situation can be defined in a manner that will permit a more effective attack. Defense mechanisms range from harmless digressions from problem solving to persistent strategems that are classified as abnormal.
7. The term *ego strength* is used to describe a characteristic of the individual who, because of previously acquired skills or successes, uses rational coping rather than defensive behavior. There are studies that show that problem-solving attitudes and confidence can be developed by rewarding behavior leading to solutions and by training programs based on success.
8. The most effective kind of adjustment involves seeing the problem clearly and somewhat calmly, finding the reasons for it, and changing conditions that enhance its continuation. This is the kind of problem solving that is sometimes called *rational coping.* Intense anxiety that impels defense may not permit immediate rational coping.

Words to Remember

Apathy
Compensation
Compromise Reaction
Defense Mechanism
Denial
Dissociation
Ego Strength
Fantasy
Goal-Directed Behavior
Identification
Introjection
Modeling
Projection
Repression
Rational Coping
Rationalization
Reaction Formation
Sublimation
Suppression
Withdrawal Reaction

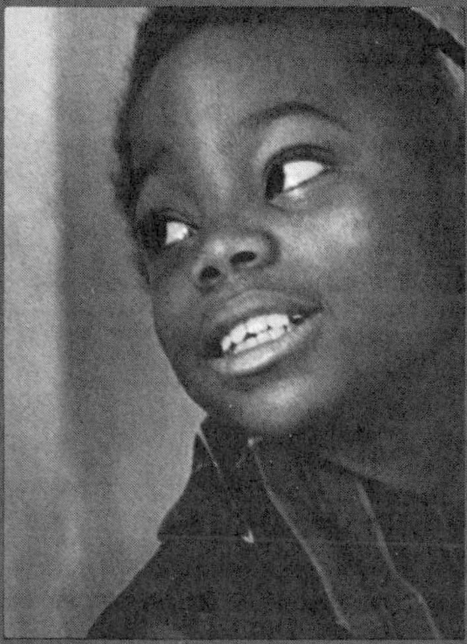

5. Learning and Behavior

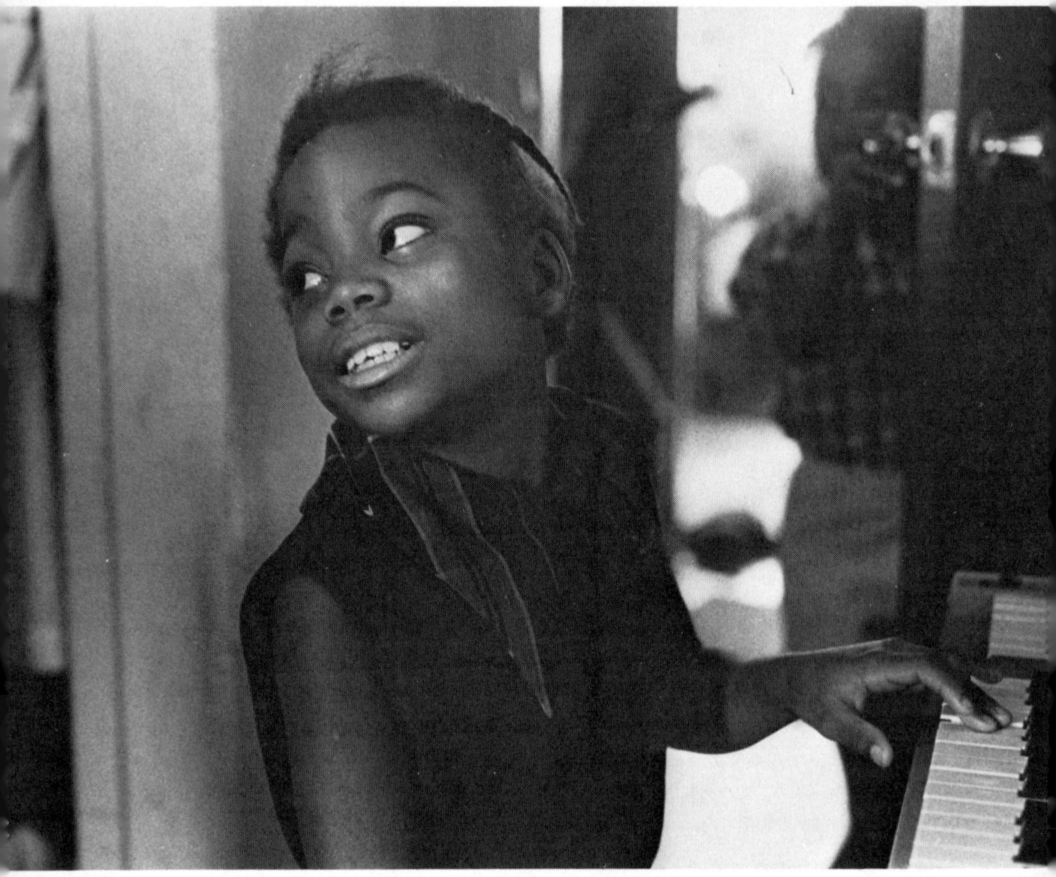

Photo courtesy of *Columbia Missourian*

Objectives

After studying this chapter the reader should be able to:

1. Define *learning.*
2. Describe respondent conditioning in terms of stimulus and response.
3. Explain two methods of modifying or weakening conditioned responses.
4. Define *operant conditioning* and describe the types of reinforcers and the ways that reinforcement can be presented.
5. Describe *behavior shaping.*
6. Identify examples of modeling in the development of complex behavior.
7. Apply the principles of learning to the production of "abnormal" behavior.

Throughout this book we discuss many problems that concern students. Among these is the inability to spend daily the three or four hours of study needed to obtain the required passing grades, or to take an active, inquisitive attitude toward courses. In social situations some students are reluctant to approach people, to introduce themselves, or to speak in public. Feelings of inferiority, self-consciousness, and lack of confidence in social situations are all problems of adjustment. Each of these problems has been learned through previous experience and—what is more important—can be extinguished or unlearned through the specific principles of learning discussed in this chapter.

The Case of Frank

As an introduction to what has been called the learning theory approach to conceptualizing and treating problem behavior, let us consider the case of Frank, which can provide clinical case material for later reference.

Frank is a graduate student majoring in English whose progress in working toward a doctoral degree was halted by severe and incapacitating anxiety about the required oral examination. Although Frank had completed the orals for his Master's degree with only moderate anxiety and had successfully undergone several job interviews, at the time of his doc-

Source: This chapter was written by William T. McReynolds, University of Missouri at Columbia, in collaboration with the senior author, Fred McKinney, of the present book.

toral orals he became tense, panicky, and unable to think or speak coherently. Frank's professors, pleased with the quality of his past work, suggested that he seek professional help.

At the time Frank made his initial contact with a psychologist he was tense, somewhat embarrassed, and genuinely fearful of the prospect of facing and freezing-up at his orals again. He related a brief personal history. He is the eldest son in a relatively prosperous but hardworking family. His childhood and adolescent development were largely uneventful. Frank did tend to be extremely shy and consequently was inexperienced with girls and dating. His relationship with his mother had always been warm and affectionate but without overattachment. Frank's father, however, tended to be distant and overcritical, often questioning many of Frank's educational and life goals. Despite his father's opposition, Frank managed to complete four years of undergraduate and three years of graduate work with the financial assistance of an uncle.

In treatment, it quickly became apparent that Frank harbored strong feelings of self-doubt and low self-esteem. He maintained a poised, formal, interpersonal style that became tenuous in the face of emerging feelings of incompetency and insecurity. In spite of these troubled feelings, however, Frank was eager to explore the nature and basis of his oral examination anxiety with the therapist and proved to be a hardworking, optimistic client. Treatment proceeded along three fronts. First, Frank learned a method of relaxation that enabled him to rid his body of all muscular tensions. On instruction, he began to use his newly acquired relaxation skill during stressful or anxiety-arousing situations as a coping strategy.

Next, Frank and his therapist explored the kinds of self-directed verbalizations or thoughts he had just before situations in which he is called on to "prove himself" and more general feelings and self-to-self statements about his general competence as an English scholar and as a person. For example, he often thought to himself:

> "I feel I am going to freeze up on that oral exam and with all the emotion be unable to talk coherently."
>
> "Even though I know the answers to some of the questions asked I'll be in such a panic that I won't be able to give them."
>
> "I've studied but I still don't know the answers to some questions they may ask."
>
> "I'm not as good a student as some in the department."

A number of positive, self-bolstering statements were formulated in the light of his real abilities and accomplishments, and Frank began to practice substituting the more favorable self-communications for the other less flattering, seemingly self-fulfilling ones. Here are examples of the positive statements:

> "Now let me look at the facts, they will be asking me questions in an area I know well."

"They themselves can't have read that much more than I have in this specialized area."

"I have covered the material as thoroughly as anyone who ever came up for an exam. Nobody is expected to know everything about a subject."

"I know the material and answer questions well when alone with my adviser, and can do it here, too."

Finally, Frank began to subject himself to anxiety-arousing oral examination situations a little at a time, first just imagining himself in the exam situation and mentally rehearsing his behavior. Later he practiced appropriate behavior in actual contrived situations patterned closely after the original and upcoming test. For example, Frank and the therapist went into a conference room similar to the one that would be used later in Frank's examination. Frank was told to sit in a manner that would make him feel most comfortable. He was to imagine his committee members sitting in the vacant chairs, across from him (the therapist occupied one of the chairs and acted as one member). Frank was to imagine their behavior and react to it. The therapist then began the examination. Frank was to practice relaxation, to practice pauses, and to use other aids which would facilitate thinking rather than panic. He practiced using statements such as "Would you repeat the second part of the question," "I don't understand the word . . . ," "Are you referring to . . ."

Progress in overcoming his fear and dread of his second examination was rapid. After three weeks of treatment Frank reported both a positive outlook toward his future as an English teacher and feelings of having overcome more general inferiority feelings. He later faced his orals successfully and was subsequently described by his professors and other observers as being noticeably more relaxed and confident.

IMPLICATIONS OF THE CASE OF FRANK

How would you describe the nature of Frank's problem and the treatment he received? Could you do so without using general personality concepts such as inferiority complex, poor self-concept, or weak ego? In what ways are Frank's problems similar to more well-adjusted behaviors such as good manners or social competence? Finally, could you make this same sort of analysis in any of the other cases described in the book?

Both the title of the present chapter and the preceding questions suggest that the basic process involved in the case of Frank is *learning*. Learning is not confined to the school or home. Many "intrinsic personality characteristics" are, in fact, learned behavior patterns. Our fears, ambitions, likes, hates, skills, sex preferences, moral beliefs, and social values—to name a few behaviors (remember that feelings and attitudes are also behavior)—are what they are because of the cumulative effects of past learning experiences. In addition some very basic temperament and character traits—such as enthusiasm, sense of humor, self-control, and obnoxiousness—appear to be largely learned traits. Thus much of the behavior that underlies the unique and identifying features of ourselves is often a matter of the presence or absence of learned responses. Learning, then, is central to adjustment. We begin looking at the processes of learning by focusing on its basic principles and concepts.

Learning Processes

Although theories of how learning takes place differ greatly, it is generally agreed that learning is the process whereby behavior is acquired or changed as a result of experience. This *definition* alone, however, does not exclude related processes of maturation and temporary states, such as fatigue and sensory-motor incapacity. Experience can produce changes in behavior through a broken arm, for instance.

The growth and *maturation* of the physical equipment of a child set the stage for learning, but some behavioral changes result directly from maturation process and are not themselves caused by learning. For example, the steady development of visual acuity in a newborn stems primarily from the maturing of nerves and neural pathways in the eyes, between the eyes and brain, and within the brain. Experience may, however, promote the maturation process. Hubel and Wiesel (1963) have shown that kittens deprived of normal vision by placing translucent covers over their eyes show visual-nervous "immaturities" as complex nervous cells decompose from lack of use. The idea of reading readiness is a maturational process in the field of education the reader may find familiar. The sexual interests of the adolescent compared with those of a younger child are due to a large extent to maturational endocrine changes. Similarly, the inactivity of the older person is due to physical changes occurring at the far end of "maturity."

Temporary states resulting in unlearned behavior changes include both sensory and motor states. Fatigue is a prime example of the latter transitory state. Behavior changes such as slowed responding and "sloppiness" that come from being tired are not attributable to learning processes. Although fatigue, and its related effect on behavior, has been a key element in Hull's (1943) theory of learning, the results of energy expenditure itself are not learned. Similarly, temporary losses of motor skills such as those resulting from a broken arm or leg represent an extreme form of unlearned motor loss. Finally, changes in peripheral sense organs resulting from prolonged or high intensity stimulation are usually attributed to sensory adaptation or habituation. For example, the momentary blindness experienced when entering a dark room on a sunny day is an example of sensory adaptation effects. Excessive light stimulation can also produce more permanent blindness and, subsequently, many other unlearned behavior changes associated with the loss of that sensory function.

Thus we may *define* learning in a slightly negative sense, as Hilgard and Bower (1966) have, as a process whereby behavior is acquired and changed through an organism's interactions with the environment when maturation or temporary states will not also account for that same behavior. We must be quick to note, however, that the obverse of this definition does not hold. Failure to observe changes resulting from experience does not mean that learning has not taken place. *Latent* or "unintentional" learning may take place without immediately observable changes in behavior. We may learn the location of many of the streets and buildings along our routes to work or school without making a point to do so. We pick up words, names of people and places, and we acquire incidental facts that are not directly related to our goals at the time. Such incidental learning may provide valuable information about our surroundings and later increase the speed or proficiency with which we learn later behavior. Observational learning or *modeling,* discussed later in this chapter, provides another example of how learning may take place without affecting observable behavior at the time. The laws of learning and the laws of performance of learned behavior are not the same.

Types of Learning

Pause for a moment and bring to mind as many different learned behaviors as you can. Perhaps the different learned behaviors seem to separate themselves naturally into two types—learned ways of doing things and learned ways of reacting to certain situations. In *learned ways of doing things* you respond purposively, changing your environment to bring about some desired ends or results.[1] Thus, dropping money in vending machines, driving an automobile, and cooking or preparing food are examples of learned, purposive behavior. *Learned reactions,* on the other hand, occur autonomically as in becoming fearful or happy when something happens. Learned behavior of the automatic type is said to result from *classical* or *respondent conditioning*. Learned purposive skills result from *instrumental* or *operant conditioning*. Both types of learning or conditioning will be considered in some detail.

[1] In other parts of the book we have used the terms *problem solving* or *coping behavior* for some of this behavior.

RESPONDENT CONDITIONING

The Russian physiologist I. V. Pavlov first discovered the principle of respondent conditioning while experimenting with the digestive system of dogs. Pavlov observed that certain digestively neutral stimuli, such as the sound of experimental machinery and the sight of the experimental room, elicited preparatory eating behavior (saliva flow, chewing) similar to that elicited by the actual taste of food. Further experimentation showed that the sound of a tuning fork when consistently paired with the presentation of food comes to elicit many of the same eating behaviors, notably saliva flow, as the food stimuli.

Food or presentation of the food has come to be called an *unconditioned stimulus,* or *UCS,* meaning that it is a change in the organism's environment to which it normally responds in a reflexive, automatic way. Salivation, the reflexive response, is called an *unconditioned response,* or *UCR.* The tone is originally neutral and does not stimulate salivation. When it acquires this new, conditioned property, it is labeled a *conditioned stimulus,* or *CS.* Similarly the dog's response of salivating to the CS is called a *conditioned response,* or *CR.* (Figure 5–1 is a schematic showing the steps in respondent conditioning.)

Pavlov and subsequent researchers have used many CSs in condition-

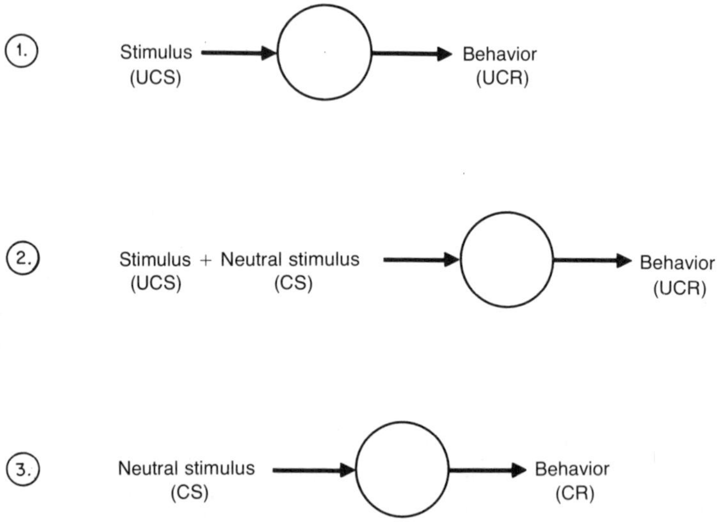

Figure 5–1 Respondent Conditioning. Step 1 illustrates an ongoing reflexive behavior pattern. In step 2 the naturally occurring stimulus (UCS) is paired with a neutral stimulus (CS). In step 3, the resultant behavior (now called *a conditioned response*) is elicited by the neutral stimulus alone—clearly a learned response.

ing other than tones, including lights, pictures, and virtually every form of sensory stimulation. A great many involuntary responses also have been conditioned including such diverse behaviors as perspiration and eye blinks.

A classic example of respondent conditioning in human experimentation has been provided by Watson and Rayner (1920). A one-year-old child, Albert, showed no signs of fear or disturbance in the presence of a white rat. Albert did, however, become extremely upset when a loud and unexpected noise—striking a steel bar with a hammer—was made. Albert then became startled, began crying, squirming, and trembling. After observing these two natural responses, Watson and Rayner began presenting the white rat to Albert and immediately thereafter banging the bar with the hammer. Not surprisingly, Albert continued to become disturbed by the noise, but this time his disturbance occurred in the presence of the rat. After only seven pairings of the rat with the raucous noise, the sight of the rat alone caused crying and distress. Albert had become "rat phobic." It should be clear that in this case the loud noise is the UCS, and Albert's reaction to the noise a UCR. The acquired or conditioned response of distress represents a CR to the CS of a white rat. The reader may be familiar with fears, anxieties, aversions, joys, or other strong emotional responses that become attached to neutral stimuli such as certain types of foods, places, and even certain people.

A student tells that he becomes highly anxious when he hears a popular song sung softly over the radio. This pattern of anxiety began when he was knocked unconscious in an auto accident; upon awakening he was in the wrecked car and the car radio was broadcasting the popular tune.

EXTINCTION AND COUNTERCONDITIONING

Were the properties of respondent conditioning to end here, ours would indeed be a simple world. A number of other basic processes merit consideration. First, conditioned responses may be weakened through an *extinction* procedure. Extinction is simply the repeated presentation of a CS without an associated UCS. In such a procedure the CS begins to lose its conditioned properties and eventually revert back to its neutral state. Many learned fears are short-lived, thanks to extinction. Think of the many fears of children—the dark, ghosts, illnesses, strangers, and so forth—that are often extinguished by the time they are in the teens.

Conditioned responses may also be lost through *counterconditioning.* Counterconditioning is achieved when a response is conditioned to a CS that already elicits another incompatible CR. Continuing with the case of little Albert's "phobia," generating pleasurable or enjoyable feelings in Albert by, say, giving him favorite foods or toys with the white rat, the CS for fear, could lead to a conditioned association of pleasure with the rat. Such a procedure has been described by Jones (1924). The conditioned fear is displaced through counterconditioning.

GENERALIZATION, DISCRIMINATION, HIGHER-ORDER CONDITIONING

Stimulation, especially as it occurs in our natural environment, rarely occurs in isolated or pure forms as in the sound of a tuning fork or even the sight of a white rat. Instead, we respond to complex stimuli such as various people; situations such as a job, a party, or an accident; and objects such as a bus, an office, or an assignment. Furthermore, different stimuli may affect us in similar or greatly different ways. To the extent that a stimulus similar in some way to a CS does *not* elicit the CR, *discrimination* is said to be operating. Albert may not become upset when a brown rabbit or teddy bear is brought into the room. Similar reactions to different stimuli may result from a process of *generalization.* When a stimulus other than, but similar to, a CS elicits the CR, in whole or part, generalization is said to have occurred. Thus, Albert might respond fearfully to both a white rat and a small white rabbit. The fear might even generalize to small white stuffed animals. Many examples of generalization occur in everyday living. A tough-grading high school teacher may have had bushy black hair and have worn horn-rimmed glasses; another teacher with a similar appearance may at first evoke the same negative reaction that the high school teacher did. A college student reports that he always looks over a group of people before approaching it. He traces this habit to boyhood days when he looked over the crowd in the playground to see if any potential bullies were there. Having received low grades in previous multiple-choice exams, another student feels apprehension and hostility as the objective exam is being passed out by the teacher.

Higher-order conditioning is somewhat related to generalization. Sometimes neutral stimuli, when paired with CSs, themselves come to take on some of the properties of those CSs. In such higher-order conditioning one CS actually serves the function of a UCS in the establishment of a second CS. In everyday experience, the consistent bearer of bad tidings is not a welcome guest. For Albert, the experimenter (originally a neutral "stimulus") who repeatedly brings on the feared rat may himself become feared. Again, in this process of higher-order conditioning, CSs function much like UCSs in first-order conditioning with neutral stimuli (e.g., the experimenter) becoming capable of eliciting the same CRs (fear) originally associated only with the first CS (white rat) and UCS (loud noise).

We have considered only the most basic processes involved in respondent conditioning. As we shall see soon, however, even these fundamental principles provide a basis for understanding behavior. Before we turn to operant conditioning, consider once again the case of Frank. Is it possible to discern CRs in Frank's behavior, possibly related to his interaction with his father? What about a CS? Did the men on his committee arouse anxiety related to earlier experiences with male authority figures? How might conditioning have contributed to Frank's main problem?

OPERANT CONDITIONING

The name most often associated with operant conditioning is that of B. F. Skinner. It was Skinner (1938) who first developed the well-known operant conditioning chamber, or Skinner box, that resulted in extensive research on this form of learning. A Skinner box, shown in Figure 5–2, is simply an enclosed compartment equipped with one or more buttons or levers that can be depressed easily by a small animal, a food chute through which food can be presented automatically, and usually a source of stimulation by sound or light. A Skinner box can be programmed so that when the lever or button is depressed, a small amount of food pellets or grain tumbles down the chute. A hungry animal very readily learns to depress the lever to obtain food. In conditioning of this nature the animal operates on his environment. In other words, the animals' lever pressing is instrumental in obtaining food. Hence, the corresponding names *operant* and *instrumental conditioning*. Lever pressing, then, is the conditioned response, and food pellets are the operant reinforcers. The important point to remember in comparing respondent and operant conditioning is that in the latter case the organism, human or subhuman, actually *changes his environment* during the process of learning and performing learned behaviors. (See Figure 5–3.) As such, operant conditioning normally deals with voluntary behavior.

Operant conditioning accounts for normal and—as we shall see—

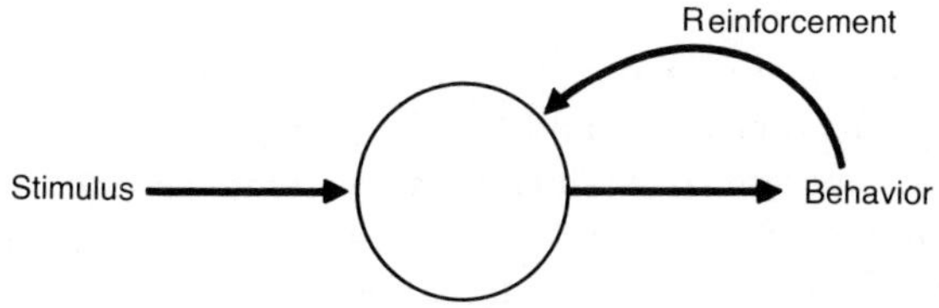

Figure 5–2 An Operant Conditioning Chamber, or Skinner Box.

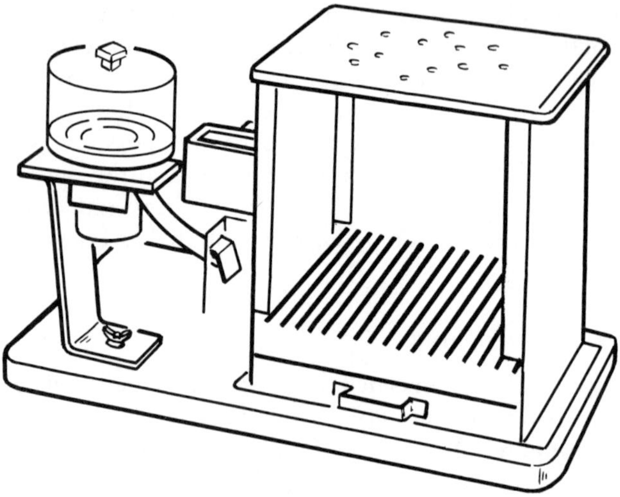

Figure 5–3 In operant conditioning, the stimulus situation leads to a behavior that operates on or changes the environment in such a way as to effect a reinforcement or facilitation of the response. Repetition of the reinforcement strengthens the learned behavior.

abnormal behavior more frequently than any other single psychological process. Much of our work and play behavior is centered around obtaining rewards or enjoyment. Clearly, however, we are not guided solely by our desire to satisfy our hunger, as in the case of a laboratory rat. To understand the operant conditioning of more complex and "remote" human behaviors, we must further describe the procedures involved. First, there are two general types of reinforcement—primary and secondary reinforcement. *Primary reinforcers* are those directly related to primary or biological needs, such as hunger and thirst. Thus, food and water are common primary reinforcers. Needless to say, however, not all forms of pleasure are directly related to biological needs. Money is a singular and often-cited example. *Secondary reinforcers,* of which money is an example, are desirable consequences that are often related to primary reinforcers but are not themselves biological in nature; money is exchanged for food and shelter. Other examples of secondary reinforcers are parental and peer approval, grades, and articles that enhance our appearance or make our lives luxurious. Most so-called "status symbols," such as fancy cars and jewelry, are secondary reinforcers that support much operant behavior. Finally, some secondary reinforcers, such as social acceptance and attention, are so pervasive in our culture that they have been called *generalized reinforcers.*

Reinforcement of spontaneously occurring or innate behavior accounts for only a limited amount of conditioning via operant procedures. Complex behavior, which appears only after much experience and training, is learned through operant conditioning. A rat's pressing a lever is one such behavior; talking is another. Must a complex behavior occur in its final, complete form to be reinforced? To teach a child to recite "Columbus sailed the ocean blue in fourteen hundred ninety-two" must we await the spontaneous occurrence of that entire, complex response so that we can reinforce it? Obviously such a process would be extremely slow and inefficient. The problem is resolved by a procedure called response *shaping*. Complex and infrequently occurring behaviors can be taught by reinforcing successive approximations to those behaviors. Such shaping capitalizes on what the organism can do to build new and more complex behaviors. Thus a rat in a Skinner box can be conditioned to press a lever for reinforcement if we first reinforce him for staying in the part of the cage with the lever, then for touching the lever with his nose or paw, then moving the lever slightly, then pushing it halfway down, and finally depressing it completely. This principle of behavior shaping is basic to much human learning.

Consider the following example of a mute and largely unresponsive hospitalized patient being shaped to speak normally. The mutism and the extreme withdrawal behavior were among the symptoms that occurred when the patient became acutely disturbed. Note also the presence of discrimination and generalization process.

> During the first week, a stick of gum was held before *S*'s face, and *E* waited until *S*'s eyes moved toward it.[2] By the end of the second week, *S*'s eyes moved toward the gum as soon as it was held up. During the third week *E* held the gum before *S*, waiting until he noticed movement in *S*'s lips before giving it to him. By the end of this week, both lip movement and eye movement occurred when the gum was held up. *E* then withheld giving *S* the gum until *S* spontaneously made a vocalization, at which time *E* gave *S* the gum. By the end of the fourth week, holding up the gum readily occasioned eye movement toward it, lip movement, and a vocalization resembling a croak.
>
> During the fifth and sixth weeks, *E* held up the gum, and said, "*Say 'gum, gum'*" repeating these words each time *S* vocalized. Giving *S* the gum was made contingent upon vocalizations increasingly approximating *gum*. At the end of Week 6, when *E* said, "Say *gum, gum*," *S* suddenly said, "Gum, please." This response was accompanied by reinstatement of other responses of this class, that is, *S* answered questions regarding his name and age.
>
> Thereafter, he responded to questions by *E* in individual and in group sessions but answered no one else. Responses to the discriminative stimuli of the room generalized to *E* on the ward; he greeted *E* on two occasions in the group room. He read from signs in *E's* office upon request by *E*.

[2] "S" is the traditional symbol for a *subject* in an experiment; "E" for the *experimenter* conducting the experiment.

> Since the response now seemed to be under the strong stimulus control of *E, the person,* attempt was made to generalize the stimulus to other people. Accordingly, a nurse was brought into the private room; *S* smiled at her. After a month, he began answering her questions. Later, when he brought his coat to a volunteer worker on the ward, she interpreted the gesture as a desire to go outdoors and conducted him there. Upon informing *E* of the incident, she was instructed to obey *S* only as a consequence of explicit verbal requests by him. *S* thereafter vocalized requests. These instructions have now been given to other hospital personnel, and *S* regularly initiates verbal requests when nonverbal requests have no reinforcing consequences. (Isaacs, Thomas & Goldiamond, 1960, p. 9).

SCHEDULES OF REINFORCEMENT

Thus far we have considered reinforcement as an event that follows every response, that is, *continuous* reinforcement. Other *schedules of reinforcement* are also possible. Reinforcement may occur only after some of the conditioned or to-be-conditioned responses. Such *partial reinforcement* may take several forms. First, every *n*th response may be reinforced where *n* is any number, say, 3 or 10. This is called *equal ratio reinforcement,* denoting that an equal number of responses per reinforcement is required throughout learning and performance. If the ratio of responses per reinforcement varies but has an average ratio, as would be the case if an average of 10 responses were required for reinforcement, but sometimes only eight or nine responses or eleven or twelve responses were required (i.e., varying around 10), the schedule is *variable ratio reinforcement.*

Instead of requiring a certain number of responses for a reinforcement we may require the passage of a certain amount of time between reinforced responses. Thus, in *fixed interval reinforcement* the first response to occur after the passage of a given amount of time, say, 30 seconds, is reinforced. Only the first response that occurs following the required time lapse will be reinforced, no matter how many times the animal responds before the interval is completed. If the interval required between reinforced responses varies about an average length of time such that responses may be reinforced before or after an average period (25 to 35 seconds), the schedule is a *variable interval reinforcement* schedule. In both types of interval schedule particular responses are being reinforced, there is just the additional condition that a response will be reinforced only after a given time period. An individual whose salary is paid on a monthly basis receives variable interval "reinforcement" (remember, the days of the months vary from 28 to 31). On the other hand, a salesman who receives a commission on the number of products sold or a laborer on the number of pieces completed operates under a fixed ratio schedule. A weekly allowance represents fixed interval reinforcement if receipt of the allowance is made contingent on good behavior. Can you think of other examples? What would a Christmas bonus based on employee productiveness be?

For our purposes, it is most important to note that extinction of operantly conditioned responses through nonreinforcement varies with different reinforcement schedules. Extinction following 100 percent or continuous reinforcement is usually rapid, the CR dropping out fairly quickly after a few nonreinforced responses. The reduction of responding during extinction of partially or intermittently reinforced responses, whether ratio or interval in nature, is *relatively slow.* The organism may continue responding after many nonreinforced trials, with the CR only gradually dropping out. The resistance to extinction following partial reinforcement is called the *partial reinforcement effect.* Some psychologists have conceptualized certain stubborn or persistent human behaviors as examples of this effect. In such cases we may hypothesize that the person has learned to be patient and to "keep plugging away," since partial reinforcement involves many "dry periods." The partial reinforcement effect helps to explain slot machine playing behavior as well as other forms of gambling.

POSITIVE AND NEGATIVE REINFORCEMENT

Earlier, two types of reinforcers—primary and secondary—were discussed. Reinforcers may be subdivided in another way, into positive and negative reinforcers, depending on certain features. A *positive* reinforcer is a stimulus or set of conditions that the individual seeks. The primary reinforcers of food and water and the secondary reinforcers of money, praise, and attention are all positive reinforcers. We often employ positive reinforcers to achieve operant conditioning. Conversely a *negative reinforcer* is a stimulus or condition that is not sought by the individual and will, in fact, be avoided in most cases. Electric shock, extreme cold, noxious sounds, and most sources of intense stimulation are negative reinforcers. Social disgrace, fear, anxiety, and guilt are also negative reinforcers that operate in our lives. It is the reduction, *subtraction,* or *withdrawal* of such "stimuli" that is reinforcing. That is, the removal of negative reinforcers is an effective operant reinforcer. Thus, we avoid underdressing in the winter, overdressing in the summer. We steer clear of situations that make us feel uneasy or anxious, and we learn how to relate to people so as not to anger them and jeopardize or embarrass ourselves.

Punishment

What about the case in which negative reinforcers are *presented* or positive reinforcers *withdrawn,* you may ask. What would these procedures be called, and what effect would such occurrences have on behavior? The effects of *punishment* are varied and complex. Most often, the immediate effect of punishment is to decrease or eliminate the punished behavior. The total behavioral effects of punishment, however, are somewhat paradoxical. On the one hand, the reliable effects of punishment in suppressing behavior are well recognized by psychologists. As long as the punishment remains in operation the punished behavior will rarely occur. The effects of punishment are not the same as extinction, however, in that *punished behaviors tend to return when punishment is withdrawn.* Although punishment produces rapid *suppression* of responses, such suppression appears to preclude extinction (since suppressed CRs cannot occur in the absence of reinforcement) and its more permanent reduction of learned behavior.

Punishment also may have certain undesirable and uncontrollable effects in producing frustration and general emotional upheaval in the punished organism. The most critical aspect of punishment in the context of behavior control is that punishment alone will not result in the learning of new behavior. Punishment may suppress old behavior, but it provides no guidelines or reinforcement for new, more desirable responses. As an example, a mother may decide to teach her child to eat with a fork by punishing him when he does otherwise. She may spank or reprimand the child when he eats with his hands or fingers, scoops his food with a knife or spoon, licks his plate, or even refuses to eat altogether. There are a number of incorrect behaviors for which he will be punished and only one for which he is rewarded. Even if he is trying to avoid punishment by trial-and-error responding, he is doomed by the variety of available wrong responses and the uncertainty of the proper one. The cards are truly stacked against him. Thus punishment may dramatically affect performance but not the learning of new behavior. For this reason, and because of the unwanted emotional effects of punishment, leading thinkers in the field of learning (e.g., Skinner) have cautioned against the excessive use of punishment to control behavior. (See Figure 5–4.)

Sometimes in helping an individual unlearn behavior he considers undesirable we have to help him learn that situations that were previously punishing (embarrassing) are subsequently neutral events. This may be accomplished by systematic desensitization, discussed in a later chapter.

Avoidance and Escape Learning

Earlier, negative reinforcement was described as the removal of a noxious or aversive stimulus. *Avoidance conditioning* provides one of the best and, as will be clear later, most meaningful examples of the operation of negative reinforcement. Consider the following experimental conditions: A dog is placed in a large cage with a wire grid floor that is electrically wired to allow an experimenter to shock the animal on his paws. A buzzer is sounded for two seconds, and if the dog is in that half of the cage containing the buzzer and a food dish five seconds after the buzzer sounds, he is soundly shocked; if after the buzzer sounds the dog scurries to the opposite side of the cage within five

Figure 5–4 Nothing Desirable to Learn Here.

Photo courtesy of *Columbia Missourian*

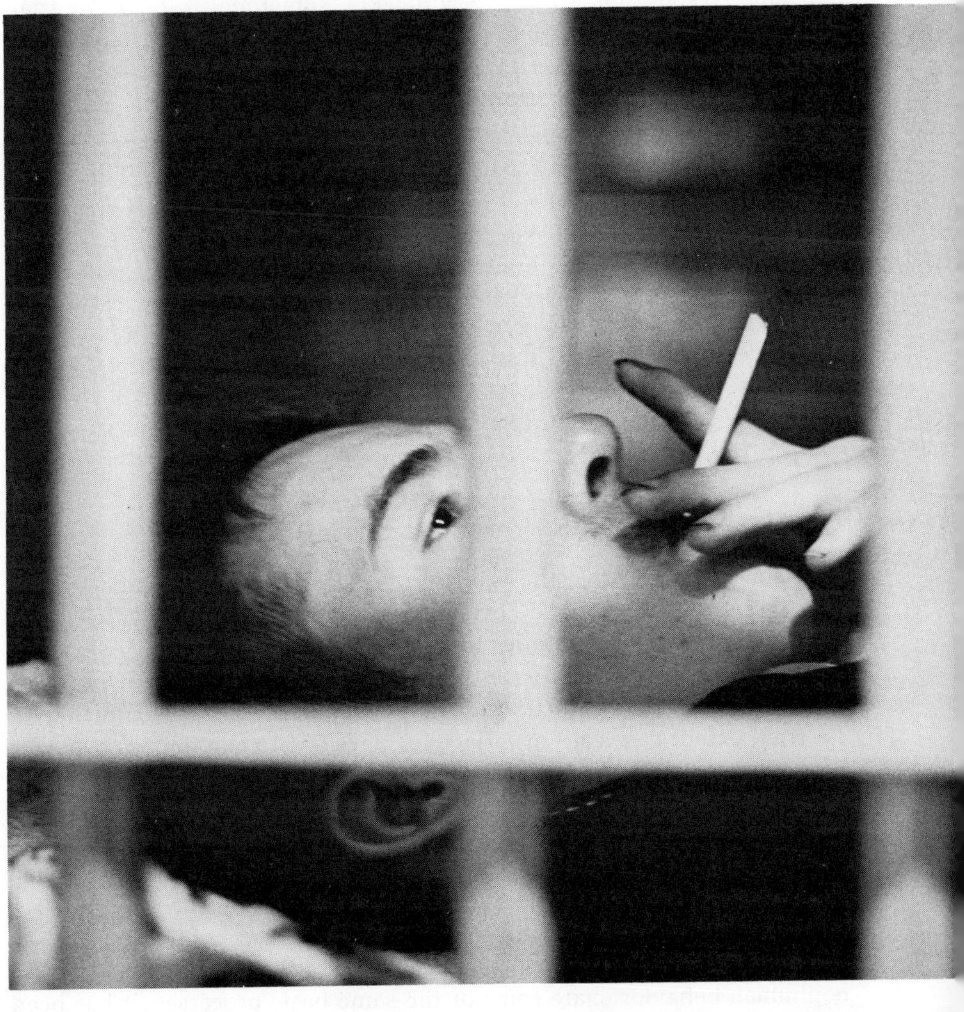

seconds, no shock is delivered. Very quickly, depending on the size of the shock and other conditions, the dog learns to respond to the buzzer by running to the safe area, thereby avoiding the shock. Such conditioned avoidance and related escape conditioning in which aversive stimulation is terminated or escaped after it has begun was first systematically studied by Mowrer and Miller (1942). Subsequently, much research has been conducted on escape and avoidance conditioning, and numerous parallels have been drawn between such experimental phenomena and more naturally occurring human behavior. The work of Solomon is especially noteworthy.

In a series of now classic experiments Solomon found that when extremely intense, aversive shock is used in avoidance conditioning, the avoidance response is learned very quickly, sometimes in only one trial. Furthermore, the conditioned avoidance response is very stable and resists extinction. Solomon and Wynne (1954), for instance, found that dogs that learned avoidance of intense shock continued to make the avoidance response years and thousands of trials later during extinction when no shock would follow the warning signal. The apparently crucial factor in this relative inextinguishability of avoidance is that an avoiding animal always makes the avoidance response, and thus never "discovers" that shock is not imminent.

This response is seen in human problems. A swimmer may never dive again after the painful and embarrassing first flop. A stage-fright experience may prevent an individual from ever again speaking before a group.

Social Learning

THE LEARNING OF COMPLEX HUMAN BEHAVIOR

In our descriptions of the principles of learning derived from laboratory research, relatively few examples of the operation and relevance of such core learning processes to human behavior have been given. The behavior of people is obviously much more complex than that of lower animals and of more primary interest in a book on personal adjustment. To what extent can learning principles developed from animal behavior be extended and applied to the problem of understanding the nature of normal and "abnormal" human behavior? When are we justified in generalizing from lower animal to human behavior?

In contemporary psychology the principles of conditioning have provided a basic conceptual foundation for understanding the nature of acquired human behavior and some of the processes involved in the acquisition of human behavior. Proceeding on the belief that human and nonhuman behavior share some of the same basic processes, it has been possible for behavioral scientists to talk about human operants and respondents. The gain at this level is in the precision of our language and in thinking about basic units of behavior and basic learning processes. By taking this conceptual or analytic approach to human behavior, behavioral scientists have found that many of the conditions, events, and phenomena involved in the acquisition of normal human behavior are similar to those observed in the laboratory. In this conditioning conceptualization of acquired human behavior, additions to basic principles and the search for additional processes have been necessary. Nonetheless the core of basic, experimentally based learning principles continues to be relevant.

Consider the case of a child's gradual acquisition of speech. It can be observed that many of the circumstances surrounding the acquisition of speech involve operant conditioning. A child may first utter the sound "da-da," as a completely accidental behavior or by way of producing a familiar, perhaps appealing sound. Proud father, quick to recognize his son's first but sincere attempt to address "Daddy," may well exclaim, "Did you hear that?" while he begins talking back to a surprised son who thoroughly enjoys his newfound attention and general approval. Such reinforcement assures the repetition of the behavior, to Dad's recurrent delight. Although the effect of subsequent "da-da" begins to wear off, "da-di" brings new approval and attention, displayed later by a full-fledged "Dad" or "Daddie." Other new baby utterances also begin to "pay off" in the meantime, resulting in a lengthening repertoire of "ma-ma," "puppy," "Teddy," "bottle," "hi," and the like. Finally, putting words together in meaningful combinations and sentences is carefully shaped by parents. The presence of basic learning principles in this example is evident, even though other considerations may also be made to account fully for speech acquisition.

The operation of learning in the development of normal behavior is also exemplified in the mother's reinforcement of dainty behavior in the girl and the father's reinforcement of large movements and rough behavior in the boy. The mother's "That's a good little girl" is often heard. Conversely, the father readily plays ball or wrestles with the boy. Again it is clear that the acquisition of normal behavior is best conceptualized within known learning processes.

Although a core of learning principles enables us to conceptualize and account for much human behavior, additional processes must also be considered in order to complete the picture. One such necessary additional process is learning through imitation or modeling. *Modeling, imitation,* or *observational learning* refers simply to the acquisition of behavior through the observation of that behavior in others. (Figure 5–5.) Much of our behavior results from our exposure to others' behavior and our observation of the consequences of their behavior. Fads,

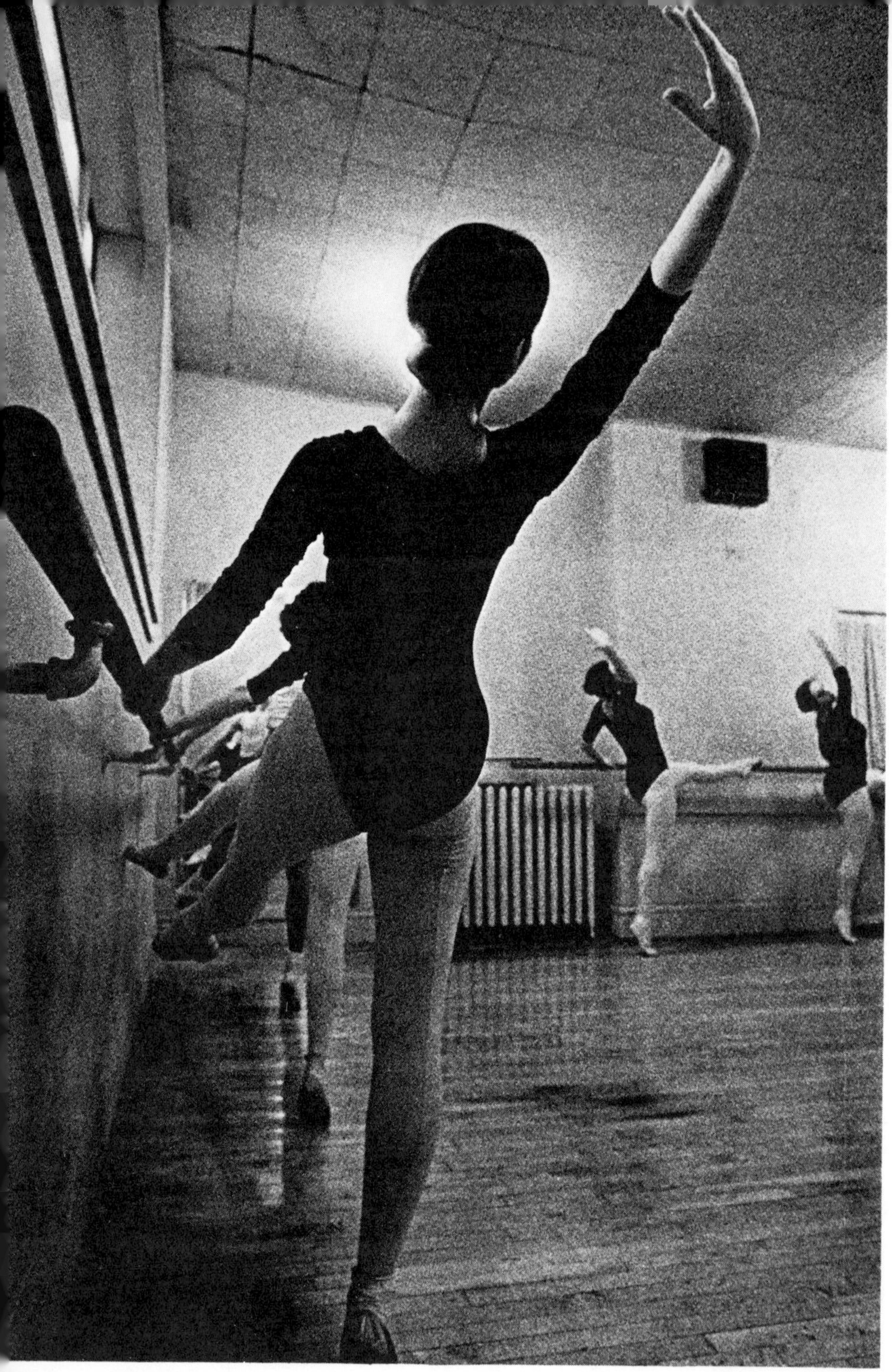

Photo by J. Brian King

***Figure* 5–5** Learning Through Modeling.

fashion crazes, and popular trends in thinking and acting result from mass behavior modeling. For example, among young people the fashion of wearing long hair may have started with the conspicuous Beatles, a young British rock band. The wearing of casual clothes, such as T-shirts and blue jeans, at a certain period of time, may have been started by local male models and spread through ads and youth magazines.

One of the first and most revealing studies of modeling was conducted by Bandura, Ross, and Ross (1963). These investigators sought to demonstrate modeling processes by showing that a group of children who observed aggressive play behavior would themselves behave aggressively when given the opportunity. Thus one group of children saw a model exhibit both physical (hitting, striking with a hammer, throwing) and verbal aggression (saying "Punch your nose") toward an inflated toy "Bobo doll." Another group observed the model behave in a restrained, inhibited manner in the same play situation. Children in a control group were not exposed to any modeled behavior. After observation of the model the children were frustrated by being deprived of a favorite toy and then observed in the playroom to determine the extent to which they would display aggressive behavior. The results lucidly demonstrate the modeling process. Children who had observed aggressive behavior displayed about twice as much aggressive behavior as children who had observed a subdued model or no model at all. These results have been extended (Bandura, Ross, & Ross, 1963) to include filmed or televised models as well as real-life models.

Model effects also produce other distinctive forms of aggression, characteristic play patterns, socially desirable responses to frustration, and speech patterns. The free use in conversation of those words "man" and "you know" to punctuate comments, and words and phrases such as "That turns me on" or "heavy" by young people in the late sixties and early seventies are examples of fads in speech. Since fads have a brief life, you may need to substitute current phrases for these dated expressions. Perhaps the truly pervasive and subtle effects of observational learning are best demonstrated in a study by Berger (1962). Berger found that individuals who observed a person receive what appeared to be painful electric shock following the sound of a buzzer and the dimming of a light, began to show arousal-related autonomic as well as physiological responses to the buzzer and light. Although the subjects *never experienced the shock themselves,* they acquired learned reactions to the shock-contingent stimuli. It is this process of identifying with the victim that appears to underlie feelings of empathy as well as the "effectiveness" of a horror show. This same process can be used to explain certain extreme fears or anxieties that exist in spite of the person's having had no unpleasant experiences with the feared object.

Doubtless the physiological accompaniments of joy and happy excitement can also be aroused by observation. Examples are seen in an audience of young people responding with their contemporaries to a popular singer or of people at a religious revival meeting.

LEARNING BASES OF "ABNORMAL" BEHAVIOR

Although systematic development of the idea is relatively new, it is clear that much so-called "abnormal" behavior results from learning processes identical to those that account for more commonly occurring "normal" behavior. Support for this notion comes from several sources. First, the conceptual gain that has come from thinking about the nature and origin of normal behavior in terms of learning principles has also advanced our thinking about "sick," "crazy," or "mentally ill" behavior. Learning formulations of mental illness have provided a new conceptual reorientation to abnormality as learned, socially undesirable behavior rather than symptoms of disease.

Whether a behavior is considered socially desirable—and hence "normal"—is dependent on the sociocultural system in which it occurs. A man who wears a skirt in our part of the world would likely be considered sick or crazy, whereas this same behavior in Scotland, Burma, or Fiji is considered both normal and socially desirable. The cheek kissing of male friends by boys in the Middle East or the mutual embrace in South America is accepted there, but in the United States these behaviors are regarded negatively. The behavior is the same in both parts of the world; the evaluation differs. It cannot be assumed that because a behavior is considered undesirable by a segment or even all of a society, the behavior developed in an unusual fashion or is symptomatic of disease. The laws governing the acquisition of behavior and social behavioral standards are largely unrelated. Behavior develops lawfully and along learning principle lines; laws can never be considered abnormal. Thus behavior is classified as normal or abnormal on the basis of the impact of that behavior on members of society (that is, social desirability-undesirability), not on the basis of the understood normal or abnormal development of that behavior. As will soon be evident, this learning formulation of "abnormal" behavior has important implications for treatment and behavior change.

Experimentally Produced Neuroses

Considerable support for the learning conceptualization of socially undesirable behavior has come from research showing that such behavior can be produced experimentally via conditioning techniques. The case of little Albert being conditioned to fear white rats and other furry objects reported by Watson and Rayner (1924) is one of the first examples of research in the area of experimental psychopathology. Other examples of the experimental production of unusual or undesirable behavior in man and animals have been reported. Pavlov's (1929) widely known discovery of "experimental neurosis" in dogs provides an immediate example in the respondent paradigm. Briefly, Pavlov, his students, and subsequent researchers have found that when an animal is forced to respond differentially to two stimuli between which it cannot discriminate, the animal becomes erratic, highly emotional, and difficult to restrain, while at the same time normal behavioral patterns are disrupted. The exaggerated emotional nature of the animal's behavior led many observers to describe the end state as "neurotic." Many psychologists (for example, Ullmann & Krasner, 1969) have drawn parallels between breakdown of discriminations in lower animals and the neurotic's inability to detect or discriminate critical interpersonal cues in his environment.

Shaping Psychotic and Normal Behavior

Haughton and Ayllon (1965) have clearly shown how operant shaping can produce what appears to be stereotypic, "delusional" behavior in a chronic mental patient. Research like this sheds light on the nature and development of symptoms. Such research and the broader field of experimental human psychopathology raises certain moral and ethical issues that psychologists have not ignored. The 54-year-old woman had been in a mental hospital for 23 years and carried the diagnosis of psychosis. Like most chronic mental patients, she led a characteristically simple life, with her days spent lying in bed or sitting in a ward with few arousing stimuli, and her only apparent satisfaction being eating and continuous smoking. The nonfunctional, seemingly abnormal behavior Haughton and Ayllon chose to produce was excessive broom holding. First, the woman was deprived of all cigarettes. Working with ward staff, then, it was arranged for her to be handed a broom in an upright position, immediately after which she was given a portion of a cigarette to smoke. Subsequently, cigarettes were given to her every five minutes if she had held the broom at least one minute in the five-minute period. Time required to hold the broom per reinforcement was then gradually extended to 120 of 240 minutes. The result can be easily anticipated. The woman began holding and carrying (but not using, since this was not part of the "required" behavior) the broom a large portion of each day. Interestingly, this conditioned behavior was seen by a panel of professional examiners to be the result of a delusional psychotic process involving complex symbolisms of what the broom represented for the patient and how the broom-carrying reflected unconscious processes. The "psychotic" broom-carrying behavior extinguished quickly when cigarette reinforcement was discontinued.

Another example of how socially inappropriate behavior can be produced through reinforcement procedures is provided by Ullmann, Krasner, and Edinger (1964). These investigators reinforced either sick or healthy talk in hospitalized patients, showing the increase of such behavior according to reinforcement conditions. Thus, when interviewers reinforced patients' sick talk, such as expressing hopelessness, discomfort, and lack of enthusiasm, by attending to such talk and responding "mmh-hmm" and "yes" to the patient, this behavior became more frequent. At the same time healthy, optimistic talk decreased. The opposite was observed when healthy talk (for example, "I'm feeling better, things are looking up") gained attention and approval. It does not seem far-fetched that similar reinforcement processes account for the chronic health complaints of people labeled hypochondriacs.

The above examples of experimentally produced deviant behavior make it clear that at least some "sick" or abnormal behavior usually considered as symptoms of an underlying mental illness can be understood simply and meaningfully as learned behavior. They also illustrate clearly that the learning processes are the same as those operative in the production of wholly desirable or admirable behavior; the condition of learning and the nature of the variables affecting *what* is learned are what distinguish the learning of acceptable from the learning of unacceptable behavior. Just how much abnormal behavior can be accounted for in this fashion is an issue that is currently being debated. It seems inevitable that other learning and nonlearning processes, such as complex verbal learning and behavior genetics, will have to be included in a learning theory of abnormal behavior. Nevertheless, even these fundamental and simplistic principles of learning have become powerful behavior modification tools in the hands of psychologists who wish to eliminate unwanted behavior. To this, the most impressive source of support for the "learning theory" conceptualization of deviant behavior, we shall turn in a later chapter.

Summary

1. We began this chapter with the case of an adult whose anxiety interfered with an important project in his life. He was treated by methods of behavior modification; the implications of the case are discussed.

2. Learning is defined as the process by which behavior is acquired or changed through an organism's interaction with the environment when maturation or temporary states will not account for that behavior change.
3. *Respondent conditioning* refers to situations in which a neutral stimulus is paired with an unconditioned stimulus (which normally brings a given response) in such a manner that subsequently the neutral stimulus comes to produce a response similar to one naturally elicited by the unconditioned stimulus. It is the process by which we acquire many fears, food preferences, dislikes, etc.
4. Conditioned responses may be *extinguished* or weakened by repeated presentation of the conditioned (neutral) stimulus without the associated unconditioned (natural) stimulus. A second method of eliminating a conditioned response is to pair the conditioned stimulus with a response that is incompatible with the conditioned response. For example, relaxation is thought by some to be incompatible with fear and anxiety, so that pairing the learned relaxation with a feared object will weaken the fear of it. This is called counter-conditioning.
5. When a stimulus similar to the conditioned stimulus arouses a conditioned response, the process is called stimulus generalization. A small child who calls the man next door "Daddy" is illustrating *stimulus generalization.* Discrimination is the contrary process—responding to the similar stimulus differently. A child who fears the dog who bit him but not the friendly little neighborhood dog is engaging in discrimination.
6. Conditioning one to perform an act in order to receive reinforcement (popularly called a reward) is known as *operant conditioning.* The individual "operates" on the environment for a satisfying consequence. Many skills represent complex operant behavior.
7. Operant reinforcers are called *primary* if they are related to biological needs. Food is a primary reinforcer; it reinforces acts that satisfy hunger. *Secondary* reinforcers, such as praise or money, have been previously paired with primary reinforcers; they are not directly biological in nature.
8. An example of operant conditioning is found in the prolonged process of teaching a mute hospital patient to talk by reinforcing with gum all actions that lead toward and finally produce speech.
9. There are various ways in which reinforcers can be presented called *schedules of reinforcement.* If the reinforcement is intermittent rather than continuous it is called *partial reinforcement.*
10. Reinforcement can occur on a time schedule; in such a case, the individual who is continuing an activity can be reinforced after

every fixed interval—*fixed interval reinforcement*. We may not be complimented all day long for a good job but only when the boss comes around, which is periodic, with a good word for one's work.

11. Interestingly, the partially reinforced responses remain with us longer and are not as easily extinguished. This may explain the persistence of both desirable and undesirable behavior.
12. *Positive reinforcers* are those the individual seeks and seldom avoids. *Negative reinforcers,* such as pain and embarrassment, the individual avoids, but if the negative reinforcer is withdrawn the behavior that precedes this will be strengthened. Acts we perform to avoid punishment are learned.
13. *Punishment* may decrease or eliminate the overt behavior that precedes it temporarily, but this punished behavior may return when the punishment is withdrawn. The obstreperous child in a classroom may not misbehave when the teacher's punishment is imminent, but let the teacher leave the room and he misbehaves again. This pattern has implications in our culture in those situations where punishment is recommended as the major means of controlling behavior.
14. *Avoidance behavior,* which is the result of aversive stimulation, is learned quickly and is highly resistant to extinction, possibly because the organism does not experience the extinction conditions.
15. For an understanding of more complex behavior, additional concepts such as modeling are needed. It has been found, for example, that children who observe aggression in a *model, imitate* it, in that their aggression increases after this observation. Also, after seeing a model shocked when a buzzer sounds and a light changes, the observer himself begins to show physiological changes in response to the buzzer and light.
16. Abnormal or atypical behavior is learned in the same manner as behavior that is acceptable to a given culture. Neuroses and other abnormal behavior can be produced in the laboratory by following learning principles.

Words to Remember

Avoidance Conditioning
Classical Conditioning
Classical Extinction
Conditional Response
Conditional Stimulus
Continuous Reinforcement
Counterconditioning
Discrimination
Equal Ratio Reinforcement
Fixed Interval Reinforcement
Generalized Reinforcer
Higher-Order Conditioning
Identification
Instrumental Conditioning
Instrumental Extinction
Latent Learning
Learning
Maturation

Modeling
Negative Reinforcement
Observational Learning
Operant Conditioning
Partial Reinforcement
Positive Reinforcement
Primary Reinforcer
Punishment
Respondent Conditioning
Response
Response Acquisition
Response Generalization
Secondary Reinforcer
Shaping
Stimulus
Stimulus Generalization
Unconditional Response
Unconditional Stimulus
Variable Interval Reinforcement
Variable Ratio Reinforcement

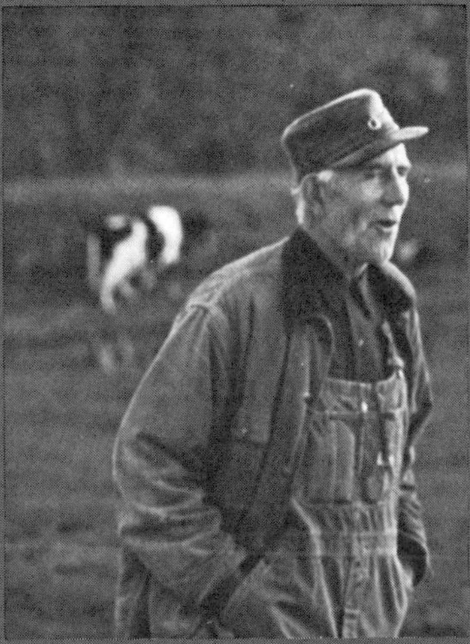

6. Self-Concept, Roles, and Adjustment

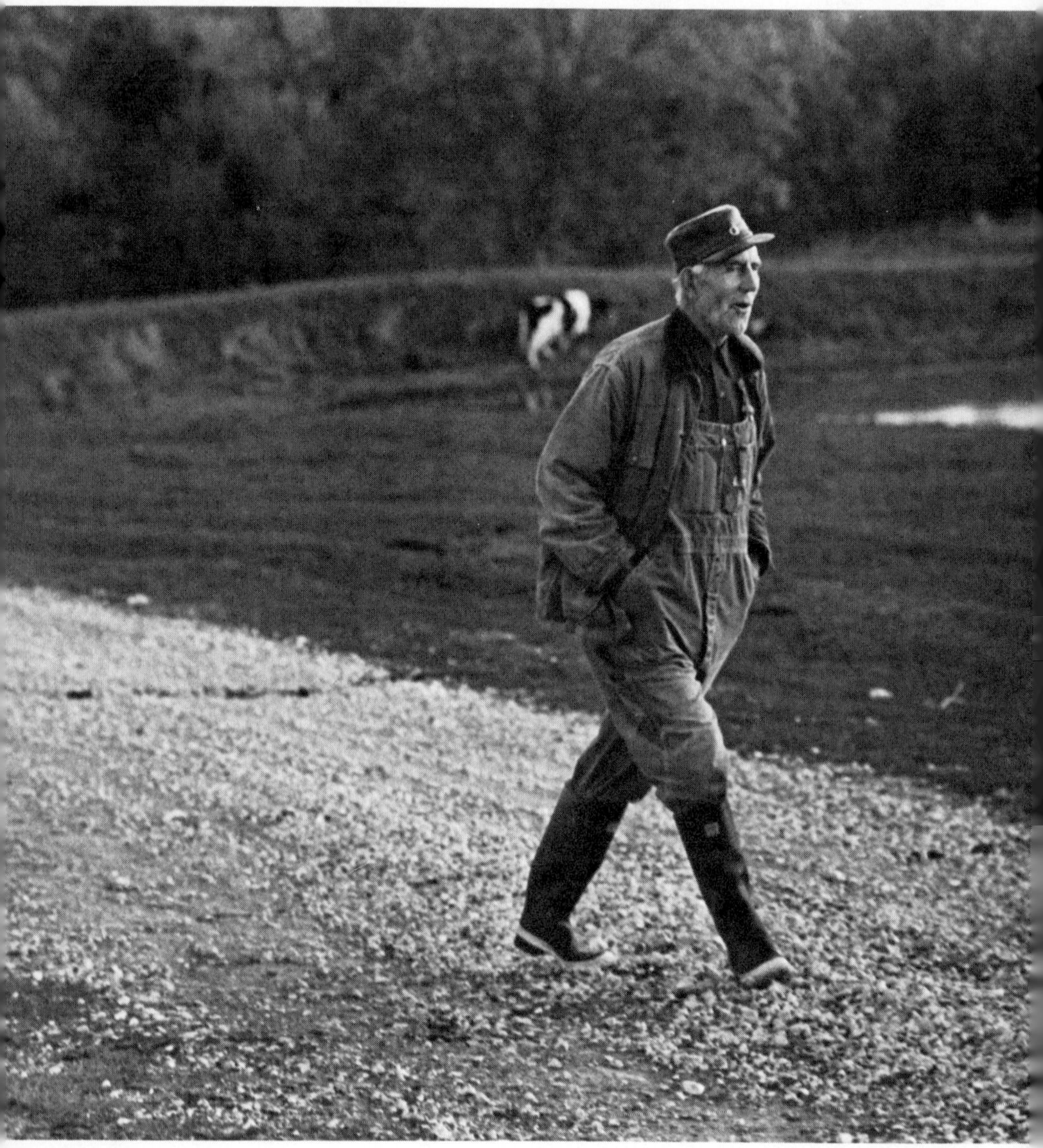

Photo courtesy of *Columbia Missourian*

Objectives

After studying this chapter the reader should be able to:

1. Define *self.*
2. Identify the interactions between role and self-concept.
3. Describe the factors influencing the acquisition of sex roles.
4. Describe adjustment problems in terms of social status factors.
5. Describe the role of race in adjustment.

Often "adjustment" is discussed as if it referred to an absolute, fixed behavioral pattern that one brings with him into each situation he encounters. After all, the "well-adjusted" person is supposed to be "healthy" and therefore *should* be able to cope effectively with whatever demands are placed upon him. Yet adjustment cannot be considered in a vacuum, for the term defines a relative state. A person is not simply "adjusted," rather he is adjusted *to* something. Adjustment carries with it the implication that appropriate healthy functioning varies in relation to specific personal and environmental circumstances. The well-adjusted individual recognizes and is able to accept his strengths as well as his weaknesses and functions within the personal and interpersonal limits of who he is, what he is, and where he is. As most readers have no doubt discovered, all men and women are not created equal: some are stronger, wealthier, healthier, more intelligent, more attractive, and more skillful than others. In similar fashion, all situations are not equal: some are mild, others are inhuman; some are restful, others are frantic; some are challenging, others are boring; some are growth-producing, others are personally devastating. Each day we face differing demands and must respond to various pressures. Whether our behavior is "adjusted" or "maladjusted" must be decided individually for each of us, in terms of our specific circumstances.

This chapter will consider how sex, race, and social class establish certain role expectations and contribute to the definition of one's adjustment. As will be seen, each of these characteristics sets limits upon the range of potential responses one can make. These limitations are currently being questioned and new, hopefully more satisfying, behavioral options are being proposed.

Aspects of Selfhood

SELF-CONCEPT

To understand the importance to adjustment of such personal characteristics as sex, social class, and age, it is necessary to consider how *self-concept* relates to behavior. *Self* is a deeply meaningful concept for the average person. Yet, although used constantly without much thought, its meaning is rather ambiguous to most people. When asked to define the term, students in a general psychology course stated that it referred to "me," "myself," and "my total person, mental, emotional, and physical." Several pointed out that one's self is unique. All agreed that the term refers to the way an individual perceives and reacts to himself as a person.

We shall define *self-concept* as the individual's enduring consciousness of his own identity as he relates to his environment. "Self" serves as an integrative concept which accounts for the sense of continuing *unity* and *organization* each person experiences. This concept also can reflect the individual's experience of *agency* (i.e., his sense of assertiveness, responsibility, and control). A strong sense of self enables a person to feel that he can get things done. The "I-me" of the individual and all that it implies are central to his complete experience and behavior, including what he might become.

It can be readily recognized that there is a continual sense of self or identity throughout life. One perceives himself as essentially the same person today as he was last week or last year, even though he may have changed in size, weight, skills, attitudes, and so forth. We are able to go back to the memory of ourselves as children as well as to go forward to our hopes and ambitions for the future. Selfhood thus continues throughout life. That which one calls "me" or "I" extends backward and forward.

An important part of a person is the relative balance of positive and negative feelings he has about himself. This is known as *self-esteem.* It may be greatly influenced by certain aspects of one's appearance, background, or skills that are considered socially important. These features become influential because they may seem to be sources of acceptance or rejection by others.

Self-image, one of Allport's (1961) seven aspects of the self, refers to how the individual conceptualizes himself and what is expected of him. It includes how he thinks others regard him, the nicknames he has been given (sometimes derogatory), how good he sees himself as a son or daughter, as a student or an athlete, in the eyes of his parents, his friends, or members of the opposite sex. Self-image relates to his sense of identity and reflects itself in answer to the question, "Who am I?"

Sometimes the self as process is called "ego." The term *ego* refers to those responses that tend to defend or enhance the self (Murphy, 1947). We are rarely neutral or static about ourselves—about what we call "me." This is especially true if we are criticized or threatened or become aware of a low status in respect to some goal. We begin to show initiative or defensiveness. These processes are what is meant by ego. The term *ego strength* has been a useful concept in attempting to distinguish those people who are able to rally from setbacks—who show inner control of their lives—from those who seem to be dominated by life events and withdraw or become emotionally disturbed. Symonds (1951) lists a group of hypothetical criteria of ego strength. They include the ability to tolerate external stress, the capacity to deal with guilt feelings and effectively inhibit antisocial impulses, a balance of rigidity and flexibility, planning and control of behavior, and self-esteem. In summary, ego strength is an index of the effectiveness with which an individual can function in his environment.

SELF-DISCLOSURE, ACCEPTANCE OF SELF AND OTHERS

If one feels insecure about whether others will accept him, he constructs a false public self (Jourard, 1971). There is then a disparity between what he is and what he pretends to be, which may result in repression of what he considers to be undesirable aspects of himself. This repression threatens personal integration or unity. Obviously, as one discloses various aspects of himself to others, particularly to intimates, he must face those very aspects. He may then be better able to integrate the negative and positive aspects of selfhood. He also learns the extent to which he is similar to other people, and this knowledge may help to remove feelings of guilt and isolation which he may have. Jourard sees a relationship between emotional health and *self-disclosure.* The open and flexible individual moves toward a feeling of security and away from the anxiety of disclosing negative features of himself. He becomes, then, less defensive in dealing with his own feelings and with those of other people.

Those who like others tend also to like themselves. Those who feel people are "no damn good" tend to see little good in themselves. Clearly there is an interaction between acceptance of self and acceptance of others. As we show our enjoyment of others, they tend to respond positively to us. Acceptance of others thus leads to more reinforcement from them, and that in turn causes us to accept ourselves even more. Unfortunately the reverse of this process also occurs.

ROLES

The typical man has mannerisms, attitudes, language patterns, grooming practices, and ways of behaving that are different from those of the typical woman, even in this period of transition of standards. Men, for example, walk and talk like other men rather than like women. Behavior patterns like these we call *roles.* A role is a *structured mode of participation in social life*—in this example, a male or female role. Each

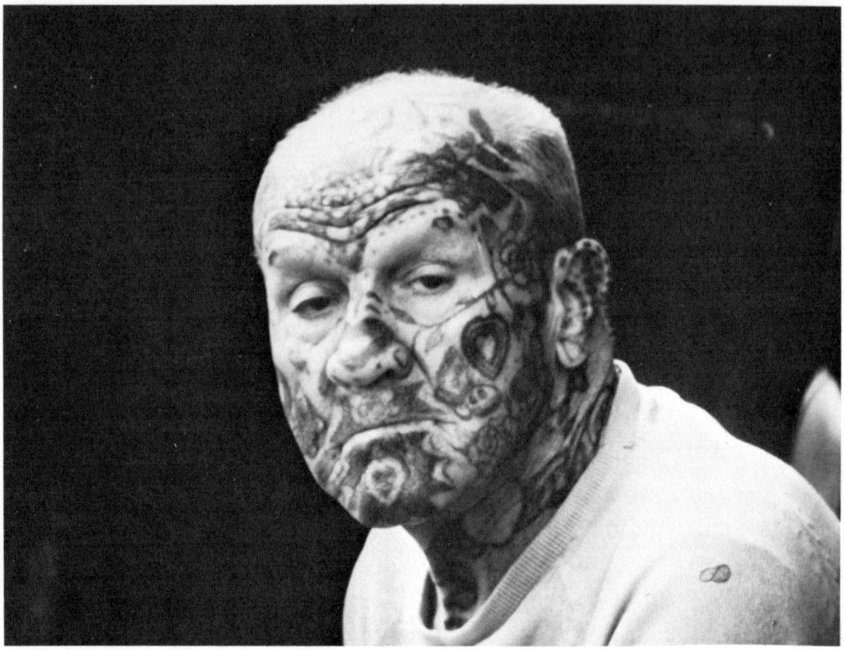

Photo by J. Brian King

Figure 6–1 A Unique Public Image.

individual has many structured roles, and will show different patterns of behavior in each of these roles. Later, we will consider in greater detail the influence of masculine and feminine behaviors upon adjustment.

The roles we perform influence our identity. As persons, we differ in how well our performance of a role meets the expectations of others in our particular subculture of society. John differs from Jack in the way he shows his maleness. John, an athlete, pursues the opposite sex with some success and meets the expectations of the fraternity subculture more fully than Jack, the poet and thinker. However, Jack has the respect of the campus intellectuals and of his teachers.

There are differing cultural standards on what is more or less desirable. People generally react to us in terms of the extent to which our personal behavior is acceptable to their standards. An emphasis on the reactions of other people is present in the *looking-glass theory* of self-development (Mead, 1934). This theory observes that children's awarenesses of themselves as persons go beyond their spontaneous discoveries as active infants. The most important aspects of their self-images arise from *how others react* to their various attributes and behavior (Figure 6–1 depicts a person very much wanting to be noticed). Other people's behavior toward them is the psychic looking glass. The very bright child who commands a large vocabulary that his peers do not understand may be laughed at, and he may come to regard this ability as negative! The energetic, vivacious, self-asserting child of authoritarian parents may actually come to perceive himself negatively. On the other hand, under conditions of acceptance in the neighborhood or family, the theory would predict that these children would perceive themselves positively. Similarly, we shall see that how we and others respond to our being male or female, black or white, rich or poor contributes significantly to the meaning of these characteristics to our self-esteem and behavior.

REFERENCE GROUPS

The growing individual is a member of many important *reference groups.* It is through these reference groups that self-attitudes develop. The family certainly represents one such important group. Jourard and Remy (1955) have shown that the child's self-image is modified by what he perceives as his parents' evaluations of him. Another reference group are his *siblings.* A second or third child of relatively average intelligence, or of average physical attributes, who follows an unusually bright or beautiful first child, may find himself inadvertently compared with his "ideal" sibling. In addition to all of the groups in the neighborhood, school, or playground, the child may find cultural ideals in our mass media with which he may identify. These models may be found in motion pictures, television, biographies, or novels. The extent to which they reinforce his reference groups positively or negatively contributes significantly to his self-esteem.

SELF-CONSISTENCY

We can all recall experiences of shame or embarrassment or some action that was incompatible with our view of ourselves. Usually when this occurs we attempt in some way to justify or excuse the behavior; we may say, "I wasn't myself." An early self-theory advanced by Lecky (1945) emphasized that behavior is an attempt on the part of the individual to maintain the consistency and unity of his selfhood. From this viewpoint, self-consistency is a major expression of motivation and, when achieved, provides satisfaction. An individual resists experiences that are not harmonious with his structure of values. Experiences, then, that are not consistent with the self-structure are perceived as threats and motivate the individual toward either problem solving or defensive behavior.

Dissatisfaction with oneself is not invariably related to maladjustment, particularly among mature adults who are highly competent socially. A study by Achenbach and Zigler (1963) indicates that wide differences between what one is and what one would like to be are often found in people with the demonstrated capacity to achieve in areas most valued in our society. Rather than being ominous in nature, high self-ideal disparity may help in attaining higher levels of development. The wide differentiation between what one feels he is and what he'd like to be may lead to self-derogation, guilt, and anxiety, all of which can motivate a person to achieve more.

DYNAMICS AS SELFHOOD

As total organisms we human beings are constantly striving to satisfy our needs and respond to an ever-changing environment. We continually move toward goals that are need-satisfying. Of all of our experiences (sometimes called the phenomenal field), that of self is the most central.

Rogers (1959) reminds us that individuals generally need to regard themselves positively. The extent of positive regard toward self depends on how others seem to perceive or feel toward us. Rogers states that some individuals can be more influenced by this need for positive regard than by the need to respond to organic drives. We have already pointed out that a discrepancy between our perception of ourselves and the ideal that we hold is disturbing. Thus experiences that are contrary to our self-concept can be distorted, not perceived, and denied awareness. For example, we may not be able to see the point of criticisms of our behavior or may fail to recognize the extent of our prejudices because we view ourselves as persons of goodwill. Continuing in this state leaves a person susceptible to anxiety, threat, and personal disorganization.

Discrepancy between self and experience may result in a breakdown of the defenses that we have used to protect ourselves against anxiety. As will be described in more detail later, a depressed or panic state results when our defenses break down. When the individual feels that he is a failure in an important area, sees little hope for change, and is unable to accept this failure or to defend himself against it by rationalization, compensation, or the like, disorganization of the self-structure may ensue. Rogers (1959), in presenting client-centered therapy, demonstrated that this disorganization can be reversed by receiving unconditional positive regard from people who are significant to us. This regard is achieved by total acceptance of the person as worthy and as someone who is encountering difficulties in coping with life problems. When anxiety and threat are reduced, the individual has less need for defenses like repression or denial and can be more accurate in his perception of events around himself and in his thinking.

An individual whose self-concept is congruent with his experiences may, when frustrated, become hostile, but the frustration is accurately perceived and his hostile behavior is appropriate to the frustrating situation. However, when frustrated individuals do not admit their aggressive impulses, they direct their hostility, not toward the source of frustration, but rather toward themselves, toward uninvolved defenseless others (the innocent bystander), or toward irrelevant situations (Byrne, 1966). That is to say, individuals who do not recognize and admit their aggressive or other negative impulses may begin to feel inadequate, inferior, and worthless, or they may use other persons as scapegoats.

CHANGES IN SELF-CONCEPT

Videbeck (1960) has shown that an individual's self-concept can be made more positive or more negative when he receives high or low evaluations from others whom he regards as having prestige. Other studies reviewed by Byrne (1966) show that self-concept fluctuates to some extent with *moods*. It also varies with *age*. It grows progressively more positive up through adolescence and adulthood until around age 60, when it begins to decline. As will be seen in later chapters, this change with age can be easily understood. The average person increases in work and social competence and receives rewarding feedbacks, such as better jobs and recognition, as he grows older. However, as his energies dwindle after middle age and as various physical complaints increase, his perceived role as an effective individual may begin to diminish as does his self-concept. This reduction in self-concept with advancing age is more frequent in the Western—and especially American—culture, which does not venerate old age either for itself or for the accumulated wisdom that supposedly accompanies it.

Basically, one aspect of adjustment relates to the extent to which one realistically perceives positive qualities in one's self. "Self-concept," "self-image," "self-acceptance," "self-esteem" are all dimensions of the process through which a person evaluates himself in his own eyes, and through the eyes of those around him. The more negative that evaluation is, the more likely will the person begin to engage in maladjusted behavior as he attempts to obtain a more satisfying self-image. Initially, negative self-evaluation or negative social feedback may serve as a catalyst for needed adaptive personal or behavioral reorganization. As attempts to reduce the negative feedback fail to achieve that goal, more extreme and less appropriate solutions will be attempted. Continued negative self-perception can therefore play a significant role in initiating and maintaining maladjusted behaviors. Such self-perception can be intimately tied to the socially defined roles one is expected to adopt because of a particular personal characteristic. As indicated earlier, three specific characteristics—sex, race, and social background—have long been cultural determinants of what a person should or should not do.

The following sections will consider some of the anticipated role dimensions of these attributes, as well as the recent reconsideration of such expectancies.

Adjustment and Sexual Roles

In our culture, men and women are expected to behave differently under similar circumstances. When danger arises, men are supposed to face it bravely while women shrink back in fear. When a newborn baby is in the room, women are expected to be motherly and want to cuddle the infant; men, on the other hand, should admire from a distance. Women can hug and kiss each other when they meet; men must never hug each other except under unusual circumstances. Overall, women are supposed to be gentle and must always be protected. Men are supposed to be aggressive and must be protectors. Yet, beyond obvious physical and somewhat more subtle physiological differences between the two sexes, how can the significant differences in behavior and attitudes expected and/or observed in the above situations be explained? Are behavioral differences between the sexes determined by biology, learning, or both? It is important to understand how sexual roles are defined and develop, for one part of adjustment depends on the cultural acceptability of one's personal roles.

SEX-TYPED BEHAVIORS

Masculine and feminine roles are typically defined in terms of "appropriate" behavioral patterns. Such patterns are called *sex-typed behaviors* and are defined as "those that are less expected and sanctioned when performed by one sex, and, in contrast, are considered to be more appropriate when manifested by the other sex" (Mischel, 1970, 8.4). Generally, women are supposed to become skillful in raising and caring for a family—for example, cooking, keeping house, serving, and caring for others, particularly children. (Figure 6–2 shows a woman doing man's work.) On the other hand, men presumably must develop skills that enable them to support a family and provide for its needs. Men, it is said, should be strong, unemotional, and dependable. Women need not be, and in fact are seen by some as attractive when they are not.

Investigations into the frequency and amount of differences in certain behaviors between the sexes have focused primarily on aggressive and dependent responses to situations. As early as 3 years of age, boys and girls differ in the amount of aggressive behavior displayed. Boys are consistently perceived to be more aggressive, more negative, and more physically quarrelsome than girls (Mischel, 1970; Sears, 1963, 1965).

Observational studies of boys and girls together have supported that boys are more likely than girls to interact aggressively with peers (Walters, Pearce, & Dahms, 1957). Similar results are reported in studies in which trained judges rate children on specific behavioral dimensions. Researchers working with groups of children ranging from 2 to 14 years of age have all found that boys are consistently perceived as significantly noisier, more aggressive, and more negative than girls (Beller, 1955; Feshbach, 1956; Tuddenham, 1952). Not only do observers rate boys and girls differently, but the children themselves agree in their perceptions of such differences. Thus boys typically see themselves as more aggressive than girls, while girls see themselves as more dependent than boys. These differences in self-reports become even sharper with age and have been consistently found in studies with young adults (Bennett & Cohen, 1959; Mischel, 1970). The bulk of findings thus far obtained therefore suggest that sex-typed behaviors in general are real and do differentiate men and women.

People, however, do not simply behave without awareness of their actions. They observe their behavior and that of others and consider the extent to which that behavior appropriately represents who they are.

Figure 6–2 An Exception to Sex Typing.

Photo by J. Brian King

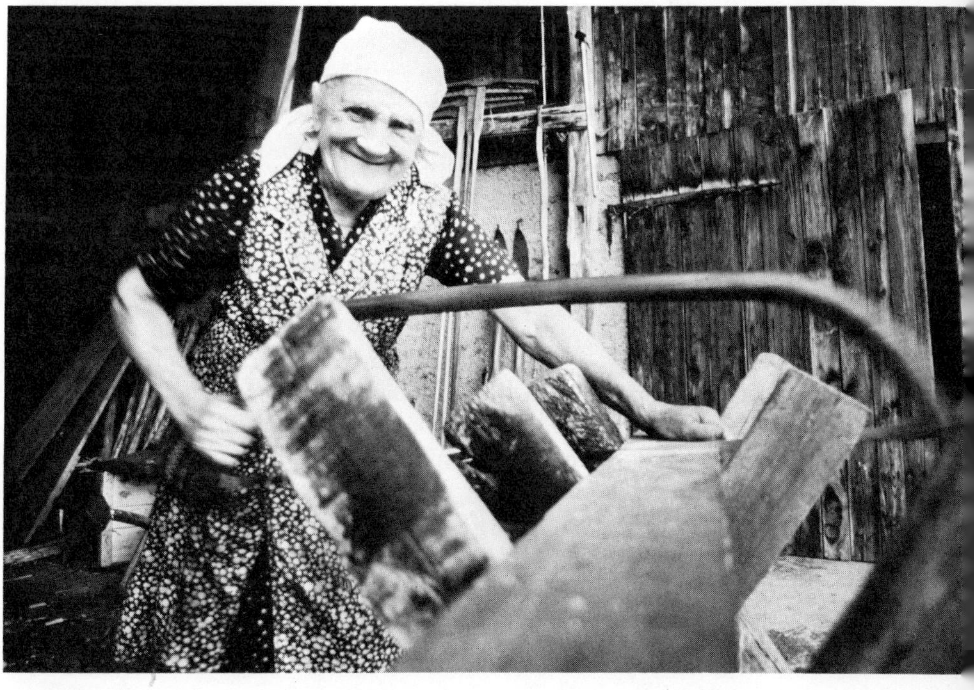

Sex-typed behaviors may therefore reflect, in part, *stereotypes* one has about how he is supposed to act. A *stereotype* reflects the expectations one has about how members of a particular group are "supposed" to act. In his treatment of sex-role stereotype, Roger Brown (1965) presents the following caricature of boy-girl differences:

> In the United States a *real* boy climbs trees, disclaims girls, dirties his knees, plays with soldiers, and takes blue for his favorite color. A real girl dresses dolls, jumps rope, plays hopscotch, and takes pink for her favorite color. When they go to school, real girls like English and music and "auditorium"; real boys prefer manual training, gym, and arithmetic. In college the boys smoke pipes, drink beer, and major in engineering or physics; the girls chew Juicy Fruit gum, drink cherry Cokes, and major in fine arts. The real boy matures into a "man's man" who plays poker, goes hunting, drinks brandy, and dies in the war; the real girl becomes a "feminine" woman who loves children, embroiders handkerchiefs, drinks weak tea, and "succumbs" to consumption (p. 161).

CURRENT CHANGES IN EMPHASIS ON SEX TYPING

It is clear that there is a social revolution for women's equal rights, taking place today, which consists of blunting the differences between the sexes. The individual differences in behaviors within groups of men and women which investigators have always noted are now widely emphasized. All measured characteristics in men and women overlap. Individuals more often now are encouraged to look upon themselves primarily as human beings with certain abilities and preferences to which they may give priority. Women may become athletes if they seem so inclined; men may enter vocations that involve care of children and similar tasks. This blunting in sex differences is favored by some, usually the young and the better educated, and opposed by others.

MASCULINITY—FEMININITY MEASURES

Given that sex-role stereotypes do exist, social scientists have attempted to measure how closely one's self-reports, self-descriptions, and preferences correspond with those of most members of one's sex. This is typically done with measures of *masculinity-femininity* in which an item is scored "masculine" if the response to that item corresponds to the one given most frequently by males, and "feminine" if the response corresponds to the one given most frequently by females. For a number of years constructors of personality tests have included items that differentiate most males from females in our culture. These items relate to interests, occupations, preferences, school subjects, emotional dispositions, personality, and overt behavior. Persons taking the test are given a score that indicates the degree of "masculinity" and "femininity" shown by their answers. Hilgard, Atkinson, and Atkinson (1967) point out that this empirical score might be called *social* masculinity and femininity and that it should be distinguished from other aspects of maleness and femaleness, such as appearance, and interest in and attractiveness to the opposite sex. This differentiation is desirable, for identification of masculinity or femininity involves a highly complex group of traits and attitudes as well as culturally typed characteristics.

One such measure, the Terman and Miles (1936) scale of masculinity-femininity (i.e., the M-F test), yields the following summary of differences in the responses of men and women:

> From whatever angle we have examined them the males included in the standardization groups evinced a distinctive interest in exploit and adventure, in outdoor and physically strenuous occupations, in machinery and tools, in science, physical phenomena, and inventions; and from rather occasional evidence, in business and commerce. On the other hand, the females of our groups have evinced a distinctive interest in domestic affairs and in aesthetic objects and occupations; they have distinctly preferred more sedentary and indoor occupations, occupations more directly ministrative, particularly to the young, the helpless, the distressed. Supporting and supplementing these are the more subjective differences—those in emotional disposition and direction. The males directly or indirectly manifest the greater self-assertion and aggressiveness; they express more hardihood and fearlessness, and more roughness and manners, language, and seniments. The females express themselves as more compassionate and sympathetic, more timid, more fastidious, and aesthetically sensitive, more emotional in general (or at least more expressive of the four emotions considered), severer moralists, yet admit in themselves weaknesses in emotional control and (less noticeably) in physique (pp. 447–448).

More and more noticeably in our culture, the strict separation of social masculinity and femininity is being bridged. It has been long realized by psychologists that there is *some degree of maleness in many women and some degree of femaleness in men.* These gradations show up on a test of the M-F trait.

Some understanding of social masculinity and femininity can be gained by scanning the scores of the Terman M-F test as they relate to vocational involvement (see Figure 6–3). This figure gives the mean M-F index of men and women in various occupations. It shows that men and women can differ widely in test scores and that this very difference relates to their selection of a vocation. The typical male journalist, artist, and clergyman, for example, does not have the same high score on the M-F test as the typical engineer, salesman, or banker. In a culture as

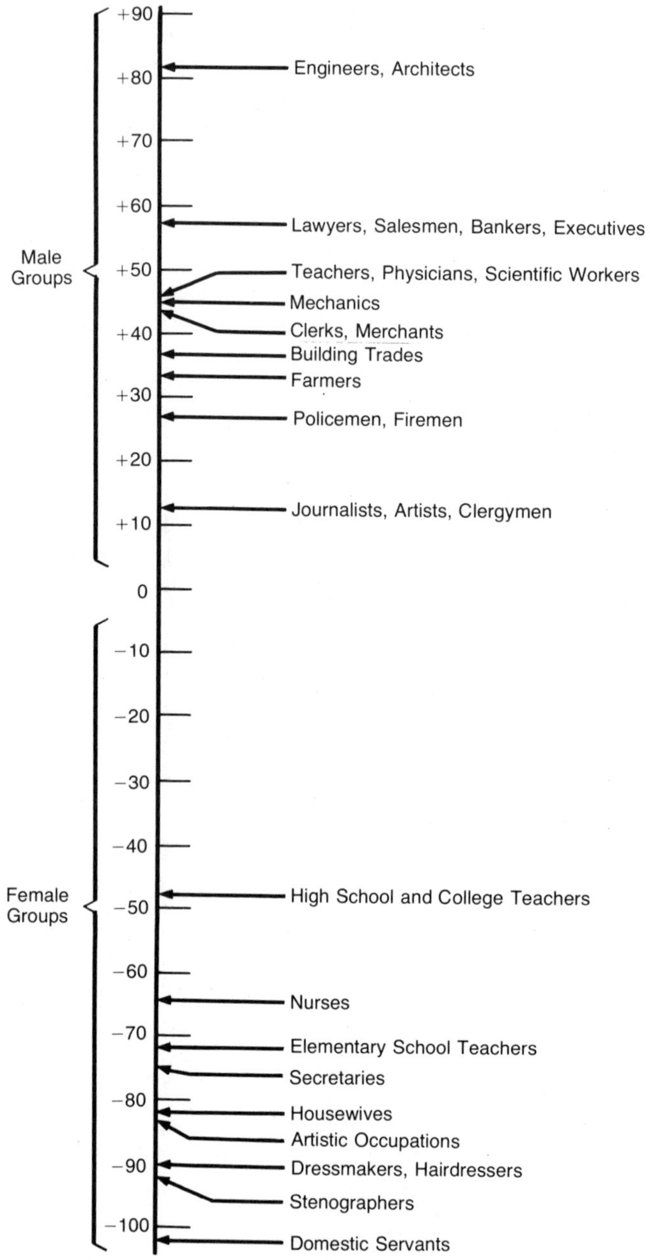

Figure 6–3 Mean M-F Index of Men and Women in Various Occupations. The positive end of the scale indicates the more masculine scores, the negative end the more feminine scores. (From A. Anastasi, *Differential Psychology,* 4th edition. New York: Macmillan Publishing Co., Inc. 1976. Reprinted by permission.)

complex as ours, with its wide individual differences, we should also expect men and women to differ widely among themselves.

The reader should be well aware that measures of masculinity-femininity such as the M-F test reflect the degree to which one's interests, attitudes, and preferences are similar to those of most members of either sex. Such measures do not, however, necessarily reflect *actual* behavior patterns or represent the degree to which one is attracted, or attractive, to members of the opposite six. These measures represent agreement with stereotypes of acceptable sex roles, not sexual orientation or sexiness. The reader is also, I am sure, well aware of the discrepancy that can exist between what one says and what one does. Nor can one assume that observations and ratings of one's masculine or feminine characteristics made early in life accurately predict one's later behavior. In a rare attempt to assess such a difficult question, Mussen (1962) compared two groups of men in their late thirties who as adolescents had expressed respectively more traditionally masculine and feminine interests. Mussen's results did not demonstrate a generalized adjustment pattern which could be predicted from early observations. In fact, Mussen's conclusion stated: "In general there seems to have been a shift in the self-concepts of the two groups in adulthood, the originally highly masculine boys apparently feeling less positive about themselves after adolescence, and, correlatively, the less masculine groups changing in a favorable direction" (p. 440).

One can therefore begin to question the meaningfulness and utility of early assessments of masculinity and femininity in predicting later adjustment patterns. As will be seen later, strict adherence to traditional stereotypes about appropriate masculine and feminine roles can have negative consequences for one's personal development. Indeed, the very acceptance and maintenance of such stereotypes has come under increasing opposition as more and more men and women are beginning to question their culturally determined roles. Sexual discrimination has now been recognized and has moved to the forefront of critical social issues. Prior to considering in more detail the contemporary push for equalization of rights for the sexes, we will review some of the hypotheses that have been proposed to explain the acquisition of sexual roles.

ACQUISITION OF SEXUAL ROLES

Why do boys acquire masculine habits and girls feminine ones? Is one's sexual role genetically determined prior to birth and gradually evolving as one's body proceeds toward mature adult development? Or are we instead the product of our environment and experience? Certainly this question is not unique to understanding the development of sexual roles, for the *nature vs. nurture* question (i.e., genetic vs. environmental determinants) has been an issue in the attempts of psychology and the other social sciences to understand human behavior. Thus the dichotomy found in this classic question has also been reflected in the work on *sex typing*, that is, "the process whereby the individual comes to acquire, to value, and to adopt for himself sex-typed behavior patterns" (Mischel, 1970, p. 18). In what follows we shall consider some proposed explanations of sex typing.

BIOLOGICAL DETERMINANTS OF SEX ROLES

One explanation of sex typing is based on the role that biology plays in the development of masculine and feminine behavior patterns. Given the major hormonal differences between the sexes, it seems reasonable to assume that these relate in meaningful ways to how men and women respond to situational demands. Investigators have found reliable relationships between various levels of sexual hormones and a person's reaction to situations, his positive and negative feelings about himself, indeed even of the incidence of automobile accidents. The reader should remember, however, that the existence of a relationship between two variables does not necessarily mean that one causes the other. For example, researchers have described the role of certain hormones in producing maternal behavior in mammals during pregnancy (Morgan, 1965). While it is known that similar hormonal changes occur in female humans during pregnancy, the wide variability of maternal responses observed in women as they prepare for the birth of a child suggests that such behavior is, at the very best, only partially a function of physiological determinants. The general assumption that all women share a maternal instinct which motivates them naturally to care for and nurture the young remains to be empirically demonstrated.

In seeking to explain differences in behavior between the sexes, much emphasis has been placed on the anatomical differences between men and women. Given their relative distributions of muscle and fat, many people have argued that it is only logical for men to engage in heavy labor and to defend the homestead while women remain behind to tend to the lighter household chores and be protected. Freud (1966), himself, perceived the human anatomy as an extremely important determinant of personality; the obvious physical differences between men and women could therefore easily account for women's relative passivity, heightened emotionality, and decreased aggressiveness.

Yet there are major problems in attempting to explain masculine and feminine behavioral patterns on a biological basis. As noted earlier, the extensive variability observed among members of both sexes leaves relatively few behaviors that can be defined as *totally* masculine or feminine. More important, what is the "natural" way for a man or a woman to act in one culture may not be so in another culture. In the United States, few women (until recently) have served in the army to fight directly with the enemy; except in rare national emergencies, few women have worked in the steel mills or at other physically demanding occupations. Indeed, labor laws have sought to protect women against exploitation by carefully specifying the hours and employment conditions that must be met by employers. During the recent conflicts in the Middle East, it was apparent that Israeli women formed an important part of that nation's army. Women in the Soviet Union and many African nations engage in the same physical labors as men. In Iran it is the men, rather than the women, who are expected to display their emotions openly (Hall, 1959). Similar reversals in the "natural" roles of men and women have been reported by anthropologists studying numerous cultures around the world. Thus, if one takes a cross-cultural perspective, the importance of biological factors in determining sex typing seems relatively minor.

IDENTIFICATION AND SEXUAL ROLES

The development of sexual roles has also been explained as a consequence of *identification* (i.e., copying, in part unconsciously, the behavior of significant others). The principal and earliest proponent of this mechanism was Freud (1966), who saw identification as an important early process through which children acquired appropriate social roles:

> According to Freud, children of both sexes develop love and jealousy relationships with their parents. Boys fall in love with their mothers and fear their fathers will punish them by cutting off their penises. At about six years of age, boys typically solve this dilemma by deciding to behave as males, to later seek out other females. Girls, meanwhile, fall in love with their fathers, and blame their mothers for their lack of penises. It does not take long, however, for them to realize they cannot replace their mothers in their fathers' affections. So most girls decide to identify with their mothers, and later find suitable males to love (Green, 1974, p. 45.)

In the acquisition of sexual roles, identification refers to more than an intrapsychic process between children and parents (Bronfenbrenner, 1960). It also suggests that children gradually begin to develop a desire to acquire mannerisms and behavior patterns similar to the same-sex parent. Identification also refers to the actual copying behavior in which children engage as they move toward being more like father or mother. A child recognizes differences in the actions, roles, responsibilities, and expectations of his parents and chooses to model himself after that parent most like himself.

Children, however, do not acquire all of their behavior patterns from their parents. Significant portions of their days are spent away from home in the presence of peers, who also play an important role in the development of sexual roles. Peers observe each other and imitate much of what they see. If the other boys in one's group display masculine behaviors, one is likely to acquire similar behaviors. Peer groups also play a very important role in determining what games one plays, what emotions one shows (and how one shows them), and what clothes one wears. Albert Bandura (1969), who has spent many years studying observational learning and modeling, has observed that an important reciprocal process occurs as peers and siblings serve as models for each other in the acquisition of behavioral processes.

LEARNING THEORIES OF SEX ROLE DEVELOPMENT

Numerous questions, however, have been raised about how such a process works and why the child would regularly continue to pattern himself after a like-sex parent, sibling, or peer. As noted earlier in Chapter 5 in the discussion on learning, much of our daily behavior can best be understood in terms of reinforcement and conditioning principles. Certain behaviors produce positive consequences and others produce negative consequences. Typically one can accurately predict that those behaviors leading to positive outcomes will be repeated. Many theorists have suggested that the acquisition of sexual roles can be understood in exactly those terms. In other words, boys acquire masculine styles because they are encouraged to display such behaviors and rewarded for doing so. (Figure 6–4 illustrates the learning of a masculine role.) Thus aggressiveness, interest in sports, and independence will all be positively received in boys, while seeking to play with dolls, for example, will be negatively received. In similar fashion, little girls are encouraged to be gentle, to "play nice with the doll," and to show their emotions openly. The reader will no doubt be able to describe the numerous indirect ways in which masculine and feminine behaviors are reinforced in children:

> "Jenny was such a good little girl today; she helped Mommy make supper."
> "Big boys don't cry."
> "Little boys don't play with dolls, go play ball with your friends."
> "No, you can't have a football, little girls don't want such things."
> "Doesn't she look pretty in her new dress?"
> "Doesn't he look like a little man in his suit?"

Thus in innumerable overt and subtle ways masculine and feminine behaviors develop in children as their parents, their peers, and, indeed,

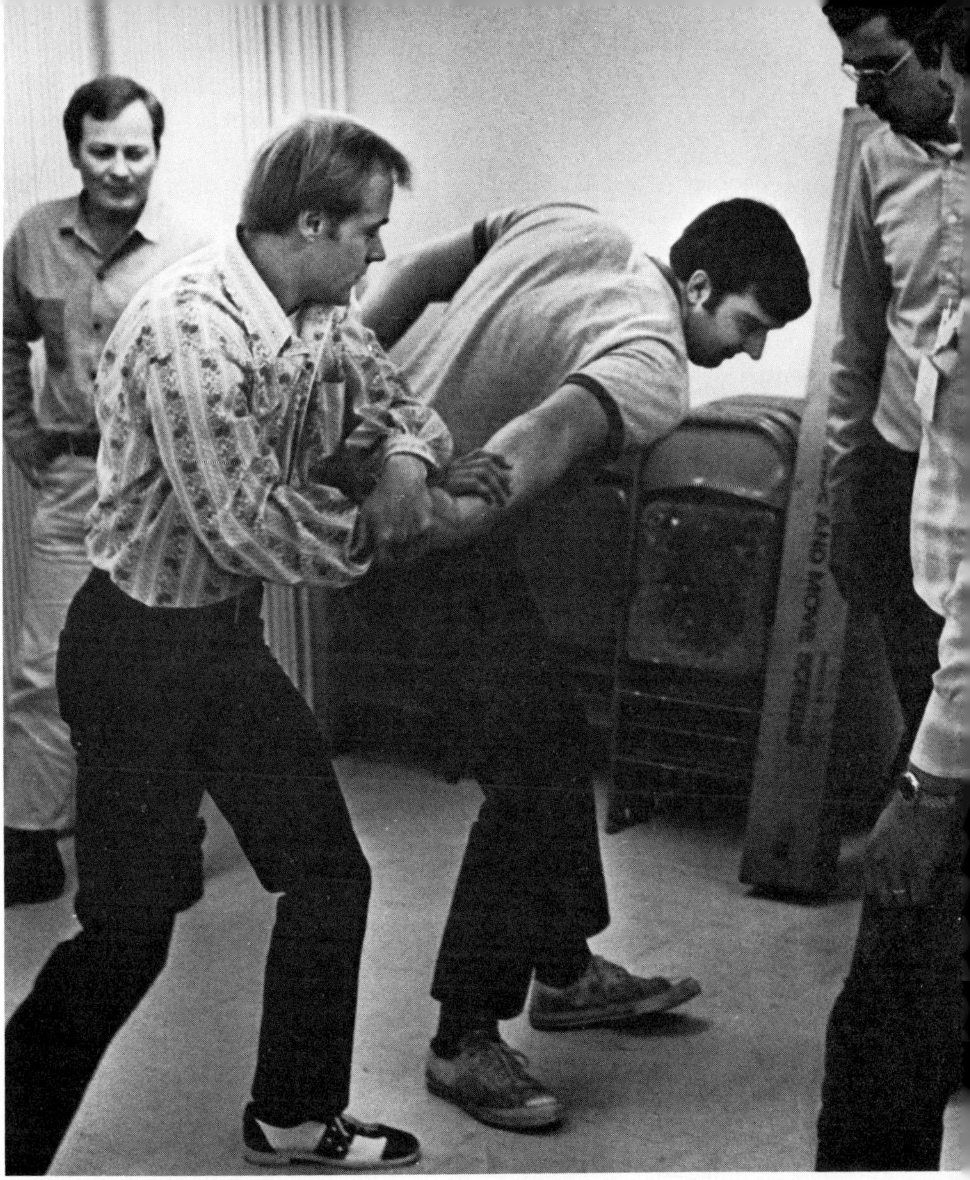

Photo courtesy of *Columbia Missourian*

Figure 6–4 Learning a Masculine Role.

even themselves perceive their behaviors and respond positively or negatively depending on their "appropriateness." In most cases the acquisition of masculine and feminine roles comes naturally and easily. The unspoken assumption is that the traditional cultural stereotypes are the "way it should be" and all involved participate in the continuation of these beliefs. Men have their roles and women have theirs; neither is comfortable nor "normal" assuming the role of the other. Yet in many ways the very existence of such roles produces adjustment problems for some people. After all, not all men are equally masculine, athletic, and independent; nor are all women equally gentle, tender, and motherly. As in all other aspects of human nature, there is considerable overlap with some men gentler than some women and some women more aggressive than some men. Problems arise when role models will not permit expression of one's natural tendencies or fulfillment of one's real potential.

Acceptance of either traditional masculine or feminine roles by a man or woman respectively has both benefits and costs. The benefits depend heavily upon the extent to which one finds acceptance and fulfillment of the specific role demands of his sex personally satisfying. For the man, there is the pride of athletic prowess, of fatherhood, of providing for a family, and of being "head of the household." There is also the cost of having responsibilities that one cannot shun without much negative feedback in our culture. There is the further cost of having to deny one's gentler feelings and constantly having to be firm and independent. Some men would enjoy keeping house, caring for plants, and cooking, although to do any of these on a regular basis while one's wife supported the family would be totally unacceptable in our society. The man who by temperament or upbringing does not fully emulate the masculine role may constantly feel compelled to prove to himself and others that he is "really" a man.

Women also gain benefits and must pay a price for accepting their role. The most obvious benefit (by appearance anyway) is the "luxury" of being cared for, of not having to work for a living, and of being treated with gentleness. The realities of the homemaker's lot limit dramatically the genuineness of some of these obvious gains. Yet the cost in terms of always having to assume a dependent, secondary role is most telling on some women. To assume some responsibility, to assert their independence, to respond aggressively to a problem are all unfeminine and interpreted as attempts to challenge the male's authority. Woman's role becomes that of an object to be admired and used by men; she is there to meet his needs as mistress, mother, and housekeeper. If she questions this role and challenges the limits placed upon her, she is demeaned, ridiculed, and if perchance, successful, immediately defined as not a "real woman." Some of the costs of the feminine role are seen in the case of Patricia described below. The reader may try to gain an even clearer sense of Patricia's experiences by imagining how the reaction to her decisions would have differed had she been a man.

The Case of Patricia

Patricia was seen in the University Counseling Center during her first year of medical school. She was an extremely attractive young woman in her mid-twenties and had been referred to the counselor by her academic adviser following (in his words) an "hysterical outburst in an anatomy lab." Patricia related well to the counselor and very quickly shared with him some of the factors which had led to her "outburst." In her own words, she explained that she had simply "been fed up" with how she had been treated and decided to openly express her frustration.

Patricia explained that since entering college she had received negative reactions from her peers and academic advisers for her career goals. Academically, she had been a straight-A student and was especially proficient in the physical sciences. She had worked very hard for her grades and rarely dated during the semester. For this, she had regularly been teased by her dorm mates, who finally decided that she was simply afraid of men. In fact, while Patricia liked men and enjoyed dating, she simply did not have time during the academic year to socialize a great deal. She became engaged to a man who was also a medical student when she entered medical school and they plan on marrying when he graduates.

Much of Patricia's early frustration arose in her premed courses. Everyone involved in those laboratory courses was both highly motivated to do well and to be very competitive. Most of her fellow students and many of her instructors saw her as unfairly taking the place of a man who might not be accepted into medical school because of her. Generally these feelings were expressed only covertly but, at times (especially when exams were coming up) they became more obvious. Patricia recalled that on the day of her Comparative Anatomy laboratory final exam she was supposed to dissect a lamb's brain for the instructor, pointing out whichever structures he named. When she arrived, she found her lamb's brain missing; the instructor's only response was that she'd have to learn to adjust to the competition of medical school. Fortunately another student offered her the use of his specimen (he was not scheduled to take that part of the exam) and she was able to complete the exam. Only because of her persistence and outstanding academic work was Patricia able to elicit recommendations to medical schools from several instructors. Once accepted, her faculty supporters issued a very stern warning that she'd better not disappoint them by getting married and dropping out. Later, after she assured them (somewhat angrily, she admitted) of her intentions to complete training, they congratulated her.

Patricia's first few months at medical school were most unpleasant. She found herself to be one of two women in the class, and her attractiveness made her the object of many derogatory comments. Most typical among these was, "Well, it's easy to see how she got accepted." While she had hoped that the constant suggestive comments and sexual propositions would decrease in a professional school, they had not. In fact, she found the instructors to be even less tolerant of her being a woman and somewhat readier to embarrass her than her fellow students. Her "hysterical outburst" occurred during a laboratory period when the instructor commented on her attractiveness and, rather than concerning himself with her lab work, propositioned her and went further by trying to touch her. "I just couldn't take that nonsense any longer," she declared, "so I just let him have it across the face."

As Patricia explained, she didn't understand why she had to work so very hard to be accepted. After all, it wasn't her fault that she was an attractive woman, a matter that had nothing to do with her potential as a physician. Why wouldn't people take her seriously and simply treat her with the respect and support given to all of her male classmates? Patricia used her visits to the counselor as an opportunity to ventilate many of her feelings. In their discussions, she reviewed her reasons for seeking a medical career and in so doing became even more committed to that choice. She gained the strength necessary to deal with the continuing difficulties throughout medical school and eventually completed her training. She has since entered an internship at a very well-known Northeastern hospital and is happily nearing her goal.

Many of the experiences and difficulties faced by Patricia have been shared by other women in and out of academic settings. During the 1960s and 1970s the frustration and anger of many women have been mobilized and has given rise to the "women's liberation movement." That movement included many excesses including public demonstrations in which brassieres were burned as a symbol of protest against man's sexual exploitation of women. Some women called for payment for all homemaking duties and demanded equal opportunities to use public restrooms. Many jokes and much ridicule have accompanied this movement, and considerable masculine anger has been stirred up to respond to "these troublemaking women" who seek to drive men from their jobs and thus deny them their masculine right to earn a living. Yet the woman's rights movement has also brought into the open serious injustices and clear evidence of discrimination against women. It has become apparent that women of equal training and expertise receive significantly lower wages than men; that being a woman is the basis for denying promotions that have been earned or for refusing to hire someone fully qualified; that being a woman makes it difficult to obtain credit, although one is financially sound; and often makes one the focus of sexual comments and suggestive overtures. The woman's rights movement has begun to make it acceptable for a woman to declare openly her ambitions, to choose not to marry or bear children, indeed, even to admit sexual feelings. This social movement has produced major changes in our culture during the past decade and will continue to do so during the present one. While its excesses are to be shunned and overlooked as a result of the early zeal of its proponents, its benefits ultimately should result in more satisfying sexual roles for both men and women.

Adjustment and Social Background

Just as sexual identity has traditionally imposed limits upon the potential range of behaviors one might "adaptively" engage in, so too have characteristics of social and ethnic background. As noted earlier, *self-concept* and *self-esteem* are important components of one's psychological status and of one's capacity to cope effectively with internal and external pressures. The reader is perhaps aware of the interrelationship between these two variables: a person with high self-esteem is able to react more adaptively to expected and unexpected demands; as one deals productively with such pressures, self-esteem is supported and even increased. One would therefore predict that adjustment becomes more difficult and tenuous for persons who face more extreme daily pressures, for those who must deal with daily assaults on their self-esteem, and for those who must live under both conditions simultaneously.

In our culture, economic success is an important determinant of the resources available to deal with the environment. Economic status determines, in large part, where a person may live, how he will dress, who his friends will be, what his children's education will be, and how effectively he can demand that his "basic human rights" be respected. The wealthy have many privileges and considerably more latitude in what they may do. When their voices are raised in protest, very few fail to hear and respond to correct the situation. Although members of the middle classes and the working classes may have to shout somewhat louder, and perhaps longer, they are also able to effect some changes in their environment through their own efforts. The poor, however, are characterized not only by a lack of financial resources but, more significantly, by an overwhelming sense of "powerlessness" (Haggstrom, 1964) when attempting to deal with external pressures. Their demands and pleas go relatively unheard, and their situation makes it very difficult for them to enlist needed help (e.g., a lawyer) to obtain satisfaction. After all, it is hazardous to complain too strongly about price gouging in the slums when few other stores will provide the credit needed to carry one until the next check arrives. While we shall speak more extensively about poverty, it should be clear that economic standing has important consequences for one's adjustment.

SOCIOECONOMIC LEVELS

While there are innumerable qualities to the American culture, one of the most basic aspects of the "American way" is the pioneer spirit. Many of our national heroes began with nothing and through hard work and close adherence to the "Protestant ethic" achieved fame and fortune. Thus a basic American ideal is the achievement of success. Those who do so are hailed and respected. They are "good guys" who have made it through their own efforts (or, at least, that's initially assumed); those who do not make it must, therefore, be "bad guys" who lack something in their personal makeup.

As a "democracy," the American culture has always been highly critical of political systems that include a caste structure. The realities of

American life (indeed of virtually all cultures), however, are that people have varying degrees of access to economic resources, comforts of living, educational opportunities, and cultural events. Extensive work has been reported in the psychological literature describing how membership in the resulting social and economic categories relate to adjustment. A basic part of this work has focused upon differentiating people into social levels. An early investigator of social structures, Sorokin (1927), defined this procedure of *social stratification* as the ranking of members of a society in a vertical series of horizontal layers or strata. He assumed that members of any culture might be placed in some hierarchy that reflects economic-cultural differences between people. Thus, for example, one might classify people *economically* according to how much money they make each year, or *socially* according to how much authority they have to effect change in their living conditions, or even occupationally according to the relative skill, responsibility, and social contribution associated with their occupations. Placement of people into a classificatory schema does not necessarily imply that all members of a given level function similarly or act in mirror images one to the other. Rather, it implies that they hold certain characteristics in common which differentiate them from members of other levels.

While one might technically separate people into as many categories as are operationally definable, most researchers in mental health have relied on a system that identifies five levels of *socioeconomic status* (SES). This latter term refers to the fact that the groups are differentiated, not only according to economic-occupational standing, but also in terms of more subjective social-educational criteria. Thus the original Hollingshead *Index of Social Position* determined SES in relation to education, occupation, and area of residence (Hollingshead & Redlich, 1958). Since this scale had originally been developed for use in New Haven, Connecticut, it was necessary to exclude residence in order to generalize the system for other communities. Given the high degree of relationship between the first two criteria and residence, it was relatively simple to redefine SES levels simply according to educational and occupational status (Hollingshead, 1957). The revised version has been the most widely used instrument for determining SES in mental health research and it still continues to discriminate groups of people usefully. Although profound educational, economic, and social changes have occurred in the last two decades, the Index remains capable of assigning people into meaningful categories according to their relative social standing.

As noted earlier, the Hollingshead (1957) Index identifies five SES levels. The general characteristics of each of these groups are summarized below, and reflect the descriptions of the original New Haven groups surveyed:

Class I, roughly 3 percent of the community, includes the "established" families who have the most wealth and power. Many of the men at this level have been educated beyond college, and are either business executives, professionals, or in political life. On the average, this group's income is the highest of all SES levels; many families, in fact, are independently wealthy. The reader can no doubt think of national or local people whose "old-line" families belong in this group.

Class II members, about 9 percent of the community, have generally arrived at this level through considerable effort on their own, as a result of their parents' work, or, most typically, both. The majority of men are college graduates, employed in salaried positions in industry, education, and the professions. Indeed, some members of this group may have higher incomes and have amassed more wealth than members of Class I. Yet the latter have so much social prestige attached to their position in the community that they are considered to be at a socially higher level. Class II members tend to have worked hard to get where they are and to place considerable emphasis upon ensuring that they and their children will remain at that level.

Class III includes that 21 percent of the community that is popularly known as the "white-collar middle class." Its members are generally high school graduates, although some of these continue their education through evening classes. Occupationally, Class III men are employed in clerical, sales, and administrative positions. Some own small shops and businesses, as for example, the corner grocery or a local TV repair shop. Members of this social group do not typically identify with labor and resist unionization (although this seems to be rapidly changing); at the same time, Class III members are not considered "equals" of the executive classes. People at this level have fairly secure jobs, although they often have little chance for continuing wage increases and advancement.

Class IV, the "working class," comprised the largest single segment (47 percent) of the New Haven sample. It included both skilled and semiskilled laborers and persons working in lower clerical and sales positions. Typically, Class IV members consider union membership as an important safeguard of their earning power and job security. Educationally, males in this group tend to have completed some high school or to have received technical training at a trade school. Often wives in this category continue to be employed following the birth of their children.

Class V, the "poor," includes that 20 percent of the population with the lowest income, the least job security, the most unemployment, and the highest concentration of minority group members. People in this group are typically poorly educated and tend to work (when work is available) at semiskilled and unskilled jobs; some have never worked. Those who do work are poorly paid and hold nonunionized positions. Class V families live in the worst sections of the community, and are frequently dependent on public assistance for medical and other human services.

ADJUSTMENT AND UPPER-INCOME STATUS

We have very briefly reviewed one basic approach to social stratification. The reader no doubt is aware that one's relative social standing as seen in the eyes of community members is as important to class assignment as is one's income. SES level therefore reflects both objective and subjective criteria which differentiate members of one group from members of the other groups. These same differences also produce different kinds of pressures on people and make available different resources for dealing with them. Adjustment and adaptive behavior is therefore relative to each SES level.

Considerable emphasis has been placed upon how SES relates to adjustment, and the bulk of this work has focused on members of Classes IV and V, the so-called "lower classes." This term, however, will not be used to refer to these groups for two reasons: (1) common usage attaches a negative value to the term that should be avoided in attempting to understand people and their needs; and (2) it is a term that the poor and the working class do not use in describing themselves. Thus the more neutral term, "low-income groups" will be used in referring collectively to Classes IV and V.

As noted, little research has been reported on the specific adjustment problems of the upper-income groups except by way of contrast with the lower-income groups. If the reader considers for a moment the characteristics of upper-income groups as described earlier, he can no doubt speculate about some of the specific pressures of their life-styles to which they must adapt. For example, particularly at the upper two levels, considerable wealth is available. Not only can such wealth bring luxuries, adventure, and pleasure, but it can also have many negative consequences. The fear of not being able to live any other way necessitates the constant need to acquire money. The executive positions held by men at this level include the responsibility for immense investments, thousands of stockholders, and perhaps hundreds of thousands of employees. Any mistake, any failure to act decisively can have devastating consequences. Thus working days often continue late into the night, and wives and families must learn to accept these conditions. Those in the medical professions may earn large fees for their services, but they must always be there when needed, always be understanding, and should never make mistakes. Consider, for a moment, the kinds of strains such professional responsibilities place upon a marriage when a spouse must always be shared with his work.

Upper-income status also poses special problems for children reared in such a background. If the parent is well known and highly respected, the child must struggle to achieve a unique identity. One's behavior must be exemplary lest the family name be tarnished. The sincerity of friendships may be questioned when one considers the advantages that accompany personal relationships. The media and popular novels have often focused on this theme—the socialite who is romanced for what she is rather than who she is. Children are pressured to define a career for themselves, a choice which becomes very painful if exceedingly high standards are set and one must earn parents' pride by mirroring their achievements. For some, the decision not to get trapped in this conflict is relatively easy; for many, it can be made only after years of frustration and self-contempt; for others it is never made and one can never live down "being a failure."

Finally, the reader has no doubt in recent years read accounts of the loneliness of being a public figure. Every comment might potentially become a quote which could affect the political or economic scene. Family problems are publicly announced and discussed. Personal weaknesses and indiscretions, which for most people can remain one's private business, are magnified a thousand times and forgotten only after a long period of time. Thus, even wealth and a comfortable living make certain demands on one's capacity to adjust.

ADJUSTMENT AND LOW-INCOME STATUS

As indicated earlier, much has been written about the adjustment problems of low-income people. While much of this literature treats Classes IV and V as a homogeneous entity, major differences exist between these groups. Miller and Riessman (1969), for example, note that the irregular, unskilled Class V worker lacks the disciplined structured working-class approach; Class V also must deal with more intense economic difficulties. In effect, living in poverty demands the constant ability to respond effectively to crisis. At all times, the poor must struggle just to provide themselves with the basic necessities of life; rarely do they have savings available for sudden emergencies. It is always necessary either to go even further into debt, or to give up something else, or simply to go without. The nature of Class V jobs makes this situation more tenuous, since layoffs and job changes occur frequently. Members of the other SES levels generally look upon the poor without sympathy and even with some disdain. As noted earlier, perhaps the most overwhelming aspect of poverty is its hopelessness and accompanying sense of powerlessness (Haggstrom, 1964).

Before considering some of the mental health problems of the low-income groups some attention should be paid to the wide variety of people who are included in Class V. This group includes those who have been poor for generations and the downwardly mobile from other SES levels. The poor include unskilled whites and nonwhites, ghetto dwellers, welfare recipients, tenant farmers, migrant workers, and many of the elderly. Subgroups among the poor may be differentiated if one considers the length of time below the poverty line, upward or downward mobility, and especially the dimensions of stability of economic level and family relationships. According to these criteria, Miller and Riessman (1969) have identified four specific categories of poverty:

1. The *stable* are characterized by both economic and family stability. This group has few economic resources but gains strength in the solidarity of important relationships. Representatives of this group might include those living on fixed incomes and pensions in inflationary times and many rural farm and nonfarm persons. Among this group are those poor who are most upwardly mobile and who have the supports necessary to take advantage of opportunities to enter better paying occupations.

2. The *strained* have similar economic stability but a relatively uncertain family situation. This group might include families in which a parent is in and out of the household, or families that have responded negatively to serious economic problems with marital conflict. Members of this group are typically at a transition point. If the family situation improves, they can often overcome their temporary economic problems and become upwardly mobile again. If family pressures increase, the family may move even further down the economic ladder following the onset of alcoholism or divorce.

3. The *copers,* as the name implies, are those families capable of coping with the problems of economic uncertainty. These people continually experience financial problems, but the family structure seems to make it all bearable.

4. The *unstable* include those persons living under the worst conditions, for they not only have little money but also find relatively little support in their families. This group typically includes the most destitute, has the highest incidence of alcoholism and broken homes, and the least chance of "breaking out."

SES AND MENTAL HEALTH PROBLEMS

Having variously characterized "the poor," we shall now consider the adjustment problems that accompany low-income status. *Epidemiological surveys* in public health medicine have sought to determine whether certain diseases are more or less likely to occur in certain segments of the population. Similar approaches in mental health have found that the relative frequency and severity of emotional problems relate quite directly to a person's economic status. In the New Haven study mentioned earlier, Hollingshead and Redlich (1958) observed that more than twice as many members of Class V, as expected, needed psychiatric treatment for some form of mental disorder. All other SES levels were underrepresented in the patient populations of New Haven and surrounding areas. These investigators therefore concluded that social class is a significant factor in the *prevalence* rate (i.e., the number of identified cases existing at a specific time) of mental illness. Further examination of patient records revealed that low-income patients, especially members of Class V, were significantly more likely to be under treatment for a serious emotional problem than were members of the upper-income groups.

While these data provide information about how one's social background relates to patient status and problem severity, it does not speak directly to the question of the occurrence of psychiatric problems in the general population. In a very well-known epidemiological study, the *Midtown Manhattan Study*, Srole, Langner, Michael, Opler, and Rennie (1962) used direct interviews by trained mental health personnel to determine the extent of emotional problems in various segments of the population. Interview material was reviewed by independent psychiatrists who, without knowledge of social background, assigned respondents along a continuum of mental health ranging from "well" to "impaired" to "incapacitated." SES groups did not differ with respect to the proportion falling into the middle categories. Differences, however, were observed for both the "well" and the "impaired" categories. Members of the upper-income groups were overrepresented in the "well" category, while members of the low-income groups were overrepresented in the "impaired" category. As noted in the New Haven study, members of the lower economic groups suffer more adjustment problems than do their financially more comfortable counterparts.

One would assume that the presence of more mental health problems among the poor would make them the target of intense treatment efforts. In fact, this is so only in terms of the number of people hospitalized with very serious mental health problems. For those adjustment problems that do not require hospitalization only a very limited amount of direct service is available. In his recent review, Lorion (1973) reported that members of low-income groups were least likely to be accepted into psychiatric treatment for individual therapy. Of those accepted into such treatment, few continued beyond five or six sessions. Those members of Classes IV and V who do get treated are also much more likely to have inexperienced therapists than are members of the upper-income levels, who can afford to pay for private care. These findings take on even greater significance when one considers that they were generally obtained from clinics in which ability to pay was supposedly *not* a requirement for treatment.

Recently mental health specialists have responded to the above findings by emphasizing the need to develop treatment procedures that take into account the everyday realities of low-income existence. After all, even if treatment is free, transportation, baby-sitting, and time-off from work may make it too costly for many poor people. While most upper-level positions permit time-off for such treatment, few Class V members can take such time without the loss of a considerable amount of their weekly salary. Their absence may also jeopardize an already tenuous employment situation. Furthermore, while there is some degree of prestige associated with visiting one's "shrink" in the upper classes, fewer members of Classes IV and V understand the need for such treatment, hence do not support a peer who seeks treatment. Recognition of such facts has led to treatments that are relatively short-term, provide immediate access to mental health personnel, and seek to respond directly to the adjustment difficulty (Lorion, 1974). Members of the lower-income groups have responded quite positively to such innovations.

The more significant need of the poor, however, is for mental health specialists to begin to consider directly the environmental conditions under which they are forced to live. In this way the causes of their adjustment difficulties can be understood and perhaps alleviated. Society will be forced to recognize how living in slums and ghettos affects people, what the welfare system does to a person's self-concept, and how constantly fighting to provide one's family with the basic necessities of life gradually wears down a man's will to keep trying. Through their studies, mental health professionals along with other social scientists will try to learn more about the living conditions that encourage alcoholism, drug addiction, and the numerous other problems that permeate low-income sectors of the city. The most effective means of overcoming such conditions can also be identified and, hopefully, put into practice.

RACE AND ADJUSTMENT

Of equal importance is for mental health professionals to begin to respond to the specific adjustment needs of blacks who have been living not only under intense poverty for decades but also under the destructive effects of unending discrimination. Since the Civil War, blacks have suffered the hatred of their white neighbors throughout the country. This prejudice has been openly and violently expressed in some sections through the forced use of separate facilities, beatings, and lynchings. Perhaps even more telling has been the *de facto* discrimination that exists implicitly in those areas that decry racial prejudice while supporting it through hiring and housing practices that require blacks to be confined to the worst sections of the community (see Figure 6–5). In this atmosphere, for many decades blacks have had to "keep their place" and

Figure 6–5 Working At What You Can Get.

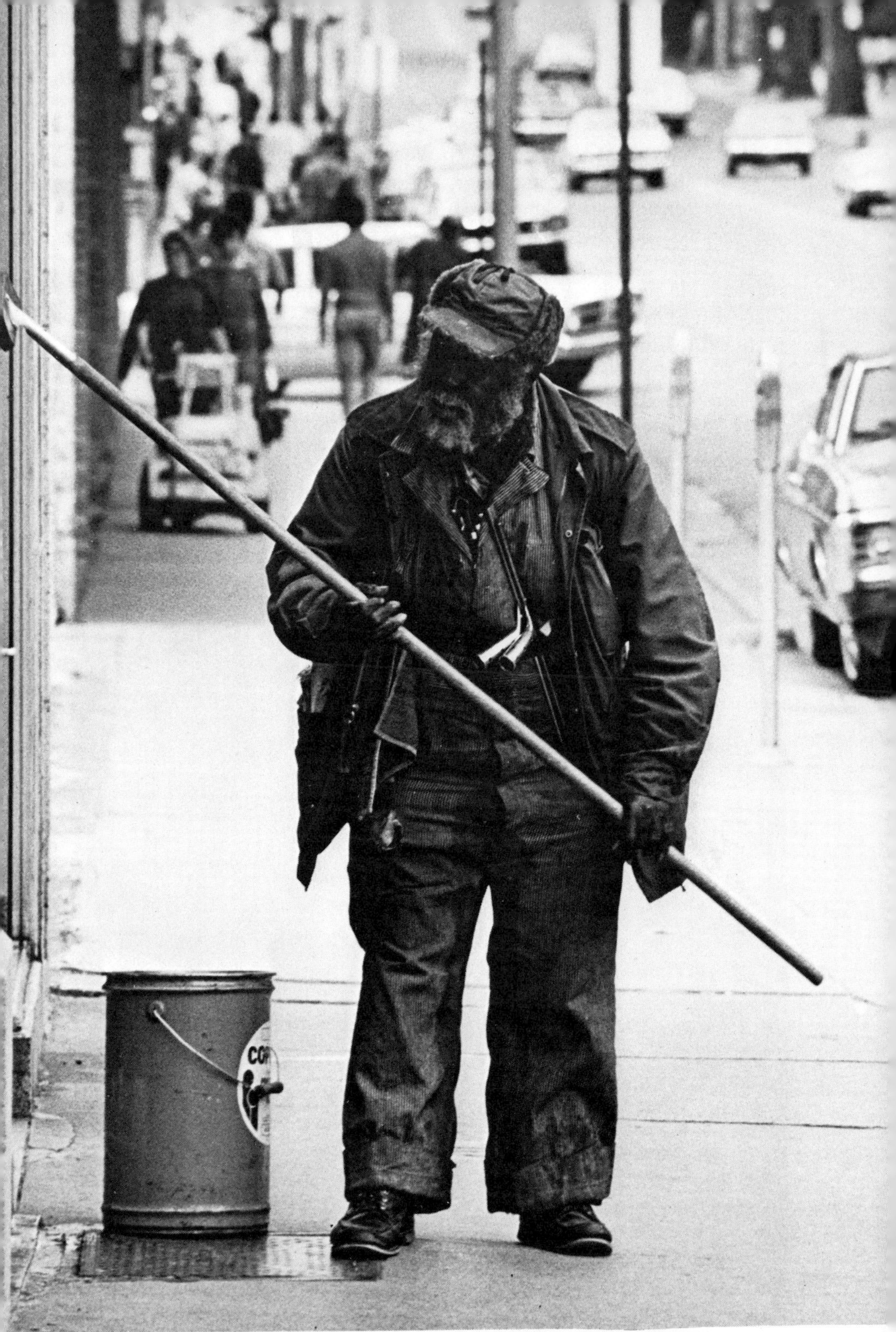

Photo by Chris T. Quillen

quietly endure lest things be even worse. Only through intense legislative debating, violent uprisings, demonstrations, assassinations, and much suffering have changes begun to appear. Many decades, however, will be necessary before true equality is achieved.

The very need to pursue the basic human right of self-respect has had incalculable negative consequences for blacks. In their consideration of black life, Grier and Cobbs (1969) note that, in the past, every legitimate expression of masculinity has been taken from the black man. He typically must struggle to obtain a job that can support his family, and is often forced to take whatever job he can get (see Figure 6–6). Often

Figure 6–6 The Ghetto Tenement.

Photo by J. Brian King

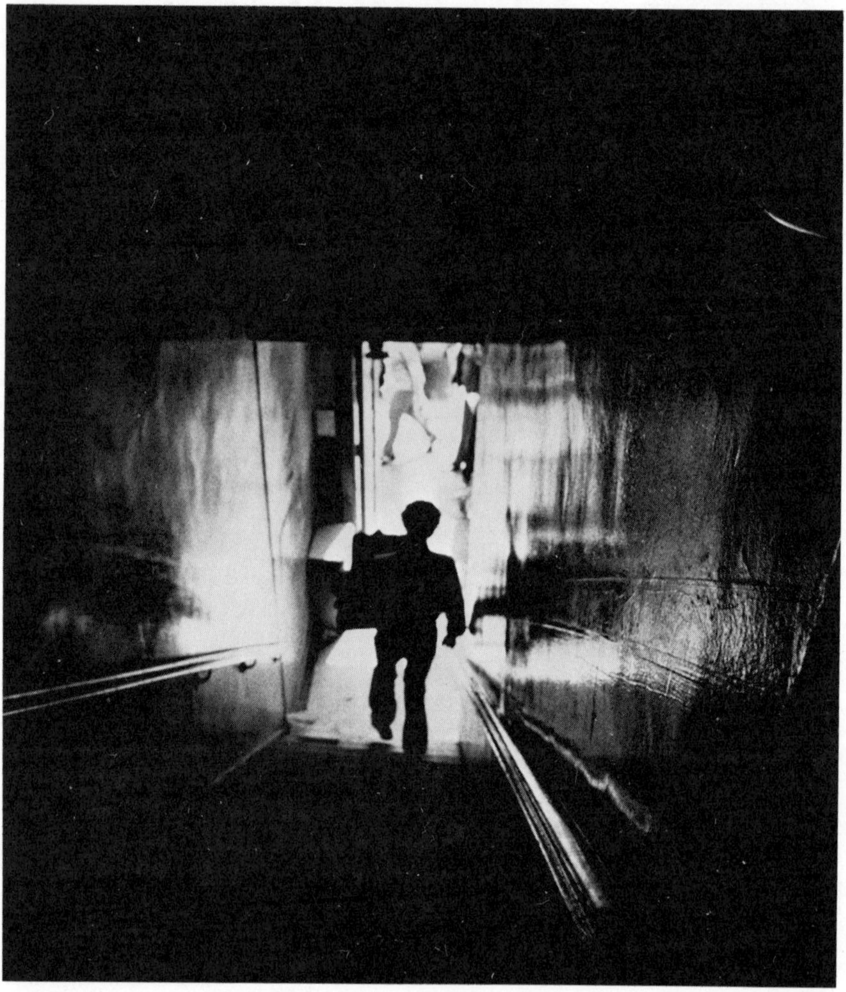

he is the last one hired and the first one fired. Until recently, the better-paying unionized trades have excluded blacks. Many available jobs are low-paying with little chance for advancement. The black man has also found it difficult to provide fully for his family even when he can afford it, since he has, in the past, been restricted to certain areas of the community and faced major obstacles in his attempts to enter the more comfortable suburban areas. The anger and frustration that accompany such constant prejudice cannot be directly expressed in most cases for that would only serve to aggravate the problem and increase the already negative situation. Thus the black man has been emasculated in many ways and left few outlets for dealing adaptively with his reactions to the life-style imposed upon him. Recent studies have suggested that many young black males are killing themselves either directly or indirectly in the face of the apparent irreversibility of their situation. Clearly many turn to crime, drugs, and alcohol as means of coping with their frustrations.

Yet at present one cannot accurately describe the adjustment demands of being a black American solely from available psychological data. Too few studies have been done and far too many critical questions remain to be answered. In an effort to clarify some of these questions, Kenneth Clark, a black psychologist and past president of the American Psychological Association, has spent many years working to understand and communicate to others some of the psychological consequences of being black and living in a ghetto. In his important book, *Dark Ghetto,* Clark (1965) noted:

> The most concrete fact of the ghetto is its physical ugliness—the dirt, the filth, the neglect. In many stores walls are unpainted, windows are unwashed, service is poor, supplies are meager. The parks are seedy with lack of care. The streets are crowded with the people and refuse. In all of Harlem there's no museum, no art gallery, no art school, no sustained "little theater" group; despite the stereotype of the Negro as artist, there are only five libraries—but hundreds of bars, hundreds of churches, and scores of fortune tellers. Everywhere there are signs of fantasy, decay, abandonment, and defeat (p. 27).
>
> Human beings who are forced to live under ghetto conditions and whose daily experience tells them that almost nowhere in society are they respected and granted the ordinary dignity and courtesy accorded to others will, as a matter of course, begin to doubt their own worth. Since every human being depends upon his cumulative experiences with others for clues as to how he should view and value himself, children who are consistently rejected understandably begin to question and doubt whether they, their family, and their group really deserve no more respect from the larger society than they receive. These doubts become the seeds of a pernicious self- and group-hatred, the Negro's complex and debilitating prejudice against himself.

> The preoccupation of many Negroes with hair straighteners, skin bleachers, and the like illustrates this tragic aspect of American racial prejudice—Negroes have come to believe in their own inferiority. In recent years Negro men and women have rebelled against the constant struggle to become white and have given special emphasis to their "Negroid" features and hair textures in a self-conscious acceptance of "negritude"—a wholehearted embracing of the African heritage. But whether a Negro woman uses hair straightener or whether she highlights her natural hair texture by flaunting *au naturel* styles, whether a Negro man hides behind a neat Ivy League suit or wears blue jeans . . . , each is still reacting primarily to the pervasive factor of race and still not free to take himself for granted or to judge himself by the usual standards of personal success and character. It is still the white man's society that governs the Negro's image of himself (p. 64).

Some of the research findings that have appeared have been sharply criticized as designed to perpetuate "myths about racial differences." For example, currently, there is much debate over the validity of reported genetic differences in intelligence between the races. One side argues that since the races differ in many other physiological ways, it seems logical and appropriate to interpret repeatedly observed lowered IQ scores among blacks as indicative of lowered intellectual potential (Jensen, 1969). Others argue that such findings simply reflect the significant gap between black and white educational resources and are thus situationally determined (Dobzhansky, 1973). The "truth" is uncertain at the present time. However, the consequence of accepting the genetic difference theory might potentially be to reinforce already existing discriminative practices. As an innocent child (see Figure 6–7), barriers are drawn for the black. Certainly this would not be consistent with the investigator's original goals. Other studies have argued about the effects of racism on children's self-esteem. Early work in this area (Clark & Clark, 1947) reported that black children attach negative values to their racial features and would prefer to be white if they had a choice. More recently, investigators have been unable to replicate this phenomenon, a consequence perhaps of recent efforts to encourage racial pride as part of the black movement.

What seems quite clear at this point is that major social changes are occurring which are redefining the black man's role in society. No longer will separate facilities and restricted job and housing opportunities be accepted quietly. The problems of ghetto life and its strangling frustration are becoming recognized and gradually faced. Throughout this period of transition, many blacks have had to redefine themselves and find new, prouder, more self-expressive identities. This fact has resulted in major adjustment problems for some who cannot easily adapt to the changing scene. They continue to feel frustration and anger, as promised changes come slowly. They refuse to trust institutions that have ignored

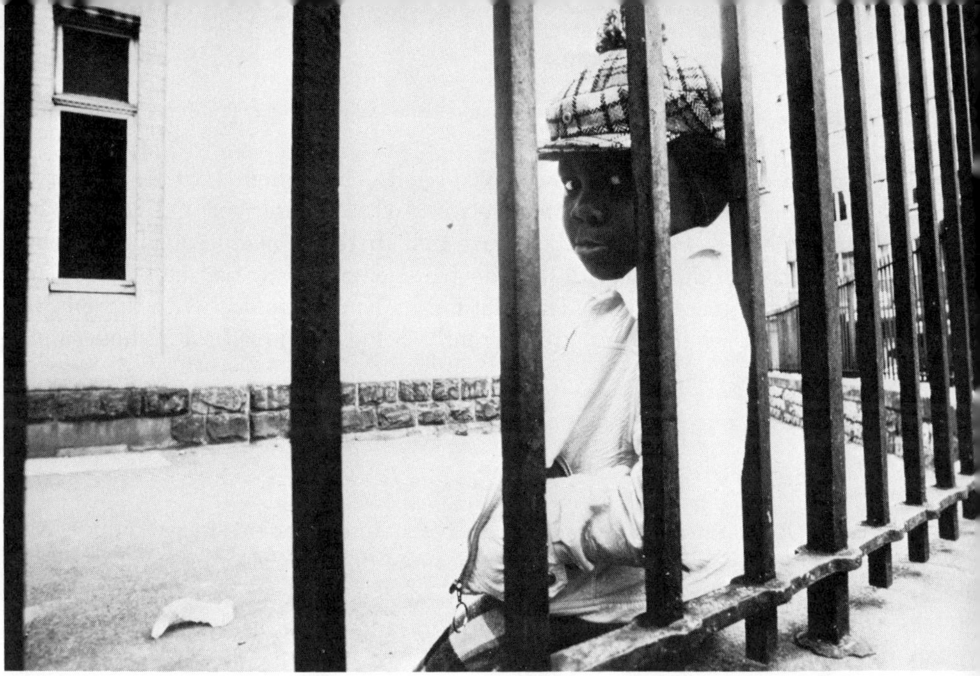

Photo by J. Brian King

Figure 6–7 Behind Bars.

or used them in the past. They refuse to accept tokenism or the role of being the "White Man's Burden" and yet cannot find appropriate outlets for expressing these feelings. Blacks recognize these problems and are now working to design for themselves agencies and care-givers who can respond to them.

CONCLUSION

This chapter has sought to demonstrate how a person's role in life and resulting self-concept can relate to his adjustment problems. As noted earlier, adjustment is a relative state defined by who, where, and what one is. Our personal circumstances determine in many ways the problems we face and the resources available for handling them. Thus one's sexual identity establishes certain role expectations and limits the options we have. Similarly, the various economic and ethnic backgrounds are accompanied by specific situational demands and have available diverse coping mechanisms. What should be clearly understood is that, in many cases, the adjustment value of a behavior can only be determined once the specific situation is understood.

Part II, which follows, will consider adjustment as it relates to yet another relative state—that of age. As will be seen, each of life's major developmental periods makes certain demands upon a person. The ability to deal effectively with the demands of one stage makes it easier to move on and confront the next period. Throughout Part II, the reader will perhaps note similarities between what is described and what he has experienced. He should be aware that there are many equally appropriate ways of dealing with the "developmental crises" we shall discuss and should attempt to consider what means he used to deal with those in the past and what means are currently being employed with those under way.

Summary

1. Adjustment is, in fact, a relative state dependent, in part, upon who one is, where one is, and what one does for a living.
2. In understanding adjustment, it is useful to consider how *self-concept* and *self-esteem* develop and relate to one's everyday behavior patterns.
3. As part of our socialization, we develop *roles* that define how we are supposed to act under certain situations. These roles provide for consistency in our behavior and in our self-perception.
4. An important role distinction in our culture is that between *masculine* and *feminine* behaviors. The development of such roles involves the acquisition of *sex-typed* behaviors and the acceptance of cultural *stereotypes.* Numerous investigators have reported significant differences between the sexes in aggression and dependency.
5. Three possible determinants of sexual role differences were considered: biology, identification, and learning. While none of these fully explains observed differences, all three seem to be involved in the acquisition of sex roles.
6. Social and ethnic background also play an important role in defining what is or is not adjusted behavior. Economic and educational differences are important correlates of the nature of one's early pressures and of the resources available to deal with these.
7. Various systems of *social stratification* have been suggested to classify people according to economic and cultural differences. The Hollingshead *Index of Social Position* is frequently used to identify five SES classes in mental health research.
8. Membership in upper- and lower-income groups results in very specific kinds of problems with which one must cope and thereby determine, in part, how one adjusts to life.
9. Poverty is a multifaceted condition defined not only by economic but also by familial criteria. It is possible to differentiate the poor along these dimensions and specify the adjustment needs of each segment of the poor.
10. Blacks not only share in the problems of the poor but also must

live with continual prejudices and discrimination which make adjustment for them specific to their circumstances and generally very difficult.

Words to Remember

- Agency
- Epidemiological Surveys
- Identification
- Nature vs. Nurture
- Reference Group
- Role
- Self
- Self-Concept
- Self-Esteem
- Self-Image
- Sex-Typed Behavior
- Sex Typing
- Social Status
- Socioeconomic Stratification
- Stereotype

Part II
Adjustment as a Function of Life's Stages

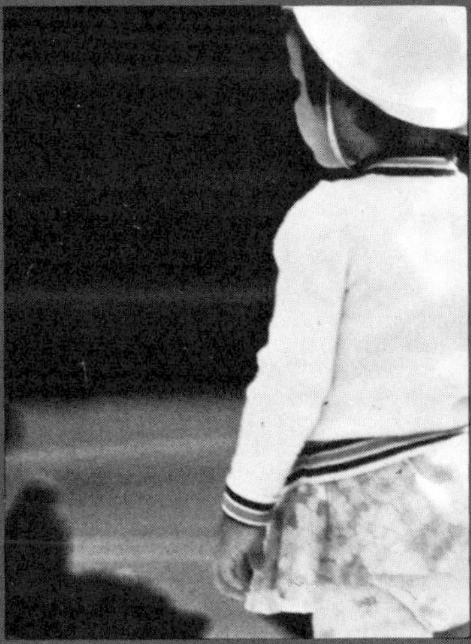

7. Adjustment to Infancy and Childhood

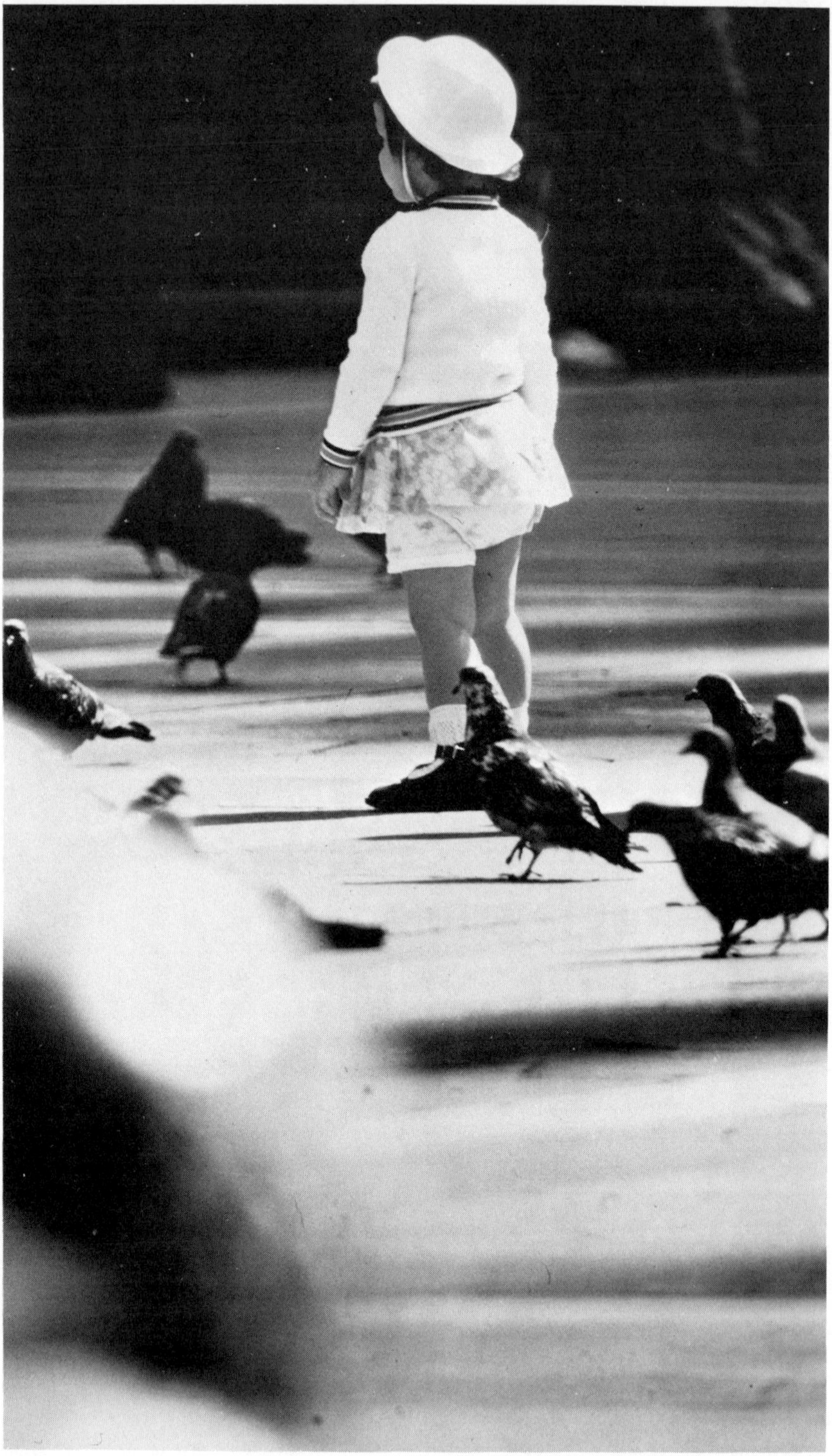

Photo by J. Brian King

Objectives

After studying this chapter the reader should be able to:

1. Define *libido.*
2. Describe Freud's theory regarding the interactions of the *ego, id,* and *superego* in determining personal behavior.
3. List Freud's psychosocial stages of development and describe each in terms of erogenous zones and need gratification.
4. List Sullivan's six developmental stages and describe each in terms of its principal characteristics.
5. List Erikson's Eight Ages of Man and the corresponding developmental task for each.
6. Describe each of Erikson's developmental tasks in terms of individual adjustment.

By now it should be clear to the reader that, whether adaptive or maladaptive, behavior is most certainly a complex phenomenon. In our consideration of adjustment, we have attempted to describe certain basic psychological processes that help us to understand behavior. Learning theory provides many useful concepts with which to understand its etiology and maintenance. Motivational and situational factors determine many of its quantitative and qualitative aspects. Through his affective and cognitive faculties, man expresses unrecognized and often unexpressible impulses. Socialization, roles, and stereotypes also play a significant function in determining behavior by prescribing "acceptable" limits within which one is expected to act. The processes mentioned thus far are all involved in the mechanics of adjustment. They serve as frameworks within which attempts to establish a resolution of external demands and conflicts can be translated into behavior. They do not however, define adjustment.

Adjustment does not refer to a specific form of behavior, nor does it imply an end-state toward which we must strive. Rather, as noted in previous chapters, adjustment refers to a process that continues throughout our lives. It is an evolving, cumulative experience. At each stage of life we have available different resources and skills which we can apply in response to prevailing demands, many of which are unique to that time. Through our cognitive faculties of memory and intelligence we have a historical dimension which permits us—indeed impels us—to attach the perspective of experience to current behavior. We are constantly building on the strengths and weaknesses of yesterday. Thus adjustment must be recognized as a *developmental* phenomenon and understood within a maturational framework. Toward this goal, Chapters 7 through 10 will review the adjustment demands of the various life stages. The present chapter will focus on infancy and childhood; Chapter 8 will consider adolescence; Chapter 9 will discuss early adulthood; and Chapter 10 will review the middle and later years of life. In reading each of these chapters, the student should attend to the ways in which the psychological processes discussed in Part I evolve and are utilized throughout human growth.

Developmental Stages

By now, the reader is probably aware that human development is a continuous process characterized by an almost infinite series of imperceptible changes. Thus, with each passing hour, day, week, or year we are in some way different from before. From such a perspective, the task of the social scientist attempting to describe and understand the chronology of maturation seems overwhelming. Such an effort would require a detailed consideration of each developmental change. The biologist, for example, would need to consider the infinite number of regenerating cells occurring each day and then specify the manner in which each affects the ongoing growth process. Yet such a microscopic analysis conflicts with the observation that a person's physical appearance does not change noticeably each day. Rather, within a limited range of variability, a healthy person's appearance remains somewhat constant over extended periods. Thus we can recognize differences between the physique of an infant and that of an adolescent; similarly, between that of the young adult and that of the elderly. This observation suggests that despite the continuous developmental process, it is possible to specify a finite number of discriminable stages through which a person passes as he matures. The specific criteria by which such stages are defined need not be restricted to physical phenomena, for man also develops cognitively and psychologically. It is important that, however defined, the stages mirror the chronology of maturation.

Developmental stages, therefore, represent a conceptually useful strategy for understanding growth in terms of specific periods in a person's life. Individuals may differ in terms of the ease with which they experience a given stage, and move on to subsequent stages. It is assumed, however, that these periods occur in a relatively fixed order. The reader should also note the *cumulative* nature of such stages, for earlier periods provide the base on which later ones develop. Transitions between stages are not sudden alterations, but rather gradual modifications of adaptive demands and patterns. The number of stages depends primarily on one's theoretical description of growth.

Since this volume is concerned with adjustment, we shall consider illustrative developmental systems that focus on the various adaptive demands made upon man throughout his life. A number of very prominent theorists have proposed conceptual systems for understanding maturation. Three of the more widely accepted of these, which clearly concern themselves with the differential challenges experienced throughout life, are the theories of Sigmund Freud, Harry Stack Sullivan, and Erik Erikson. We shall briefly review the first two and then consider, in some detail throughout the following chapters, Erikson's developmental theory.

Psychoanalytic Theory of Development

Sigmund Freud is widely known as the founder of psychoanalysis, a method of treating personal and emotional problems to be described in some detail in Chapter 13. Freud's psychoanalytic theory from which the treatment method evolved was one of the earliest and, to this day, most controversial views of the maturational process (Freud, 1966). He proposed that psychological development was stimulated by a form of psychic energy which he called *libido*. Although associated primarily with the sexual drive, libidinal energy referred more generally to the stimulation arising from incomplete satisfaction of the survival and propagation instincts including hunger and thirst, as well as sex. The reader should understand that the sexual instinct described by Freud included not only that related to genital stimulation but also that aroused in all bodily areas that can experience irritation and pleasure. These areas were labeled *erogenous zones*. According to psychoanalytic theory, during each maturational period, different erogenous zones are prominent. Interactions with oneself, others, and situational demands are mediated primarily through behaviors related to a specific period's libidinal focus. Thus the major adjustment task of each stage is to achieve some acceptable satisfaction of the libidinal desires arising within the currently relevant zone.

Were man to live alone, instinctual gratification would be a relatively simple matter. Depending upon whether one were hungry or thirsty, one could seek out whatever objects were necessary to meet that need. Sexual arousal could be dealt with by self-stimulation. Man, however, cannot live in isolation, for he has an instinct for survival. His sexual urges motivate him to reproduce and thereby to live with others. Because of these needs, the size of social groups expanded from primary to extended families, to tribes, to the more contemporary units of towns, cities, and nations. It then became increasingly necessary for instinctual satisfaction to occur within culturally approved limits. In recognizing

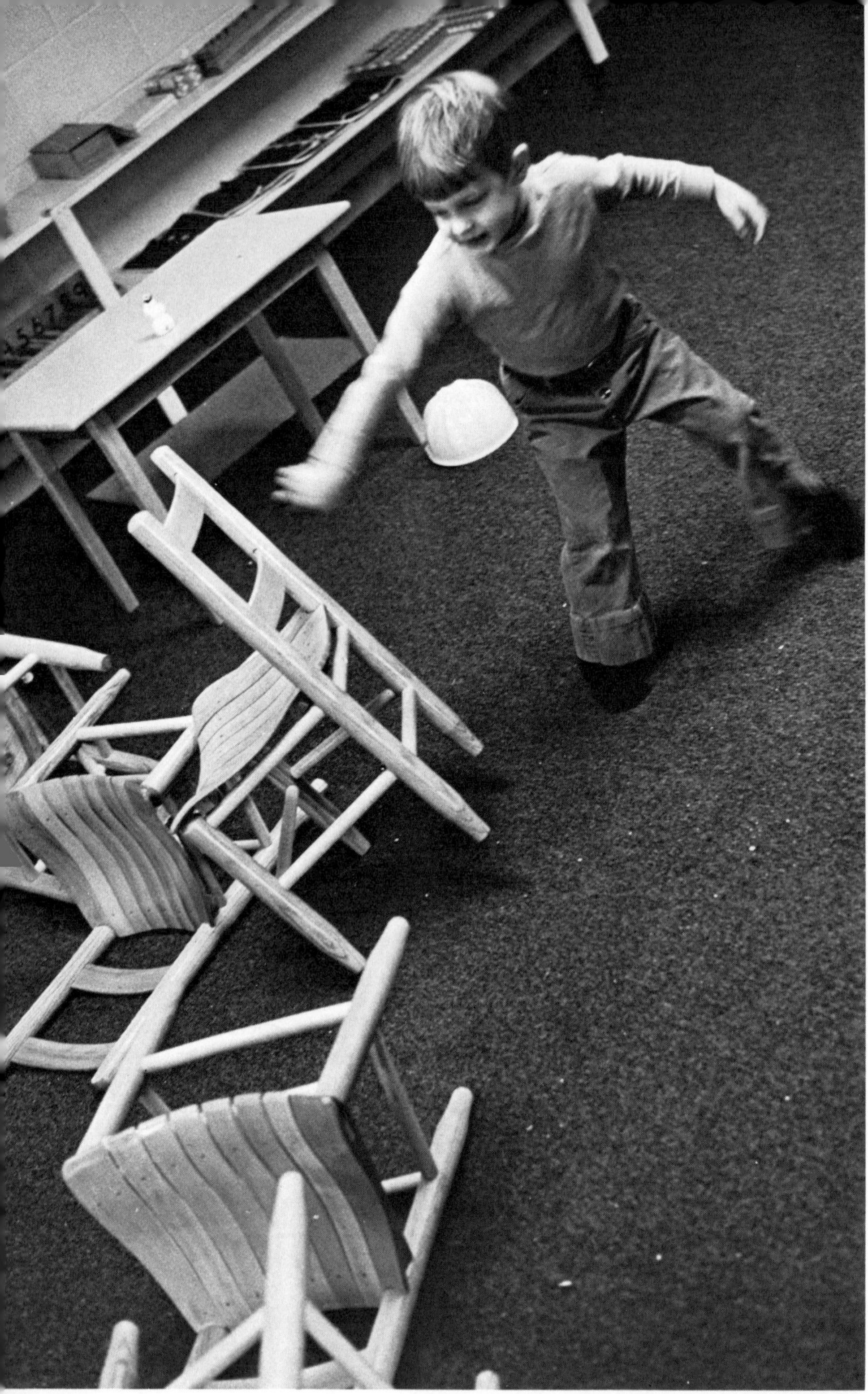

Photo by Chris T. Quillen

this fact, Freud postulated a tripartite structure of personality for the control of instinctual expression and the effective performance of one's social responsibilities.

THE STRUCTURES OF PERSONALITY

The most primitive structure is the *Id*, which "consists of everything psychological that is inherited and that is present at birth, including the instincts. It is the reservoir of psychic energy and furnishes all of the power for the operation of the other two systems" (Hall & Lindzey, 1957, p. 33). The Id refers to one's innate impulses including libidinal urges, as well as the destructive feelings of hostility and aggression. When tension arises in the Id, it seeks immediate direct discharge regardless of cultural or situational circumstances (functioning according to the *pleasure principle*). (See Figure 7–1.) Thus a young child experiences hunger and demands food; he has bladder or bowel urges and relieves himself. When an immediate solution is not present, the neonate has at his command the mechanism of *primary process* (i.e., fantasy) whereby he can imagine an object that will satisfy him (e.g., mother's breast or the bottle) and temporarily gratify himself in that way. Since fantasies do not satisfactorily meet physical needs, the child continues to seek a direct solution to his urges.

In doing so, the developing person becomes aware of the importance of interacting with the outside world. He learns that the fantasied image is insufficient and only real food will satisfy the needs. A second structure, the *Ego*, evolves as that portion of personality that mediates between internal instinct (i.e., the Id) and external reality. For example, it might delay Id satisfaction until an appropriate object is available. The child will cry or communicate his hunger in some manner until the mother arrives. The mechanism proposed by Freud by which one becomes actively involved in appropriately satisfying needs is labeled *secondary process* (which operates within the *reality principle*). According to Freud's theory, instincts or physical drives arise in the Id and, if possible, are immediately gratified. If, as is more likely, the situation is inappropriate for instantly meeting the need, the Ego is the mechanism that tests external reality and actively manipulates it until conditions are such as to permit satisfaction.

Working together, the Id and Ego would seem to be a logical team resulting in the efficient direct satisfaction of human needs. Yet as people formed societies, it became increasingly necessary to limit the expression of certain impulses, especially those involved with sex and

Figure 7–1 Giving Vent to the Id.

aggression. Such limits were expressed through civil and religious laws, taboos, and customs. Freud, living in Victorian Vienna with its strict morality, perceived moral principles as harsh masters of impulsive expression. In fact, it seemed as if the goal of such explicit rules was to eliminate rather than to moderate instinctual expression. Thus Freud saw such restrictions as equally important to reality in understanding the extent and form of impulsive expression. He therefore postulated a third structure reflecting the impact of man's conscience on his behavior.

This final structure of personality to evolve is the *Superego*—"the internal representation of the traditional values and ideals of society as interpreted to the child by his parents and enforced by means of a system of rewards and punishments imposed on the child. The Superego is the moral arm of personality; it represents the ideal rather than the real and it strives for perfection rather than pleasure" (Hall & Lindzey, 1957, p. 35). The Ego relates the expression of impulses to reality; the Superego, on the other hand, attempts to control rigorously the expression of libidinal (i.e., sexual) and aggressive desires by having the Ego choose moral rather than practical solutions to needs. Psychoanalytic theory postulates that all behavior represents the operation of one or more of these structures. Adjustment problems arise when the Ego is unable to resolve differences between Id and Superego demands satisfactorily.

PSYCHOSEXUAL STAGES OF DEVELOPMENT

As discussed previously, libidinal urges are centered in various organ systems throughout life. These developmental periods are labeled *psychosexual stages.* Initially, the mouth is the principal focus of libidinal activity during the first year, or the *Oral Stage.* At this time of life, the infant is primarily concerned with the pleasures associated with eating. Observations of children at this age provide evidence of their almost insatiable need to have something in their mouths: food, their thumb, blanket, and so forth. Everything the child touches eventually reaches the mouth. During the later part of the first year, teeth appear and the child adds biting and chewing to his oral exploration skills. Since mother or some other adult is typically the main provider of nourishment, the child becomes dependent on his caretaker and learns to rely on others to satisfy needs. Freud argues that during this stage a number of personality traits associated with oral incorporation may evolve, such as dependency, inquisitiveness, verbosity, and greed.

During the second year of life or the *Anal Phase,* the primary erogenous zones center around the anus and eliminatory mechanisms. The young child experiences, for the first time, the strict external requirement that he establish control over his impulses. Toilet training begins, and both pleasures and conflicts arise in relation to elimination. The child must learn the socially appropriate manner in which to satisfy the impulse to eliminate. Depending on the reaction of others to his behavior at this time, the child can also develop a number of enduring character traits during the anal period. For example, Freud suggests that overly harsh toilet training may establish a pattern for future cleanliness or disorder. Similarly, experiences at this time of life may presage later retentiveness or generosity.

With the resolution of the demands of toilet training, and continuing physical growth, sensitivity centers in the genitals, and the sex organs become the next major erogenous zone as the child enters the *Phallic Stage*. It is at this stage of life that Freud hypothesized that the young child begins to fantasize a sexual relationship with the opposite-sexed parent. He termed these feelings the *Oedipal Complex* for boys and the *Electra Complex* for girls. In each case positive feelings develop for the opposite-sexed parent and competitive hostile feelings for the same-sexed parent. Since these fantasies cannot be satisfied in real life, the appropriate solution is for the child to ultimately identify with the same-sexed parent and repress (i.e., put out of consciousness) the phallic urges for the opposite-sexed parent. This process was reviewed in some detail in Chapter 6 for it has been presented as one theory explaining the establishment of sex roles.

Following the dynamics of the first three stages of development—termed the *pregenital*—Freud felt that with the relative reduction in the rate of biological development the child entered a quiescent period, the *Latency Stage*, during the fifth or sixth year. This period was to last until puberty when sexual urges would again present a source of conflict and anxiety. During the early years of latency, Freud assumed that the child experienced few libidinal instincts and perceived this time as a period of happy innocence. Schoolwork, play, and growing up filled the child's time, and little of any great psychological consequence occurred. When the sexual impulses awakened with puberty, the child reexperienced the impulses of the phallic stage. If successfully handled at that time, the renewed urges were generally sublimated with little difficulty, and the adolescent was able to enter the next stage.

Freud called the final developmental period the *Genital Stage*. During this part of life, a person enters adulthood and assumes the normal responsibilities of that time. He goes beyond himself to give and receive from others. When asked what one should expect of a normal man, Freud is said to have responded: "Lieben und arbeiten"—to love and to work. In his analysis of that statement Erik Erikson (1963, p. 265) commented:

> It pays to ponder on this simple formula; it gets deeper as you think about it. For when Freud said "love" he meant *genital* love and genital *love;* when he said love *and* work, he meant a general work productiveness which would not preoccupy the individual to the extent that he loses his right or capacity to be a genital and loving being.

Thus mature man is able to achieve complete sexual satisfaction through his relationship with another and is able to go beyond himself in his work to care for the needs of others.

Sullivan's Interpersonal Theory of Development

In his theory of personality, Harry Stack Sullivan (1953) disagreed with Freud's emphasis on the centrality of the sexual drive in human development. While acknowledging the importance of biological factors to growth, Sullivan proposed that man's social-interpersonal experiences were critical to maturation. Sullivan viewed such social-psychological events as the determiners of personality development and postulated characteristic human interactions for each of the six stages, which he identified as occurring prior to adulthood.

SULLIVAN'S DEVELOPMENTAL STAGES

The first period is *Infancy,* which lasts until the child begins to use intelligible speech. Similar to Freud, Sullivan agreed that the oral zone was very important during this time of life. In Sullivan's system, however, its importance is a function of the interpersonal feelings that arise as the infant is being nourished. Thus initial interactions with others may be positive or negative depending on the care and satisfaction that accompany feeding. Sullivan also believed that the subtle feelings of parents were communicated to the infant through a process he called *empathy.* In this way and through more overt interactions with caretakers, infants form images of the good parent (one who is comfortable and satisfying) or the bad parent (one who is tense and unsatisfying) depending on the prevailing mood present during feeding and cuddling. Sullivan also indicated that important cognitive changes occur during this period. The infant passes from the *prototaxic* mode of thinking in which all experience is processed as mere sensation without meaning or relationship to any other experience to the *parataxic* mode in which the infant begins to cognize causal relationships between events. Often in the parataxic mode the causality presumed to exist between experiences is actually in error, their only real relationship being that of temporal or spatial contiguity. Nevertheless the infant does begin to establish some sense of cause and effect in his actions and to relate more consciously with those around him.

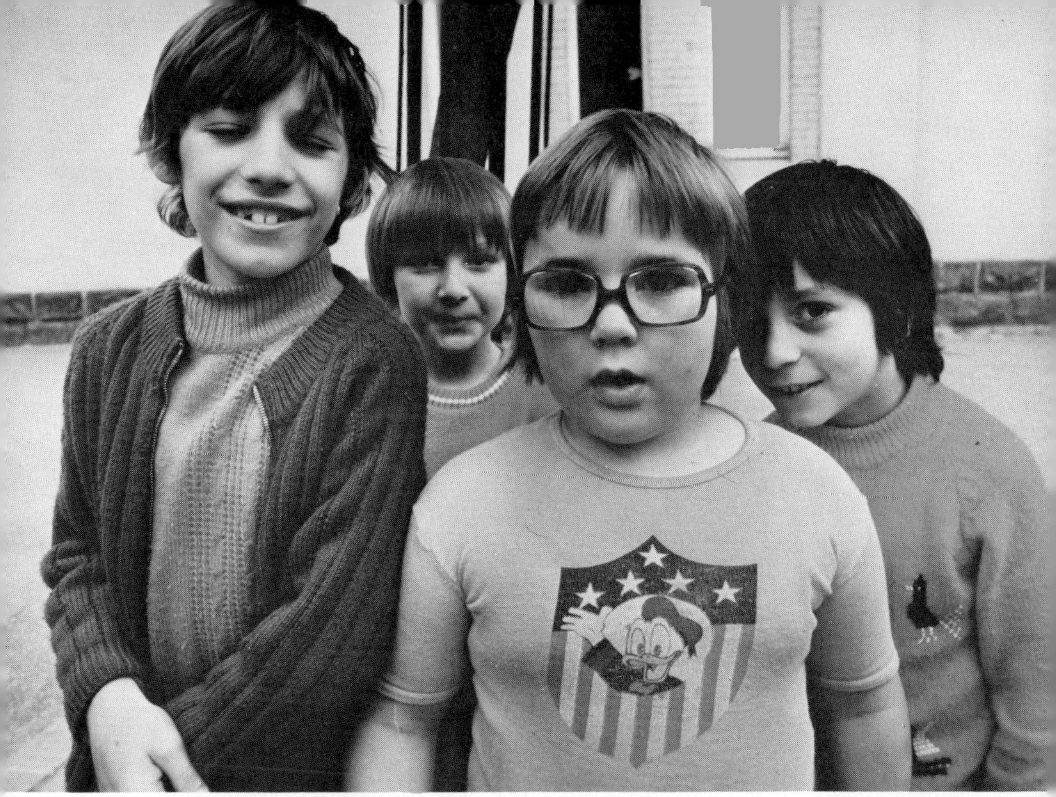

Photo by J. Brian King

Figure 7–2 The Juvenile Era.

As he acquires use of language, the infant passes into *Childhood*. During this stage the child begins to differentiate between the sexes and to adopt a socially defined sex role. Additionally, linguistic ability coincides with further cognitive reorganization as the child passes from the parataxic to the *syntaxic* mode of thinking. This form of cognition allows the child to use verbal and nonverbal symbols and he becomes capable of logically organizing the meaning of experiences. The child's newly emerging cognitive abilities enable him to play at make-believe and thereby extend beyond the limits of actual experiences. Childhood is also a time, Sullivan notes, when we first become aware that relating to others can result in painful as well as pleasant consequences. This awareness Sullivan labels the *malevolent transformation* and leads a person to be somewhat cautious in relating to others. Depending on the severity of one's negative interpersonal experiences, it may also predispose one to shun all but a few known, "safe" people and thereby become a social isolate. For most children, however, the malevolent transformation is merely the recognition of a social reality.

Once the child begins to go beyond himself and relates to playmates he enters the *Juvenile* stage. (See Figure 7–2.) This period extends throughout the elementary school years, and is characterized primarily by the events associated with educational experiences. Thus peers become important partners in learning about cooperation, competition, and companionship. Through the school, the juvenile learns to respect outside authority and to subordinate his personal desires to those of the group. He begins to internalize controls and to establish long-term goals. Later in this stage the juvenile will begin to seek out a more intense peer relationship. With the establishment of an intimate friendship, the juvenile enters Sullivan's fourth developmental stage—*Preadolescence.* This is a relatively brief period, with the principal event being the development of close interpersonal ties with another of one's age group.

Preadolescence is followed by the period of *Early Adolescence* during which the attention previously given to same-sexed peers begins to be directed toward the opposite sex. The early adolescent is experiencing puberty with all of its physical and psychological concomitants. He is now aware of genital arousal and takes an interest in dating. Early adolescence is that time of life in which the teenager gradually learns to adjust to his changing physical makeup and to his evolving physical needs. With time, he enters *Late Adolescence,* which Sullivan describes as a somewhat extended final apprenticeship into adulthood. Having satisfactorily adapted to his sexuality, the young adult also assumes the social, familial, and occupational responsibilities that characterize maturity.

Erikson's Eight Ages of Man

In his classic work, *Childhood and Society,* Erik Erikson (1963) extended the psychosexual stages proposed by Freud by delineating some of the social implications of each of those periods of life. He called these the *Eight Ages of Man.* He proposed that one consider human growth as a positive phenomenon in which health becomes an entity unto itself rather than the absence of illness. Psychosexual development occurred in parallel with psychosocial growth, and at each point in life the individual was faced with the task of establishing a new equilibrium between himself and his social world. The successful accomplishment of this task provided the individual with additional psychological resources for dealing with life. In his conceptualization of the maturational process, Erikson assumed that the resources gained at earlier stages continued to be available and to serve as a basic foundation of strength throughout adjustment. Recognizing too that not all men can successfully meet the demands of maturation, he outlined the negative consequences of failure. These negatives involve psychological traits that persist throughout life and are incorporated in later attempts to meet the challenges of growth. Erikson went beyond Freud in maintaining that development does not end with the attainment of adulthood and genitality. Rather, he recognized that men and women face very specific pressures and challenges during adulthood, middle age, and retirement. It is this very breadth of Erikson's system that makes it an appropriate model for those concerned with the developmental demands of adjustment. Indeed, the essence of Erikson's theory is his attempt to describe the health-producing cycle of human maturation.

Since we shall consider Erikson's stages in considerable detail, we shall outline them only briefly here. The initial period of development is the oral-sensory period occurring during the first year of life. The infant's primary task is the development of a sense of *basic trust* in people. The second year brings the muscular-anal period, and with it the young child must develop a sense of *autonomy* instead of *shame and doubt* in his interactions with his parents. Between three and five years of age, the child's major task is to develop *initiative* rather than *guilt* in his contacts with others. From the sixth year to the onset of puberty, *industry* versus *inferiority* can be initiated through neighborhood and school groups. Adolescence is a time when *identity* instead of *role confusion* (i.e., not knowing who he really is or should be) is developed through peer group associations, dating, and the selection of certain people as models. Early adulthood is a period of intimacy and solidarity versus *isolation.* This trait can grow from relationships with friends in competitive, cooperative, and amorous relationships. Middle adulthood is a time for a productive sense of *generativity,* which is the concern for establishing and guiding the next generation; it can also involve creativity and productivity. Persons unable to achieve this sense experience *stagnation.* The final stage is that of maturity and late adulthood when the well-adjusted person experiences a deep sense of personal *integrity* and satisfaction rather than the painful *despair* that accompanies those who fear the approach of death.

Studies at various stages of development, by and large, give credence to this model of development. Whether the time limits defined by Erikson hold precisely or whether the traits mentioned are always developed in a precise order are questions that will have to be answered by future research. Similarly it will be necessary to establish that the proposed negative characteristics result from an unsuccessful response to the demands of a given stage. Nevertheless, the traits that Erikson mentions are all important for mature adjustment, as the reader will observe in the following chapters.

The reader may wonder which of these systems is *the* correct one. The present state of knowledge of the behavioral sciences makes us unable to answer that question. For now, proponents of each system attempt through their theorizing, research, and therapeutic approach to clarify human behavior and to provide a matrix within which adjustment and maladjustment can be understood. To facilitate the reader's comparison of these systems, Table 7–1 outlines the major points of Freud's,

TABLE 7–1
Developmental Stages of Freud, Sullivan, and Erikson

Age	Approx.	Freud	Sullivan	Erikson
	Developmental Period	Oral Stage	Infancy	Oral Sensory
0–1	Principal Characteristic	Focus on oral incorporation and stimulation	Prototaxic to parataxic cognition; empathy and verbal skills	Basic trust vs. mistrust
	Developmental Period	Anal Stage	Childhood	Muscular-Anal
2–3	Principal Characteristic	Toilet training with resulting conflicts over expulsion	Parataxic to syntaxic cognition; beginnings of peer relationships	Autonomy vs. doubt
	Developmental Period	Phallic Stage		
3–4	Principal Characteristic	Awareness of genital sensation and development of Oedipal feelings		
	Developmental Period	Same as above		Locomotor-Genital
4–5	Principal Characteristic	Superego formation with resolution of Oedipal conflict		Initiative vs. guilt
	Developmental Period	Latency Stage	Juvenile Preadolescent Era	Latency
6–11	Principal Characteristic	Socialization and education as libidinal urges diminish	Formation of intimate peer relationships	Industry vs. inferiority

	Developmental Period	End of Latency Stage	Early Adolescence	Puberty and Adolescence
12–14	Principal Characteristic	Renewal and resolution of Oedipal conflict	Development of interest in heterosexual attachments and deeper interpersonal relationships	Identity vs. role confusion
	Developmental Period	Genital Stage	Late Adolescence	
14–18	Principal Characteristic	Sexual drive basis of mature and intimate relationship; sublimation of libidinal energies to productive tasks	More active pursuit of heterosexual relationships	
	Developmental Period	Same as above	Adulthood	Young Adult
18–25	Principal Characteristic		Establishment of a close heterosexual relationship with mature acceptance of responsibility	Intimacy vs. isolation
	Developmental Period	Same as above	Same as above	Adulthood
25–60	Principal Characteristic			Generativity vs. stagnation
	Developmental Period	Same as above	Same as above	Maturity
60+	Principal Characteristic			Ego integrity vs. despair

Sullivan's, and Erikson's developmental stages. Although each theorist differs in his conception of the underlying determinant of the developmental process, there is considerable similarity in the sequence of stages through which they see development occurring. In part, this is an artifact reflecting Freud's overwhelming influence on social scientists. Yet in large part, the congruence among developmental theories reflects the actual discriminable nature of these periods of growth.

The Adjustment Demands of Development

The remainder of this chapter and the following three chapters will consider in some detail the adjustment demands experienced at the major periods of life. As noted earlier, the theoretical framework within which this material will be presented is Erikson's (1963) "eight ages."

Infancy: Basic Trust vs. Mistrust

During the first year of life much happens to an infant. Major physical changes are obvious. Basic sensory modalities are exercised and intoduce him to the world. Initially totally helpless and dependent on others, the infant gradually acquires useful skills as he becomes able to voice pleasure and need, to grasp at wanted objects, and to move around and explore. During this phase of life the reactions of others to his needs are especially significant. The "others" must respond, for without them he can only experience continuing need. Yet the manner in which they respond will affect how the child interacts with other people later in life. It is at this point in life that Erikson sees the infant as forming a fundamental conception of the social world around him. If needs are met and discomforts removed, the world seems secure. If the grown-ups in one's life provide warmth, comfort, and much enjoyed cuddling, a sense of *trust* develops with respect to relating to people. When such conditions are not met, the child becomes suspicious and hesitant about interacting with others—a general *mistrust* of human relationships is formed. Although neither is indelibly fixed to personality throughout life, the healthy, well-adjusted infant has an obvious advantage in being able to engage others openly and confidently.

PHYSICAL ADJUSTMENTS OF THE FIRST YEAR

The birth of a child is a truly awesome event to observe. As it leaves its mother's womb, the infant appears tiny, wrinkled, and totally helpless. Suddenly it finds itself expelled from an environment that was completely comfortable and that met all needs automatically. The cold of the outside contrasts sharply with the nearly 100° watery capsule that suddenly changed with violent contractions. No longer can the child be totally dependent on another, for he must immediately take that first breath to take in oxygen, and in so doing utter the first cry. From then on, during the coming year the gentle, quiet, seemingly unpreoccupied child will in fact be hard at work developing a host of physical abilities and responding to a number of physical needs.

The most immediate need we have already described—oxygen. Until birth the infant received all that he needed of this vital element from his mother. From birth on, his respiratory system must function efficiently. Indeed, within a short time, the neonate has stabilized the proportion of oxygen and carbon dioxide in his blood to within acceptable limits and, barring any major disease or mechanical dysfunction, can pretty much ignore that need for the rest of his life. At birth the infant must also activate various thermoregulative systems within his body. The sudden drop in temperature at delivery is dramatic. Aided by the heat lamps and wrappings present in most delivery rooms, the neonate gains time to adjust to the new changes. Once again normal physiological functioning will assure that within a short period of time most infants will be physically able to withstand normal variations in temperature without negative consequences.

Once recovered somewhat from the trauma of birth, the neonate also experiences the exhaustion of the rigorous ordeal of leaving the womb. Sleep is an important part of the newborn's day. Initially he will require almost 20 hours of sleep per day and be awake for only the 4 remaining hours. As he gains strength the infant will gradually increase his working hours, so that by the end of the first year he will be awake for more hours than he sleeps. Within a few days of birth the infant will regularly demonstrate his reactions to some of his more well-recognized needs. Although unable to eat a great deal, the neonate is certainly able to eat often—typically requiring nourishment every 4 hours. During the first few months the number of feedings will decrease until it matches the modal 3. Correspondingly the amount ingested each time will increase. Simultaneously, the infant's bladder and bowel functions initially operate with a rather high frequency (in fact, many a new parent fervently believes that his offspring holds a world's record in that event) and gradually decrease during the first year as the child's storage capacity increases in preparation for the demands of toilet training.

The physical advances occurring during the first year are indeed significant. The major sensory systems all develop in acuity, and locomotion begins. The infant gains the ability to communicate on a simple level with those around him. These advances are considered in detail in the excellent text *Child Development and Personality* by Mussen, Conger, and Kagan (1969). These authors have also provided a very useful outline of the significant changes occurring during the first eighteen months of life in their Stages of Infancy (pp. 156–157):

> The newborn period is considered to cover the first 5 to 7 days. At this time, the infant is recovering from the physiological trauma of delivery and is just beginning to establish an equilibrium with his environment.
>
> The second period of infancy lasts from 1 to 8 weeks of age. The reason that 8 weeks is designated as the approximate end of a phase is because several important changes occur at this time. The infant becomes markedly more visually attentive to the world around him, his vocalizations increase dramatically, and the amount of time he spends crying is markedly reduced.
>
> Between 8 and 12 weeks another set of important events occurs. First, the infant's behavior suggests that he is beginning to appreciate depth and to perceive objects in three dimensions. Before this, the baby reacts with the same amount of smiling and the same duration of looking to two- and three-dimensional forms of human faces. Between 3 and 4 months, however, he will look longer and will smile and vocalize more frequently at a three-dimensional form. In addition, the three-month-old will begin to lose interest to repetitions of same stimuli. This phenomenon is called habituation.
>
> The next stage lasts from about 4 to 7 months and is characterized by increased smiling to human voices and faces, the peak of such smiling occurring between 3 and 5 months of age. . . . The second major event occurring during this period is the coordination of eye-hand movements and coordinated visual-motor reaching, which usually occurs at 5½ months.
>
> The next period lasts from about 7 to 12 months and is characterized by frequent displays of anxiety in response to surprising or unexpected stimuli, anxiety about the presence of a stranger being only one instance of this reaction.
>
> This period lasts from about 12 to 18 months and involves the onset of walking, and increased mobility, as well as the beginning of language comprehension and expression. The infant can now understand simple requests, can use language to obtain desired goals and can react to objects on the basis of their symbolic names rather than only on the basis of their color, shininess, or capacity for being sucked or slapped.

It is important for the reader to understand that the age ranges described above and to be discussed in later sections are not fixed. Each child develops at his or her own pace, and parents are often unnecessarily alarmed when their child is unable to locomote as easily as or babbles somewhat less than a comparably aged peer. They must recognize that major individual differences exist between children and that the vast majority develop appropriate physical and mental skills by the end of infancy. Some proceed more slowly or more quickly than others. Some appear to be making little headway and suddenly a number of slowly developing processes seem to consolidate, and the child progresses markedly in several areas. The new parent who is concerned about his child's progress should compare his child's functioning to that of other children who are 4 to 6 weeks older or younger. If the parent continues to be concerned, he or she should then discuss this with the pediatrician who regularly examines the child.

PSYCHOLOGICAL ADJUSTMENTS OF INFANCY

As the child develops physically throughout the first year, he employs his newly emerging skills in his daily interactions with those around him. With the emergence of attentional and cognitive processes, the infant becomes aware of a highly significant component of his environment—other people. Very quickly he responds to their reactions, and their responses to him establish a relationship between them. Their smile and the warmth experienced as they hold him, communicate to the infant that others can be sources of great satisfaction. Perceptual processes become discriminating enough to identify mother as a primary care agent and perhaps father also, depending on the extent to which he is involved in early child care. Thus the presence of mother becomes a positive event, and if she is regularly there to solve the problem when hunger arises or wetness occurs, the probability that the child will be basically confident and trusting in later human relationships is quite high. The opposite is equally likely if the significant human in one's life tends to be unconcerned and unpredictable about responding to the infant's needs. This state of early dependency was described long ago by Josselyn (1948, p. 36):

> During this early infancy period, the child is completely dependent upon his environment for his safety and comfort. He needs other people in order to have his physical requirements met. His dependency on others, if satisfactorily fulfilled, allays anxiety—an anxiety that has its roots in his own physical inadequacy to deal with the unknown. This unknown is often a noisy, uncomfortable, threateningly large, inexplicable, reality world. Anxiety, if present, is manifested by a state of general physical tension. This need to be dependent is very strong in the first year of life but lessens gradually as the child becomes physically capable of meeting his own needs and of handling external situations to a greater extent by his own abilities.

Thus an infant develops a very special, close relationship to its mother. The determinant of this need is not, however, totally clear. Is it simply because mother provides all of the positive reinforcements the child seeks and thereby, through generalization, becomes herself reinforcing? If so, the extent of the mother-child relationship should be a direct function of the frequency of feedings, diaperings, and cuddlings, with some consideration given to the satisfaction level associated with each of these. For example, some mothers may be more comfortable holding a child than other mothers and therefore the former may be more relaxed and satisfying "rockers and cuddlers." Although little direct research data currently exist on this issue, interesting related findings have been reported in studies of infant monkeys.

"LOVE" IN INFANT MONKEYS

As part of a research program on the effects of the separation of infant monkeys from their mothers, Harry Harlow (1959) and his co-workers ran a number of studies at the Primate Laboratory of the University of Wisconsin during the mid- and late 1950s. Those studies of interest here involved the reactions of infant monkeys to artificially constructed *surrogate* mothers (i.e., mother monkeys made out of wood and metal wire). Two sets of identical surrogate mothers were prepared, except that one was covered with terry cloth, whereas the other was only a bare welded-wire cylindrical form. Both "mothers" were able to nurse their infants by a bottle which had a nipple protruding from the "mother's" breasts. Harlow discovered that infant monkeys fared equally well with either mother in terms of amount of nourishment consumed and weight gained. The major difference, however, was that those infants with the terry cloth–covered "mother" spent significantly more time cuddling and clinging to it than did the infant monkeys with the wire "mothers." Harlow concluded from this that in infant monkeys, and by extension human infants, the attachment with the mother gratified a need for bodily contact. To investigate this conclusion further, Harlow performed a series of related follow-up studies.

In the first of these both "mothers" were present, and infant monkeys originally nursed by one or the other "mother" were subjected to a fear-arousing stimulus. Regardless of their early experience, the infant monkeys overwhelmingly chose the cloth "mother" for relief from fear. They would hug the terry-cloth form and cling very tightly to it. At times the infant monkeys would chance approaching the upsetting object, but would consistently return to the cloth "mother" for "additional courage." In an "open-field" test, the infant monkeys were placed in a large room with numerous strange objects. With the cloth "mother" present, they would initially go to "her" and cuddle for a time before exploring the environment. In the absence of the cloth "mother" or in the presence of the wire "mother," the infant monkeys would demonstrate fearful behavior such as crying, crouching, and thumb sucking. A later study demonstrated that motion in the cloth surrogate increases her attractiveness somewhat, but heating it does not. Additionally, Harlow reports some evidence suggesting that monkeys deprived of early opportunities for affection have later difficulties establishing relationships.

This series of studies demonstrates, in part, the scientific utility of comparative research. Ethical considerations would never permit such studies to be carried out with human infants. Harlow's work does, however, provide important insights into the formation of attachments early in life. In many ways the behavior of infant monkeys toward strange objects or persons is quite similar to the behavior observed with human infants. They demonstrate similar needs to feel assured of the mother's presence. Also, as it turns out, they demonstrate similar difficulties in establishing later ties with others if early attachment experiences are absent.

INFANTS WITHOUT MOTHERING

Some of the consequences of not having a close personal tie early in life have been demonstrated in studies on the effects of institutionalization on human infants. Basic research in this area was performed during the 1940s by René Spitz (Spitz & Wolf, 1946), who reported that in institutions where care was inadequate and inconsistent, a significant portion of the children at first cried regularly, but within six months became quite indifferent to those around them and appeared to simply withdraw from their environment. This condition was labeled "marasmus." Studies of other infants residing in institutions in which physical care was clearly inadequate reported that after four months the institutionalized infants showed significant deficits in the amount of time spent vocalizing and an inability to adjust physically to being held by an adult (Provence & Lifton, 1962). Overall, these children seemed to lack the interactional skills observed in most children by that age.

The aforementioned studies certainly represent extreme situations. One would expect that under more typical family situations children would readily develop the necessary social skills. The reader should, however, keep in mind that quantity of maternal caring is by itself insufficient. A basic sense of confidence and ease in interpersonal situations develops when the infant experiences positive interactions with the significant adults in life. Sullivan hypothesizes that a young child senses emotion through empathy. Although as yet unproved, this suggestion does correspond to the often noted perception that an infant seems to sense whether or not it is wanted and loved. If the answer is positive, the infant gains valuable personal assets that he can use as he enters the next phase of development.

The Second Year of Life: Autonomy vs. Shame and Doubt

During the infant's second year he continues to grow physically and to develop psychologically. The almost total state of dependency that characterized his first year now begins to decrease gradually. Maturation is a hazardous state, for it requires the infant to place his basic trust in those around him. In his pursuit of independence he must now discover whether or not they will permit him to exercise his newly emerging abilities and thereby begin to do things for himself. Erikson identifies the infant's needs during this period with the acquisition of a sense of *autonomy* about himself. At this age the child seeks to manipulate the world around him and to establish some control over his person. Those who fail to do so, develop—in Erikson's view—a sense of *shame* toward their accomplishments and *doubt* in their abilities.

PHYSICAL ADJUSTMENTS OF THE SECOND YEAR

Among the major physical developments occurring during the second year are significant increases in locomotor and vocalization skills. The infant becomes much more mobile, and his innate curiosity motivates him to explore the many facets of his environment. Additionally, his ability to understand instructions, as well as to communicate his desires, increases during this period, thereby adding to his sense of control and mastery over the things around him. Neurological gains are also critical during this period, for they provide him with the capacity to exercise voluntary control over his bladder and bowel functions. This advance is particularly important, for a basic task the young child must accomplish at this age is to become toilet trained.

With his added mobility, the two-year-old child will seek to experience many new and wondrous aspects of his world. He will seem to "get into everything," and each closet, drawer, and cupboard will hold an inviting mystery. Not only will his exploration lead him into possible mischief, but also into potential danger. The child of this age does not anticipate physical harm and sees no danger in knives, scissors, or sharp objects. Any liquid is appropriate for tasting and any object small enough to be placed in the mouth will be appropriate. In his eagerness to go from one place to another, the child is sure to trip and fall many times and occasionally will experience scrapes, bruises, and cuts. Parents must be prepared for such doings and must be comfortable in permitting the child some freedom to have minor accidents without regarding them as major traumas. To most falls the child's initial reaction will be fear expressed by crying. If calmly reassured, most children will quickly forget the incident and continue their play. If the parent regularly overreacts to such events, the child will have great difficulty developing self-confidence. Naturally parents do not allow a child to taste poisons or manipulate sharp objects. But assuming the truly dangerous items are out of reach, encouraging and permitting the child's exploration can have positive consequences for his intellectual and psychological development.

PSYCHOLOGICAL ADJUSTMENTS OF THE SECOND YEAR

The child's pursuit of autonomy must somehow mesh with his parent's need that he become socialized. His unbounded curiosity, his desire to locomote in whatever direction he pleases, his willingness to give in to whatever impulse arises—all of these must gradually be limited by the local bounds of values, attitudes, and propriety. The specific restrictions placed on a given child will be relative to his socioeconomic background, his religious affiliation, and whatever cultural norms his parents accept. However, their task at this time—as most parents see it—is to provide the child with some basic rules of what is or is not acceptable behavior. Some contemporary parents find the notion of socializing a child abhorrent and claim that to do so would deny the child's basic individuality. They therefore raise their child to be "free." What they fail to recognize is that this approach also represents a form of socialization and that, although perhaps fewer in number, the limits such parents impose upon the child do provide him with a set of guidelines for future life. Often such "rule-free" procedures fail to appreciate the later problems the child will encounter when forced to interact with the larger society.

Whether or not he is prepared for it, the child will encounter a new force to contend with during the second year—his parent's prohibitions. Heretofore his needs have been met by his parents, and only positive experiences have been shared with them. As the child begins to explore, however, and as his parents begin to socialize him, it will be necessary to set limits on behavior and to communicate displeasure with some of his activities. The reader who is a parent perhaps recalls the first time he or she corrected a child. The youngster's response was probably at first shock followed by apparent heartbreak. Josselyn (1948, p. 50) has attempted to clarify the meaning of this experience for the child:

> Disapproval by the parent has elements of real danger for the child. To the small child, anger and love cannot occupy the same space at the same time. When the small child loves, he loves; when he hates, he hates. He hates anything or anyone not complying with his expressed or unexpressed wish. He assumes the same lack of ambivalence on the part of the parent. Ultimately, his gradual awareness of his own ambivalence toward his parents and his recognition that he actually can feel hostile toward the person he loves help him to realize that parents can love even though they are angry. This development can be traced more readily in his reactions to inanimate objects than in his relationship to parents since there is less confusion and anxiety in the normal child's relationship to inanimate objects. Early in the child's play life, if a toy does not conform with his wishes, he will attempt to destroy the toy. Later, the emotionally maturing child will not destroy it but, recognizing a positive value that transcends the immedi-

ate frustration, will abandon the original aim in the play, or will substitute another toy, returning to the original toy for some game in which it can function adequately. This capacity for tolerance and understanding, however, is a later development. Until the child is able to recognize and accept the limitations of the toy in terms of the reality of its structure, and to see that the toy does not fail him completely by restrictions of its own use in certain areas, he rejects, hates, and wishes to destroy the toy. In his early experience of prohibition by the parent, he reacts to the parent with the same kind of resentment. He also assumes the same attitude on the part of the parent toward himself as he has toward his toy and fears the implied rejection, until he has experienced repeatedly the love of his parents in spite of their condemnation of his behavior.

TOILET TRAINING

The event around which much tension between parent and child is often experienced is toilet training. Previously, the procedure was simple for the child. Whenever either bladder or bowel were full, they would be involuntarily emptied and, shortly thereafter, mother would relieve the child of any related discomfort by cleaning and changing him. With the onset of training:

> this sequence must be rearranged. The connection between bowel stimulus and the evulsion response must be weakened. The child must learn to suppress the evulsion response to the bowel drive stimulus alone. It must then insert other responses in the sequence. At first it must learn to call to the parents. It must later learn to insert walking, unbuttoning, and sitting on the toilet chair while it is still suppressing the urgent evulsion response. Only to a new pattern of cues—the bowel stimulus, the cues of the proper room, the sense of freedom of clothes, the pressure of the toilet seat on the child's thighs—make the evulsion response occur without anxiety (Mussen, Conger, & Kagan, 1969, p. 262).

That few three-year-olds and far fewer older persons have not mastered these skills attests to the universal potential for their acquisition. For the child experiencing it, however, toilet training is a significant challenge, indeed.

The child's initial reaction to toilet training is often one of puzzlement. Considerable attention is paid to his excretory functions. Parents seem very much to want him to produce this "gift" for them and yet when he does, they very quickly do away with it. The child initially shares none of the parents' revulsion toward feces. He perceives his excretum as his own creation and wants very much to preserve it. It is not unusual around the time of toilet training for a child to try to hide his feces or to smear them around a crib or playroom. If he has angry, hostile feelings toward his parents, he quickly discovers that he can express these feelings through his bowel functions. When pressured to produce a movement, he can frustrate them by refusing to go. Once the pressure is eased, he can have an "accident" and need changing. The child may also, in more serious cases, feel so anxious about toilet training that diarrhea will develop and he will effectively lose his ability to control his eliminative functions. Temper tantrums in reaction to toilet training are not uncommon. The child may sense that learning to control himself is of utmost importance in his parents' minds and, fearing their rejection should he fail them, may become so upset by the process as to find it very difficult to accomplish the goal they wish for him.

When and how toilet training occurs depends on a number of variables including the child's social background. Studies have shown that lower-income mothers tend to toilet-train their children earlier than do middle-class mothers. Generally, in most cases, with both lower- and middle-class parents it was found that those children who began training later (especially when 18 months or older) required less time than those beginning earlier. Specific training procedures have received relatively little attention in research studies, although basic learning theory would suggest some combination of positive reinforcement for appropriate elimination behaviors and negative reinforcement for messing or wetting. Most parents seem to watch for some indication that the child needs to urinate or defecate and then encourage the appropriate response sequence. In this way, they are able to reinforce the child and also establish an association between feeling a need to eliminate and following the desired procedure.

Overly severe or premature toilet-training techniques have been found to relate to a number of negative consequences for children (Mussen, Conger, & Kagan, 1969). A significant proportion of children having such training experiences needed some form of psychological treatment during their childhood. Others seemed to develop very negative personality characteristics such as obstinacy, aggressiveness, or by contrast, excessive timidity. Psychoanalytic theorists hypothesize that a child's experiences during toilet training and the anal period will have considerable influence upon his later tendencies toward cleanliness or messiness. The important thing for a parent to appreciate is the difficulty of the task being demanded of the child, and to expect that accidents will occur with some frequency early in training. With patience and consistent reinforcement for attempts to accomplish the desired behavior, most parents should be able to succeed in helping their children through this period.

NEED FOR AUTONOMY

Erikson, therefore, reminds us of the essential meaning of this period for the young child. He or she is aware of newly emerging skills and appears to have an innate drive to try these out (Figure 7–3). The one-

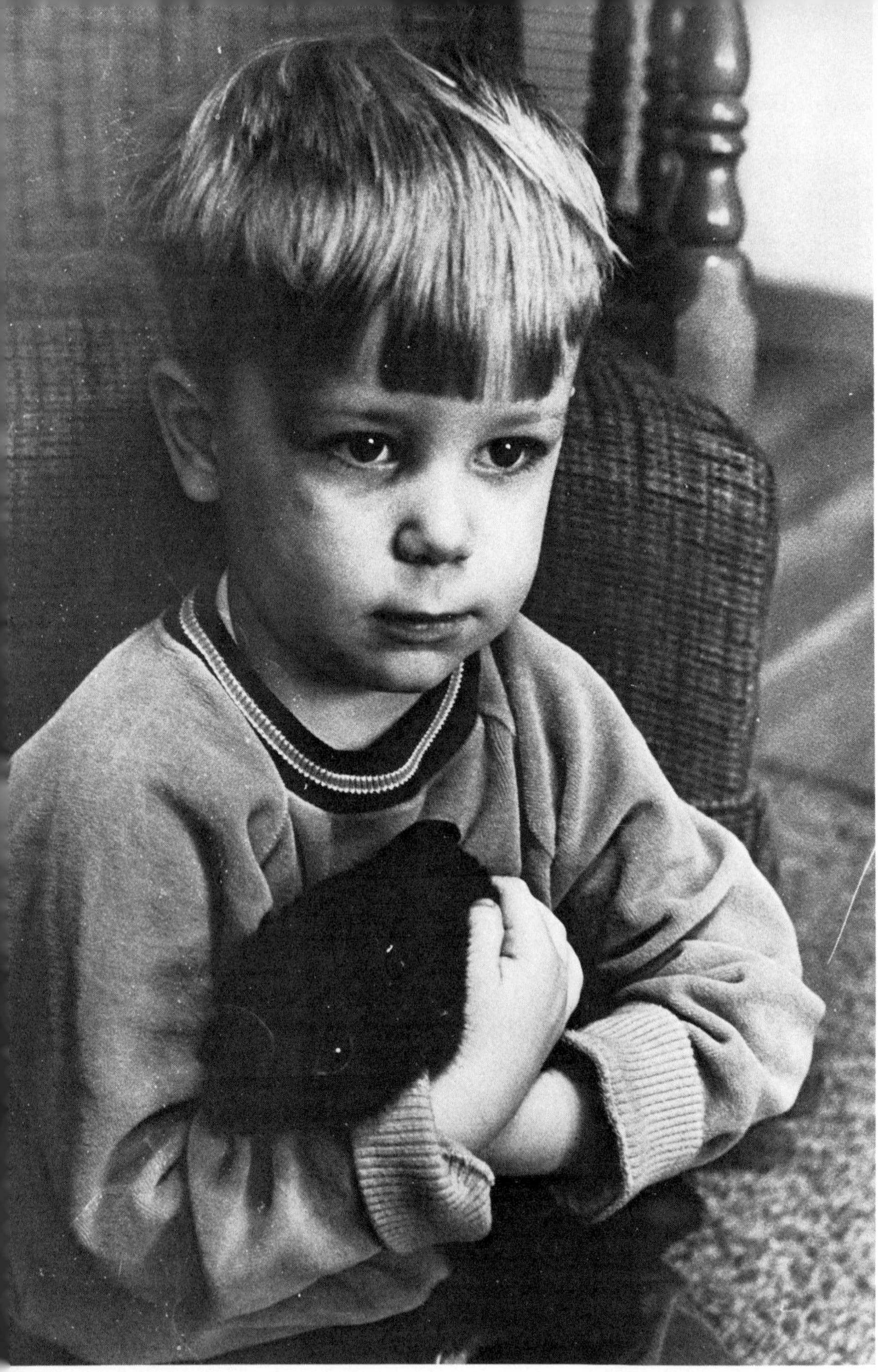

Photo courtesy of *Columbia Missourian*

Figure 7–3 A Time for Initiative.

or two-year-old insists on doing things for himself. No longer will he simply open his mouth to be fed. Instead, he wants his own utensils and, oblivious of the resulting mess, tries to feed himself. Erikson defines this as a need for autonomy and that concept seems to reflect accurately the observed pursuit of self-reliance. If parents insist on making their children dependent and refuse to encourage their growth, their children will doubt the value of their own capacities. If parents do not appreciate the products of their children's efforts, however crude or uncoordinated they may be, and tease them about the worth of their efforts, the children are likely to feel ashamed of themselves. If, instead, the parent allows a child to find himself and to control those aspects of himself of which he is capable, then the child can pass on to the next stage with both a sense of personal confidence and a continuation of his basic trust in others.

The Preschool Years: Initiative vs. Guilt

Erikson conceptualizes the primary task of the second year of life as the development of a sense of competence and autonomy. The child seeks the assurance that he can accomplish a task through his own efforts. He will struggle to "do it himself" and, if his parents appreciate and encourage this need, he will build yet another component upon his evolving personality. During the period between three and five years of age, the preschooler will begin to *initiate* many of his own activities. Thus far, much of his behavior has been a response to external stimulation or an imitation of the actions of others. By contrast, the preschooler is cognitively, physically, and psychologically ready to engage in activities of his own choosing. He can run, climb, ride a tricycle, and enjoy a wide variety of playthings and can select which he will do. Erikson (1963, p. 255) notes that: "Initiative adds to autonomy the quality of undertaking, planning and 'attacking' a task for the sake of being active and on the move." If the child of this age is permitted the freedom to engage in activities of his own choosing (assuming, of course, their safety and social acceptability), he will develop the positive quality of feeling confident of his ability to initiate behavior. If, instead, he is restricted or ridiculed in his choices, he will experience a sense of *guilt* and thereby become very reluctant to pursue a personally chosen course.

Sexual Development and Initiative

Although Erikson does not emphasize the importance of the child's emerging sexual sensations to the exclusion of other aspects of the child's psychosocial environment, he does consider emerging sexuality to be an important motivating agent for some of the child's experiences during this time of his life. Similar to Freud's theory of psychic energy, Erikson perceives the child's experience of these sensations as a stimulant to engage in more independent, even aggressive behaviors. The reader will recall that according to Freud's theory, the preschool child must struggle to deal with the anxieties associated with the Oedipal conflict. Erikson agrees that at this stage of life the child pursues closer attachment to the opposite-sexed parent. Furthermore, when older siblings are present, this period is often marked by demonstrations on the part of the preschooler of intense rivalries with those who threaten to hold a more favored position with mother or father. The preschooler may express these conflicts by engaging in fantasies about his overwhelming strength and his capacity to achieve whatever he wishes. Thus can he deal with his potential rivals, immune from retaliation, even though relatively little has changed in the family relationships. Freud (1966) had also hypothesized that the preschool male fears retaliation from his father because of the former's attachment to the mother. This fear Freud labeled *castration anxiety* and proposed that it and its parallel in girls (*penis envy*) are the underlying motives for identifying with the like-sexed parent and the assumption of sex roles. Chapter 6 considered a number of processes by which such roles develop. Thus both theorists perceive infantile sexuality as phenomena genuinely related to personality development.

In fact, children of this age do experience pleasure from genital stimulation and not uncommonly engage in both masturbatory and sex-play activities. As the child becomes more generally interested in his genitals, he or she will display considerable curiosity toward the differences between boys and girls and (if the occasion occurs) children and adults. Questions about why such differences exist and how babies are born are frequent at this age. Some children will engage in "playing doctor" and thereby look at and even touch each others' genitals. The parents' reaction to sexual behavior and curiosity plays an important role in determining the later sexual attitudes of the mature person. Ideally parents will respond openly and comfortably to children's questions. They will hear what the child is asking and limit their answers to the child's level of understanding and curiosity. Thus, for example, the four-year-old's question of "where do babies come from?" can be quickly answered with "from inside mommy's tummy" rather than with an illustrated lecture on male and female anatomy and the mechanics of procreation and birth. Similarly, peer sex play or individual masturbation should be treated as any other socially unacceptable behavior rather than labeled as "dirty," "sinful," or "physically harmful." Ideally the child learns from his parents to control the expression of his sexual urges and acquires an appreciation and acceptance of his sexuality rather than a generalized reaction of disgust and guilt concerning such feelings.

THE DEVELOPMENT OF CONSCIENCE AND GUILT

One of the important socialization processes occurring during the preschool years is the development of conscience. In Freud's view this occurs as part of the resolution of the Oedipal conflict. Identification with the same-sexed parent includes the unconscious adoption of the moral standards of that parent, that is, the Superego. Since it is not a conscious process, the resulting control provides almost automatic security against a resumption of the anxieties associated with the sexual longings for the opposite-sexed parent. Erikson notes, however, that this very fact makes the Superego extremely rigid and uncompromising. Thus the conscience of the young child can be a harsh master indeed. (See Figure 7–4.) Children of this age often tend to follow parental instructions to the letter and can be much more exacting than was ever

Figure 7–4 Contending with Conscience.

Photo courtesy of *Columbia Missourian*

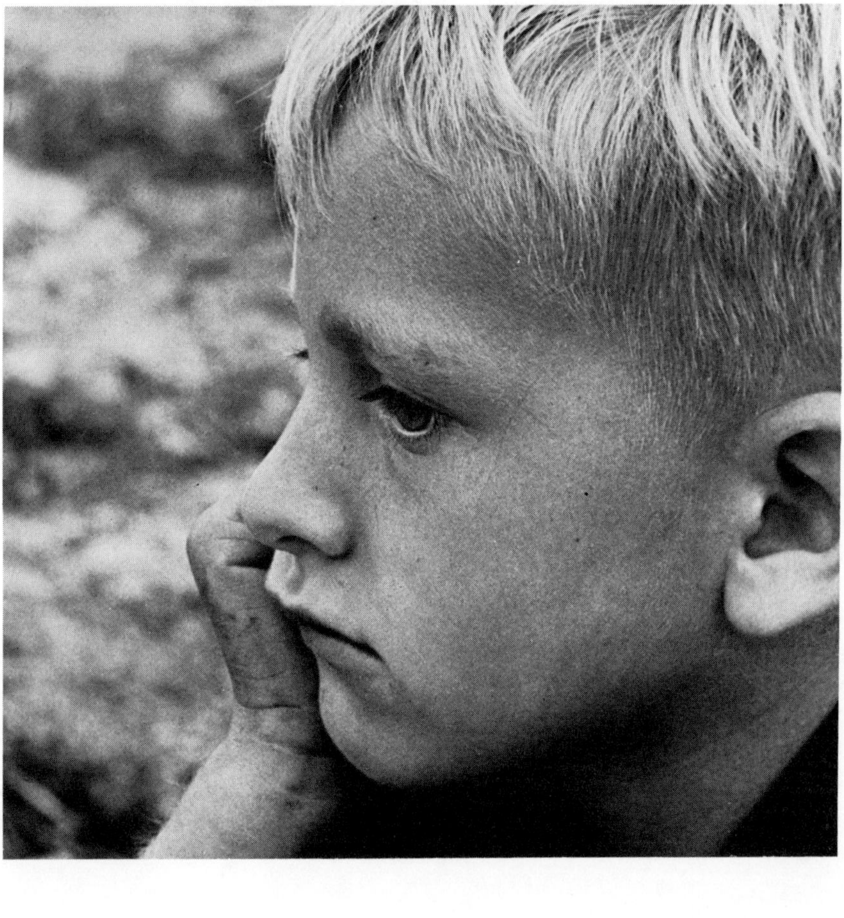

intended by the parent. At the same time, by behaving according to what the child perceives as the parents' mandate, he becomes more like them and gains positive feelings in his new closeness to them. In both Freud and Erikson's view, therefore, identification is a central process underlying moral development.

BEHAVIORAL MODELS OF CONSCIENCE

Learning theorists propose that conscience develops much more directly in terms of a child's reinforcement experiences (Hoffman, 1970). According to this view, a child's behavioral patterns gradually begin to conform to those of his parents because they reward his adherence to them and punish his transgressions. The specific rewards used would typically be the child's concern that parental anger or disappointment represented a potential loss of their love and acceptance. Thus a simple "good boy" or "I'm glad to see you being nice to other children" can be very positively reinforcing to a young child. Moral development is but another example of basic discrimination learning in which the child, through experience, associates certain positive consequences with particular behavior patterns, and negative consequences with other behaviors. Developmental psychologists have studied this process at some length and report evidence supporting the learning theorists' view. For example, in an extensive five-year study of cheating and dishonesty in children, Hartshorne and May concluded that neither honesty nor dishonesty were unvarying characteristics of children but rather were a function of situational circumstances (Hoffman, 1970). Furthermore, the generalizability of their honest or dishonest behavior appeared to be a function of the similarity of later situations with those in which learning initially occurred. In a later series of experiments, Aronfreed (1968) demonstrated that the extent to which children are likely to deviate from a learned behavioral pattern depends, in part, upon the latency between when the initial transgression was made and when it was negatively reinforced. If the child was punished very early in the act, he was then much less likely to repeat that behavior in private at a later time. On the other hand, children punished late in the response were more likely to be tempted to transgress in private than were the former group.

Studies reported by Bandura (1969) suggest that another mechanism in the development of morality is the *modeling* process whereby the child observes desired behaviors on the part of peers, siblings, or parents. Research in this area indicates that an important determinant of whether or not the observer initiates the perceived behavior is the consequence of the act for the model. If the latter is rewarded in some way for his action, the probability that it will be adopted is high. If, instead, the model is punished for his actions, it is likely that the observer will not repeat that particular behavior. Learning, in this instance, seems to occur through some form of vicarious reinforcement. This process also provides one explanation for how people develop certain behavioral patterns, even though they themselves have never previously been involved in a situation demanding such behavior. These results suggest that learning principles are important, at least initially, in the development of "moral guidelines."

PIAGET'S THEORY OF MORALITY

Yet another point of view is presented by cognitive theorists who argue that moral development occurs through the evolution of definable conceptual stages of thought. Jean Piaget (1932), a very important French developmental psychologist, asserts that the basic elements of morality are the individual's acceptance of rules of social order and his sense of justice. To identify how these processes evolve with age, Piaget performed a series of experiments with children of various ages in which he discussed with them their understanding of the rules for a children's game. The children's responses suggested that initially—that is, during the period of *moral realism*—the child adheres very strictly to the rules and can accept nothing but total adherence. The older child, by contrast, is able to perceive regulations from a more relative perspective and thus considers them as a product of social agreement. Thus, once he enters the later stage—that of *autonomous morality*—the child accepts rule changes and understands that rules can be altered in response to human needs and situational realities. The reasons for the child's initial rigidity can be explained cognitively in terms of his inability to take the perspective of another (labeled *egocentrism* by Piaget) and his inability to distinguish clearly between fantasy (e.g., dreams) and reality. Furthermore, the young child at the preschool age has an almost inflexible respect for adult authority and does not conceive of the possibility of questioning that authority.

That children do begin to display signs of conscience during the preschool years is an oft-reported observation. Parents will proudly share with friends their amusement at seeing their three- or four-year-old child begin to approach a forbidden object and then stop with the admonition "mustn't touch." Less clear, however, is the specific process whereby such behavior develops. Cognitive development, social learning principles, and identification—all seem to explain some but not all aspects of the phenomenon called conscience. There is also some evidence that certain moral behaviors are not only situationally determined but also seem to reflect a more general personality trait. Further research on this issue will clarify the manner in which each of the above processes contributes to moral development.

PRESCHOOL SOCIAL ADJUSTMENT

Part of Erikson's concept of autonomy in the preschooler includes a significant increase in the child's interaction with those around him. During the first two years of infancy, relatively little social behavior is observed. When together, very young children typically engage in *parallel play* in which each one acts independently of the other. Often parents observe that very young children simply take a desired object from each other as if quite oblivious that the other was playing with it. In fact, such is the case. The egocentrism discussed earlier extends to many parts of a child's life and cognitively the child focuses only upon his own experience. By the end of the preschool stage, the child is much more likely to react to peers and engage them in more cooperative forms of play. With increases in socialization, the child will also begin to demonstrate a variety of sex-typed behaviors discussed in Chapter 6 including dependency, aggression, and competition. As one would expect, the extent of observed emotional dependency between a preschooler and his parents is, in part, a function of age, with noticeable decreases as the child matures. The size of this decrease is partially a function of parental attitudes toward encouraging independence in their children. Those parents whose personal needs are such that they must maintain close contact and control over their children are likely to establish dependence in their children which will characterize later social relationships. Equally serious, however, is the parent who demands too high a level of independence and scolds the child of this age for "being a baby" and "not acting your age." In reality, preschool children are still babies and need support and reassurance from their parents. If forced to become independent too early, the child may later have difficulty establishing any kind of lasting, sharing relationship with another. As in most things, balance is the key, and the ideal response to a child's expressed dependency needs is to accept his immaturity and balance parental comfort and support with positive encouragement of autonomous behaviors.

Aggressive and competitive behaviors reflect for Erikson the child's pursuit of autonomy. The child seeks to express himself and reacts with aggression when frustrated and prevented from doing so. He also begins to perceive others as rivals for desired objects or parental attention and acts out to defeat their claim to his goal. The parental reaction to such behaviors will determine, in part, the extent to which they will continue as part of the child's response repertoire. A child who experiences little parental acceptance and attention may discover that they pay considerable attention to him when he acts aggressively. Although they may be verbally or physically reprimanding the child, the increased attention he receives may be sufficient to reinforce repetitions of the unwanted behavior. Similarly, negative reinforcement of aggressiveness along *with* positive reactions to nonaggressive behaviors can aid the parent in instilling control over aggressive impulses in the child. Individual differences in parental attitudes toward such behaviors therefore relate significantly to their maintenance in a child's response patterns. Parents from all social backgrounds should anticipate that their children will display such behaviors and should accept that, within reasonable limits, that is a normal part of development. Maturation and healthy adjustment are reflected in the capacity to control the expression of such impulses when they arise.

PRESCHOOL EDUCATION

The preschool years are a unique time in life because it is perhaps the only period relatively free of responsibilities. When school begins, children must begin to learn and work toward specific goals. Part of their day is very strictly regimented and such will be the case during the next 10 to 12 years and very likely even longer. During the years between ages 3 and 5, the child's major task is simply to be a child. Erikson's concept of autonomy is very centrally concerned with such freedom, for it reflects the child's need to explore, fantasy, and experiment. Increasingly, however, these years are becoming transformed into a preparation phase for eventual entry into the school system. Nursery schools are seen as agencies designed to introduce a child gradually to the social and intellectual demands of elementary school. It also provides an opportunity for the child to adjust to separation from mother and to the necessity to respect the needs of others in seeking to have one's own needs met. Proponents of nursery schools also suggest that these settings are an important means of helping an overly dependent or immature child learn more age-appropriate behavioral patterns.

Although not extensively researched, the effects of nursery schools have been evaluated somewhat (Mussen, Conger, & Kagan, 1969). Such studies have reported rather inconclusive data relative to the academic consequences of nursery school experiences. Although nursery school children typically begin the primary grades at a slightly more advanced level than nonnursery school children, the latter appear to catch up within a reasonable period of time. A group for which that question has been particularly important has been children from low-income and minority group backgrounds. Recently, much attention has been paid to *Headstart*, the government-sponsored preschool program to help underprivileged children profit from traditional educational settings by providing them with a "headstart" on intellectual tasks (see Figure 7–5). Vast sums of money and much enthusiasm accompanied the introduction of this aspect of the "war on poverty." After nearly a decade, the program is presently threatened with extinction because of its inability to demonstrate positive educational consequences of its intervention. Payne,

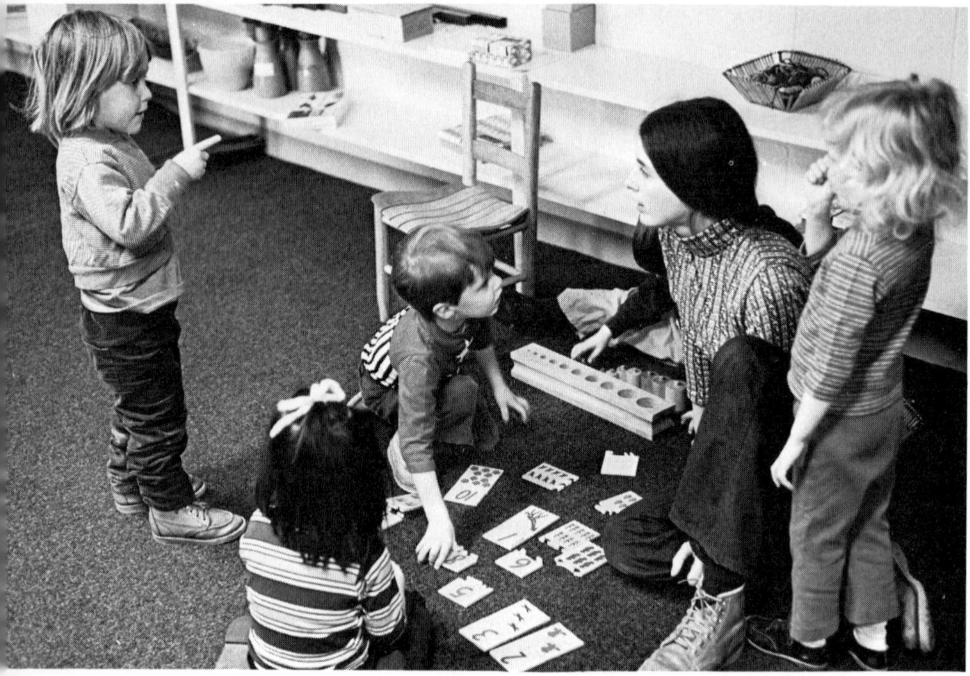

Photo by Chris T. Quillen

Figure 7–5 Learning in the Preschool Years.

Mercer, Payne, and Davidson (1973) argue, however, that to date the procedures for evaluating the program have been inadequate and thus not a fair test of its potential benefit. Studies of other remedial programs for disadvantaged preschoolers have reported positive effects (Jason, Clarfield, & Cowen, 1973). The observed differences between the educational benefits of preschool programs for children from various social backgrounds may reflect the realities of their situations. For low-income children, more systematic attempts to tailor preschool programs to their specific needs appear necessary if they are to have an equal chance to benefit from their later education.

For most nursery school children, the major benefit appears to be the facilitation of social adjustment. The experience of being with a variety of other children in a structured situation appears to stimulate the development of a number of positive social traits. Children who attend such programs appear more comfortable meeting new adults and peers, expressing their ideas, and initiating their own activities. These results do not necessarily suggest that all preschoolers need specific programs to develop such traits but, rather, that only some children do benefit in these ways. Thus, in some cases at least, attendance in a nursery school program can help a child deal successfully with the developmental demands of the period he is negotiating.

Childhood: Industry vs. Inferiority

The fourth of Erikson's developmental periods begins at age 5 or 6 when the child enters school and continues until the onset of adolescence and puberty. Freud (1966) described this time in a person's life as the latency period because following resolution of the Oedipal conflict, the child appeared to enter a relatively quiescent phase with few major psychological conflicts. Freud assumed that this period was much less anxiety-provoking than those preceding or following because libidinal urges appeared to be absent at this time. Problems that a child would encounter at this time reflected *fixations* (i.e., to earliest unresolved developmental periods) rather than an inability to cope with any new demands made upon a child of this age.

Erikson disagrees with the view that childhood is a neutral period and argues that it, too, has unique psychosocial demands that the developing child must attempt to master successfully. Each stage experienced thus far has provided the child with very specific strengths and weaknesses for dealing with himself and his social environment. Each of these is built, in part, upon its predecessors in such a way that the well-adjusted individual has available more assets with which to confront current demands than does the less adjusted individual. For example, the infant's basic trust in others supports his striving for a similar view of himself (autonomy) which in turn, supports his attempts not only to respond to but also to initiate activities. By contrast, the negative consequences of each of these stages make the challenges of succeeding stages more difficult, since past attempts to confront oneself or others have been negative. Difficult does not, however, imply impossible. Erikson insists that development is not an inflexible process. The infant who successfully acquires basic trust does not have an absolute guarantee that all will go well. Likewise, the child who fails to achieve basic trust is not doomed forever to maladjustment. Developmental demands are identified with particular periods because those happen to be the times of life when such demands are most likely to be central and the individual is best prepared to meet them. If, however, one does not have the personal strength or, equally important, the support of other persons or of the situation to meet the demands of a stage of life, Erikson proposes that that demand may be met at another time or place. Thus a very close personal relationship during childhood or adolescence may provide the basic trust in people lacking it until then.

It is important that the reader understand this aspect of Erikson's theory, for the demands of the "latency" period strongly test the psychosocial benefits acquired thus far. The child begins at latency his "entrance into life" (Erikson, 1963). The psychological and social de-

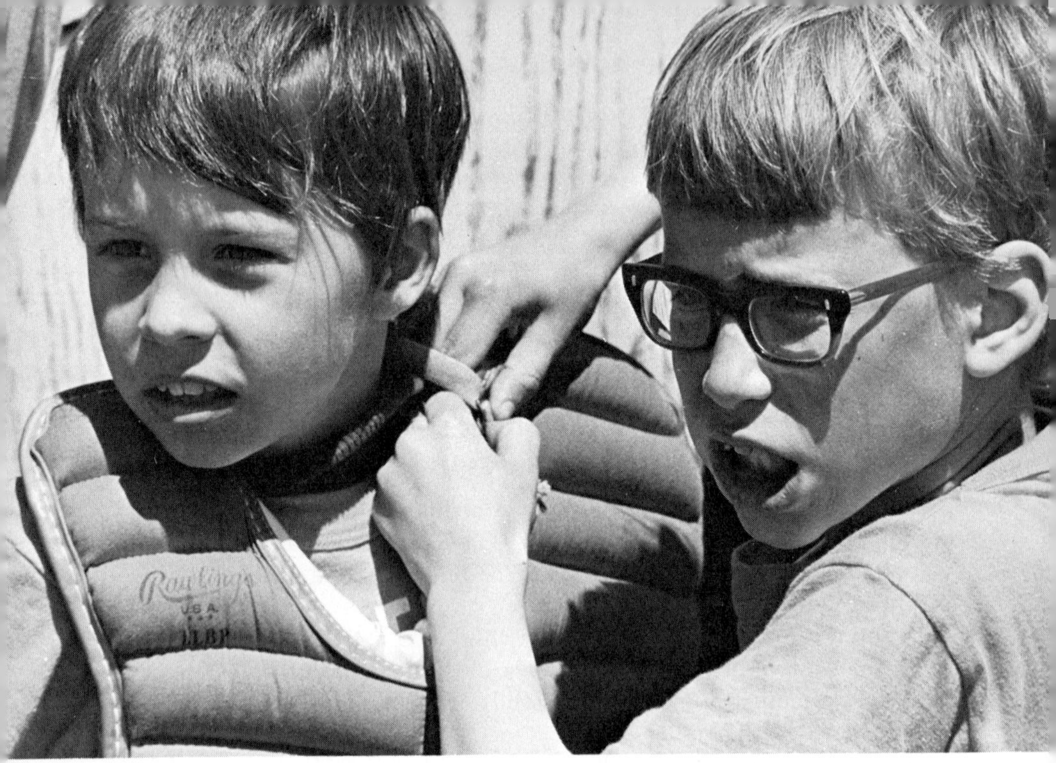

Photo by Chris T. Quillen

Figure 7–6 Cooperative Play.

mand of this period is the achievement of *industry;* a failure to do so results in a sense of *inadequacy* and *inferiority.* By industry Erikson refers to the need for the child to begin to focus his efforts toward the attainment of a goal and the turning out of a product. In preparation for the later maturational demands of adulthood, the child must learn at this time to use his skills and abilities to make something. Industry is important not only as a personal trait but also as a social one (see Figure 7–6). The ethos of Western civilization emphasizes the production of goods and the profitable use of one's time. Much of one's personal and social value is a function of the effectiveness of his efforts. The consequence of not becoming productive and industrious is to feel inferior to others and to doubt the value of himself, his skills, and his right to relate to others. The individual who leaves this stage with a feeling of inadequacy and inferiority will experience considerable difficulty with the demands accompanying life's later stages.

A HISTORICAL NOTE

Childhood as a unique phase of life was not always so recognized by man. The art, literature, and folklore of cultures existing prior to the seventeenth century portray children as small adults. The clothing worn by children was comparable, except in size, to that worn by adults. Children were expected to assume their share of the burden of meeting the physical needs of the family. Thus they worked in the fields, or in the shops, or were apprenticed to craftsmen in order to learn a trade. Once they were no longer infants, children received few of the special protections they now receive. Thus adult topics such as financial, marital, or sexual matters (if discussable at all) would be discussed in the presence of children. Following the seventeenth century, however, cultural changes, particularly the emphasis on education and the innocence of childhood, led to a significant discrimination between infancy, childhood, and adulthood. More recently, the latter phase has been further subdivided so that we now recognize the uniqueness of adolescence and maturity in later life. The institution most responsible for defining childhood as a special period of growth seems to be the school. Once it became important to acquire an education, the labors of children became secondary to the acquisition of the three R's. Gradually, increasing emphasis was placed on the necessity for recognizing the unique social and psychological needs of children. They were dressed in their own way, permitted to be irresponsible within certain limits, and protected from the immoral, violent, and disturbing happenings of the world. Currently, the period of childhood has received even more attention with extensive emphasis on educational innovations in elementary school teaching.

ADJUSTMENT DEMANDS OF SCHOOL

The child's struggle between industry and inferiority will occur primarily in his school-related experiences. His ability to succeed in the academic arena is multiply determined by factors such as his innate intellectual capacity, socioeconomic background, and emotional adjustment to the classroom. As adults, we tend to forget what school days were like for us. The tasks that are part of being a "good student" seem minor in relation to those that accompany a career and a family. Yet for the young child, the demands are very real and, when viewed objectively by adults, burdensome indeed. Josselyn (1948, pp. 76–77) recognized this fact in her description of a child's average school day:

> He is suddenly expected to be able, for six hours of the day, to control his behavior in order to conform to the school situation. He must arrive at school on time, properly dressed and properly fed. He must sit quietly for three consecutive hours or be active, according to the dictates of the teacher. This period may be broken by a short recess when he is supposed to be able to make a complete social adjustment to a group of confused children of his own age. Then he must get home on time for lunch, inhibit any of his

desires to relapse into his former play in order to return to school on time, and then for another two hours resume his pattern of conformity to an unnatural situation of quiet and study. Six hours of the child's time are therefore occupied by regimented activities, a regimentation that is foreign to his past experiences. The physician decrees that the growing child should have at least ten hours of sleep at night. This, theoretically, allows eight hours of freedom for the child. Often, however, parents decide the child should have music or dancing lessons, should practice certain hours, or should study a school subject in which he is retarded. Certainly, says the parent, he should develop some sense of responsibility and learn to help maintain the home he enjoys. So little domestic tasks come into the picture.

American homespun philosophy prescribes that adults should work eight hours, sleep eight hours, and be free for eight hours to do as they wish. The average home, however, does not concede the same right to the child. His hours are much more occupied with the demands made by others than are those of adults.

Thus, the child must assume considerable responsibility in his role as a student. If he cannot meet all of the academic demands of school, he may be labeled a "slow learner," an "unmotivated student," or a "learning problem." Since education is a cumulative experience, the child who fails to develop a basic skill such as reading or arithmetic at the appropriate time will face continuing difficulties with school. Throughout his school career, the child will be struggling to catch up with his classmates and, if unable to do so, may ultimately stop trying. Academic failure does not occur in isolation, for it is often accompanied by feelings of inadequacy, rejection, or ridicule by peers, and pressure from parents to "get down to work." Thus the child who cannot succeed in school finds that his failure pervades much of his daily life.

The determinants of school failure are multiple as is seen in the following descriptions:

Peter, a handsome seven-year-old has very limited intellectual ability and is unable to keep up with the pace of normal classrooms. Psychological evaluation of his cognitive functioning has indicated that his I.Q. is below 70 and he is, therefore, diagnosed as mentally retarded. He does, however, reveal sufficient strengths to be able to profit from a special education class in which there are fewer students and a highly trained teacher who has specialized in working with intellectually deficient children. In this class, Peter will be able to proceed at his own pace and will be given considerable individual attention in his instruction. Although he will never attend college, Peter will be able to acquire basic reading and math skills sufficient to provide for himself as an adult.

John, on the other hand, also has difficulty with his school subjects but when tested psychologically proved to be of average intelligence. Further evaluation with very specific tests designed to identify perceptual difficulties revealed that John had a perceptual handicap. Such conditions are often labeled as a minimal brain dysfunction to reflect the fact that they appear to be due to a minor aberration in the informational processing mechanisms of the brain. Thus, perceptual input may be erroneously interpreted or the person's ability to make a correct response may be somewhat impaired. In John's case, he was unable to learn to read due to his perception of the letters of the alphabet as reversed. For example, he would confuse "b" and "d" or "g" and "p." To solve John's problem also required a special education class only this one focused upon *learning* disabilities. With a carefully planned program designed to meet John's individual perceptual needs, the learning disabilities teacher will try to help him to compensate for his deficit and thereby be able to use his innate ability.

Ann Marie represents a third kind of academic problem. She had been an outstanding student in the first and second grade. She was able to read at an advanced level, appeared to enjoy school, and was very popular among her classmates. Her behavior changed dramatically when she was in the third grade. Ann Marie rarely had her homework finished on time and paid little attention to the teacher during classtime. She became quite moody and would often be very sad and withdrawn. Gradually, her classmates began to ignore her, for she continually refused to play with them. When she did agree to play, it was only a matter of time before she began to argue with and physically abuse her playmates. Ann Marie's teacher and principal became worried about the dramatic change and asked that the school psychologist evaluate her and that the social worker meet with her parents. The psychologist learned that Ann Marie was a child of superior intelligence but now felt very little motivation toward schoolwork. He realized that this was related to the indications of anxiety and very strong negative feelings expressed by her in her drawings and in the stories she made up for him. Further information about Ann Marie's problems was obtained by the social worker in her home visit. During the summer, a second child had been born and Ann Marie now had to share her parents' attention with her infant brother. Her mother acknowledged to the social worker that both parents had been giving considerable attention to the newborn and may have been ignoring Ann Marie. As the mother explained, she's always been such a perfect child that it's become easy, I guess, to take her for granted. Both school professionals met with Ann Marie's parents, teacher, and principal to explain their findings and suggest solutions. They proposed that the parents help the child learn to accept her new brother by assuring her through their words and actions that she had not become less important to them. They also suggested that the teacher help in this effort by giving Ann Marie a limited number of individual tutoring sessions to help her catch up with her peers and by reinforcing her positive behaviors.

Each of these children experienced difficulties meeting the academic demands of the classroom. The causes of their problems differed as did the required help. The cases described do not include another type of adjustment problem often seen in schools, although much less emphasized. This difficulty is seen in the child who is "no problem at all." In truth, however, the child is too perfect and overly submissive to the demands of the classroom. Rather than obeying rules because the child accepts and understands them, the child is simply too overwhelmed by his fear of the teacher, his peers, and school in general to do otherwise. Such a child is unable to socialize with other children and, during recess periods, is often found alone in a corner. He does not misbehave in class because he barely behaves at all. This type of school adjustment problem reflects very serious underlying emotional problems and often requires the intervention of a mental health professional.

Finally, the reader may also be aware of a not uncommon school problem observed in children referred to as *school phobia.* In such a case, the child is intensely frightened by school and leaving home and becomes very upset if required to attend classes. Behaviorally, the child will present all of the signs of extreme fear when faced with the prospect of going to school. These symptoms typically disappear when the child is permitted to remain home. Such a solution is unacceptable because both reason and law demand that children be educated. School phobias are often treated by child therapists who help the child understand and gradually overcome his fear until he is able to attend classes regularly.

The consequences of school-related failures, whether academic or social, have already been noted. Research by a number of psychologists and educators has demonstrated that early failure predicts later problems. If left unattended, some forms of school maladjustment do not simply go away by themselves but rather build upon themselves and are manifested in a variety of ways throughout a child's educational career. The pervasiveness of school adjustment difficulties is documented in the findings of a recent survey prepared by a task force of the Joint Commission on Mental Illness and Health in Children. In this report, Glidewell and Swallow (1969) reviewed a number of studies on the incidence of school maladjustment in children. They found that approximately 30 percent of all elementary school children had such problems. In some inner-city settings, this figure ranged as high as 50 to 70 percent. Their overall findings also indicate that nearly one-third of the children having problems are in need of some form of immediate professional help.

PSYCHOTHERAPIES FOR CHILDREN

Later in this book, we will consider the meaning of the adjustment problems of adulthood which are the focus of psychotherapists. Thus personality disorders, neuroses, and psychoses will be reviewed in some detail. Not surprisingly, children also experience psychopathological states requiring intervention. Such difficulties are sometimes school-related and sometimes not. *Childhood neuroses* are occasionally manifested as anxiety or depressive conditions but most often are expressed through behavioral dysfunctions such as aggression, delinquency, and difficulties with parents. The more serious psychological difficulties in which the child is unable to relate to reality are called *childhood psychoses* and, fortunately, are found much less frequently in children than are neurotic difficulties. Psychotic conditions are typically manifested by serious impairments in interpersonal relationships, a lack of awareness of one's own identity, intense preoccupation with an object to the exclusion of other elements of the environment, and abnormal perceptual experiences called *hallucinations.* The child may or may not display anxiety in relation to these conditions. Anthony (1970) recently reviewed the literature on this topic and designated two broad categories of childhood psychoses: *childhood schizophrenia* marked by hallucinations, bizarre behavior patterns, and wide variation in emotional responses (most often observed in children above eight years of age); *childhood autism* is observed in younger children (at times less than one year old) and is primarily characterized by an overwhelming detachment from people and self-destructive behavior. Autistic children seem to exist in a world of their own; they rarely acknowledge the reality that another person is with them and attempting to interact.

Treatment approaches for the childhood psychoses have had limited effectiveness thus far. These include the institutionalization of psychotic children along with medication wherever it appears indicated. Improvement rates for childhood psychoses have not been high and, although they may return home for periods of time, a significant proportion of childhood psychotics will continue to return to institutions throughout their lives. Recently, a dramatic treatment for autistic children has been proposed by Lovaas and his colleagues (1965) in which he has been able to develop language skills in autistic children through the use of the principle of learning and reinforcement theory.

Children with neurotic difficulties are often seen in individual or group treatment by a child psychiatrist or psychologist. The purpose of these approaches is to help the child to recognize some of his negative feelings toward himself, his parents, or significant others in his life and to learn appropriate means of expressing these feelings. Since children are much less verbal than adults, the child therapist typically will encourage the child to express his feelings through some medium such as play, drawings, clay modeling, and storytelling. Thus the child who is unaware of his anger toward his father can express it by burying a toy adult in the sand or drowning it in water. Similarly the child may draw an adult male figure and then cover it over with red or black paint. The therapist will attempt to interpret such feelings to the child, letting him know that they are acceptable as long as they can be expressed symbolically through words. The child's anxiety is related, in part, to his fear that he may, in fact, actually do some of what he is feeling and thereby kill his father or injure another. Other therapists will avoid interpreting a child's feelings, allowing him to become aware of them gradually by himself. Group approaches are employed when the child needs help developing social skills and discovering that his feelings and fears are shared by others. All forms of child psychotherapy seek to increase the child's self-esteem and to make him able to recognize and express his emotions more effectively. The results of such treatments are generally positive, with most children showing a reduction in their initial problems following therapy.

CONCLUSION

Human development is not a simple task. It demands constant vigilance and much effort. Erikson's contribution to understanding adjustment resides in his ability to conceptualize the nature of the psychosocial demands of each stage of life in such a way that they are not only scientifically useful but also face valid. They make sense to people from many social and educational levels. They seem to fit the way life is and the way people see each other. This chapter has reviewed some of the adjustment demands of the four developmental stages between birth and adolescence. The next three chapters will discuss the pattern and demands of growth throughout the remaining periods of life.

Summary

1. Adjustment refers to an ongoing maturational process whereby an individual modifies his behavior to meet the changing demands throughout life.
2. Development may be efficiently studied as proceeding through a fixed series of definable stages. Sigmund Freud, Harry Stack Sullivan, and Erik Erikson have each proposed a system for understanding maturation.
3. Freud viewed development as motivated by libidinal energy which becomes focused on specific bodily areas, labeled erogenous zones, during growth. The demands of adjustment cause the *Id* to function in coordination with the *Ego* and *Superego* in gratifying instinctual needs.
4. Freud perceived development as proceeding through the oral, anal, phallic, latency, and genital stages. Each of these presents specific challenges to the individual attempting to respond to instinctual drives within the limits of situational constraints.

5. Sullivan discounted the importance of basic biological and sexual drives in development. He emphasized man's social-interpersonal experiences as the major determinant of personality development.
6. Sullivan described six stages of human development: infancy, childhood, the juvenile era, preadolescence, early adolescence, and late adolescence.
7. Erikson expanded the work of both Freud and Sullivan by outlining the positive and negative developmental consequences of maturation from birth through senility. In his system, Erikson acknowledges the importance of biological and psychosocial determinants of growth.
8. The chapter discusses in some detail Erikson's theory of the adjustment demands of the first twelve years of life.
9. The major developmental task of the first year is for the infant to acquire *basic trust* in other people. Failure to do so results in a general *mistrust* of human relationships.
10. During infancy, numerous physical changes occur in perceptual, cognitive, locomotive, and verbal abilities. The infant gradually adapts to the eating and sleeping patterns of his family and becomes more mobile.
11. The primary personal relationship of this age is between the infant and his mother. Extensive research studies with infant monkeys and children reared in institutions verify the significance of a warm, loving relationship to later development.
12. During the second year of life, the basic developmental task lies in the acquisition of a sense of *autonomy* rather than *shame* and *doubt* toward oneself.
13. Autonomy refers to the child's need to manipulate the world around him and control his actions. In pursuing this goal, the child is likely to experience his parents' disapproval, initially a very upsetting event.
14. Toilet training regularly occurs at this stage of life. The manner in which parents teach their child these skills may have many future repercussions for the child's later personal and social characteristics.
15. During the preschool years, the child will seek to *initiate* his own behavior. If he is not allowed to do so, he may experience much *guilt* and be reluctant to pursue a personally chosen course.
16. The preschooler must learn to share his opposite-sexed parent with others in resolving the *Oedipal* crisis occurring at this time of life.
17. During this time of life, *conscience* begins to develop as a result of identification, learning, and cognitive processes.
18. The pros and cons of preschool education have been extensively debated during the past few years. Cognitive benefits seem most appropriate and likely for low-income children and social benefits for middle- and upper-income children.

19. During childhood proper, from 6 to 12 years of age, the primary goal is to develop *industry* and productivity, rather than a sense of inferiority.
20. Childhood itself was only viewed as a unique period of life following the seventeenth century. Prior to that time, children were treated in many ways like adults.
21. School makes major adjustment demands on children. Surveys have reported that up to one-third of the nation's children have difficulty adapting to the educational and social demands of school.
22. Children may suffer from serious psychological problems such as neuroses and psychoses. Child psychotherapy appears to reduce the consequences of the former. Institutionalization and medication have had less impressive effects on the latter.

Words to Remember

Anal Stage
Autism
Autonomy
Basic Trust
Developmental Stage
Ego
Egocentrism
Genital Stage
Id
Industry
Latency Stage
Libido
Malevolent Transformation
Marasmus
Oral Stage
Parataxic Thought
Phallic Stage
Pleasure Principal
Primary Process
Prototaxic Thought
Psychosexual Stage
Reality Principle
Secondary Process
Superego
Syntaxic Thought

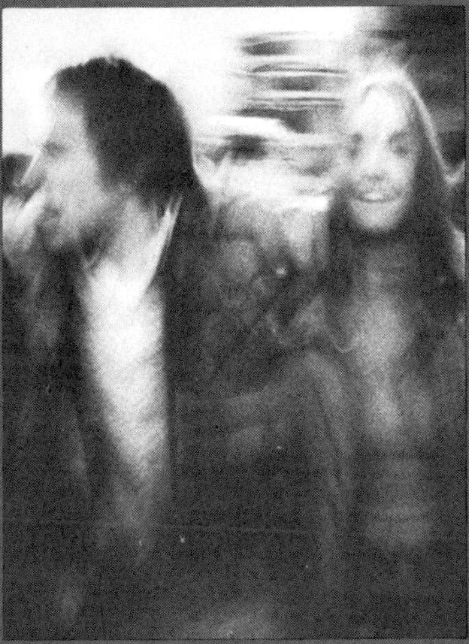

8. Adjustment to Adolescence

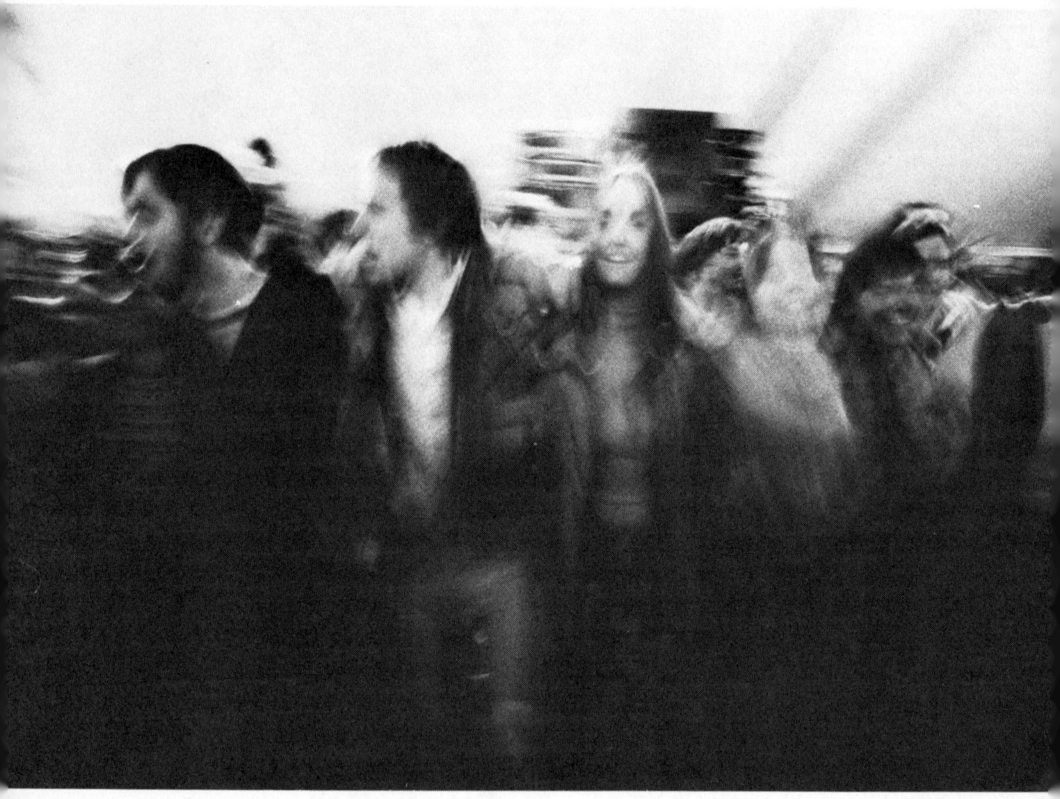

Photo by J. Brian King

Objectives

After studying this chapter the reader should be able to:

1. Define adolescence in terms of its biological and developmental stage factors.
2. Describe the roles of conformity, popularity, and peer relationships in adolescent social adjustment.
3. Discuss potential adjustment problems caused by the adolescent's sexual development.
4. Identify the role of self-identity in successful adolescent adjustment.

Becoming a teenager is an important step in a youngster's life. It carries with it a sense of "growing up" and of acquiring many long-sought freedoms. During the years between childhood and the assumption of adult responsibilities, a child passes through a wide variety of enjoyable, challenging, disquieting, and confusing experiences. The child continues his education, but entry into junior and senior high school and later into college offers increasing flexibility in the determination of one's training and development. During these years, the child becomes more involved in and influenced by peer groups and begins to define himself in their terms.

Adolescence is also a critical developmental period, for it marks the point in growth where one must develop an *identity* independent of one's family. The newfound freedoms, ever-changing peer groups, increasingly more personal and intimate relationships, and numerous demands to adjust to internal and external pressures must somehow all be integrated into a meaningful whole by the developing adolescent. For Erikson, the primary developmental conflict of the adolescent years centers upon the distillation of one's teen-year experiences into a relatively consistent identity which defines who one is, where one is going, and how he hopes to get there. The inability to achieve a blending of the numerous aspects of one's personal and social existence results in a sense of *role confusion,* a discontinuity between one's evolving physical, psychological, and interpersonal needs and abilities. The purpose of this chapter is to review the adjustment problems associated with the maturing adolescent's developing sexuality and increasing social needs.

The pressures and conflicts of adolescence can hardly be defined solely in psychological terms. The slow, steady pace of physical growth which was experienced during childhood is abruptly terminated by the onset of *puberty.* At this time, major hormonal changes occur in both boys and girls associated with noticeable (and sometimes disquieting) bodily changes. During puberty (from the Latin *pubertas* referring to the onset of manhood) the heretofore dormant reproductive organs mature, awareness of sexual impulses increases, and procreation becomes possible. Typically, puberty is marked by the *menarche* (onset of menstruation) in girls and the appearance of pubic hair in boys. The age at which each occurs in boys and girls varies widely but in most cases it takes place somewhere between 11 and 15. Related physical events occur during this period including the development of the mature female figure in girls and the appearance of facial hair and masculine musculature in boys.

The manner in which each of these physical events is received by the maturing adolescent relates in large part to how he or she adjusts to the social and sexual demands of that period. For some adolescents, physical maturation is very upsetting. They feel overwhelmed by the perceived intensity of their newly awakening drives and experience considerable anxiety in interacting with their peers. This is often the case for adolescents who mature very late and who therefore experience feelings of inferiority, self-doubt, and, unfortunately all too often, the ridicule of their peers. For most, the changes are somewhat disquieting but are accepted as an expected and appropriate part of becoming an adult. As noted earlier, the problems of adjusting to the sexual and interpersonal demands of adolescence are highly interrelated; successful adaptation to one facilitates adaptation to the other.

This chapter, therefore, considers the adjustment demands which adolescents face as they begin to establish their identity, initially through peer contacts and eventually through dating behavior and the resolution of their interpersonal needs, moral values, and evolving sexuality.

Social Adjustment in Adolescence

The high school and college years can be a period of high socialization, increased autonomy, and great openness to change in social behavior. Typically at this age a person becomes closely attached to friends and joins recreational and social groups. Through such contacts, he continues to develop social skills and attitudes, especially those accepted by the primary group with which he is most closely affiliated. Despite wide differences among high school and college students in their preferences for individuals and groups and in their social competencies, they are, in general, gregarious. Moreover, the structure and atmosphere of most campuses make it much easier to affiliate with a wide range of groups than it is at any other time in life. Yet at the same time, on campuses, as nowhere else, there is a high concentration of members of a single age group, and peer pressure to form friendships is intense. For most people this pressure is welcome and satisfying. For the shy, timid, or otherwise socially inhibited individual, the demands of this period can be highly upsetting. In adolescence one is inevitably more influenced by his accepted contemporaries than by any other group. In fact, peer pressure for some kinds of behavior frequently comes in conflict with the expectations of one's family. Since it affords some of the security which the family provides in childhood, peer acceptance is vitally needed. Yet when it must be gained by opposing cherished beliefs or at the cost of weakening long-held relationships, the adolescent experiences much anxiety and turmoil.

In general, social adjustment has the same dynamics as any other kind of adjustment. We suggest that the reader consider for himself what his personal social needs, conflicts, and problems have been. The exercise of defining his own purposes may help the reader to become conscious of his social goals and of the frustrations and conflicts he has experienced in his efforts to reach these goals.

Generally, adjustment consists of finding the social-interpersonal environment that will best bring satisfaction, develop new skills, and modify old attitudes. Specific answers to the questions one asks about helpfully maturational goals will help to define one's needs; some answers may be suggested in the sections that follow. Once goals are clear, activities and attitudes can be learned, and will be effective if properly reinforced. The people who are sensitive and in easy possession of social skills have developed these traits throughout their lives by becoming part of whatever groups are available and by learning through observation, reinforcement, and trial and error what adjustments in their personal makeup are necessary to mesh smoothly into the new group. On the other hand, where these skills are lacking, entrance into a new group is awkward, uncomfortable, and at times unsuccessful. As a result, rejection by the group may arise. In response, the person withdraws from people and may develop social aversions rather than social skills.

Studies have shown that the most sensitive persons are those who are most readily equipped to *learn* about people. Sensitive people are very curious about others and thus become deeply involved with them. They are discriminating and therefore able to sense each person's unique traits and strengths. Focusing on these aspects of others often results in a reciprocal warmth and acceptance. For this very reason, sensitive people are likely to be open rather than defensive when with others. They tend to be frank about themselves and are willing to approach people, to ask questions, and to express their own feelings. They can do these things because they have been rewarded in the past for these same behaviors.

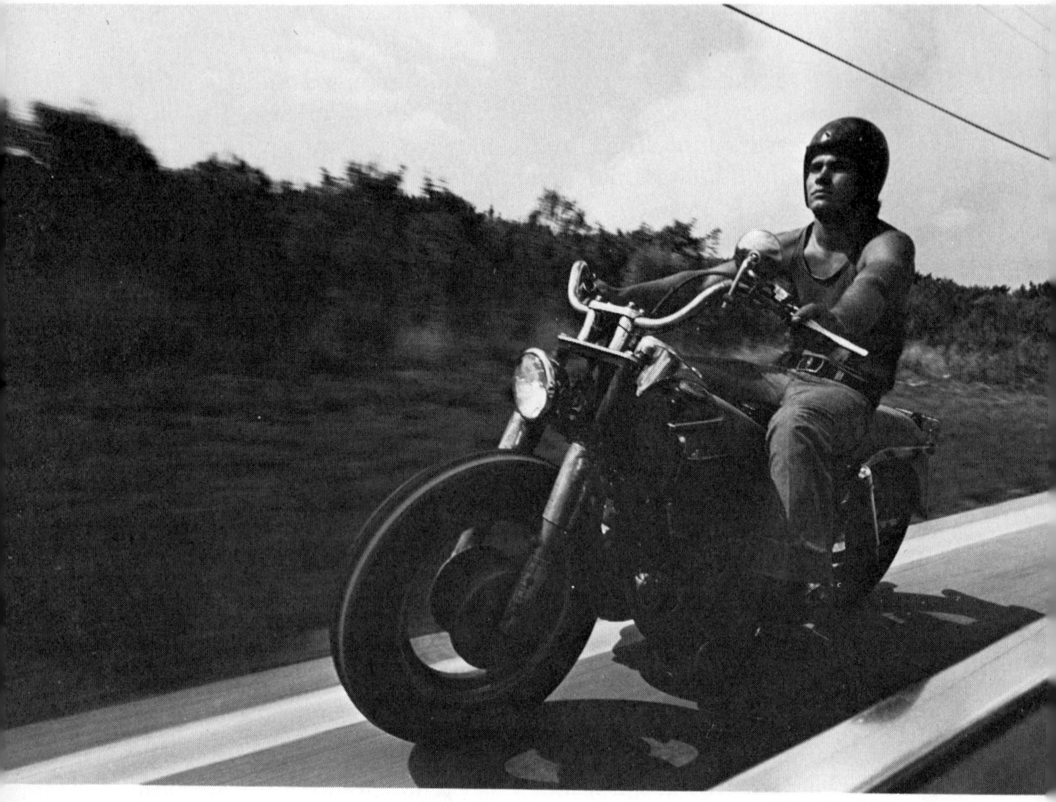

Photo by J. Brian King

Figure 8–1 Rebellious But Conforming.

CONFORMITY

The answer some people give to somewhat difficult social problems is: "Fit in with the group—conform; don't fight it." Strict conformity to group norms, however, results in uniformity and rigidity of human behavior, a condition infrequently found among most individuals. Typically some degree of conformity and individuality is found in members of all groups. Wide individual and cultural group differences are found concerning the degree of conformity expected of members. For example, a conservative, homogeneous group, as in a small German or Irish community, may put great emphasis on close adherence to tradition. On the other hand, an artistic, theatrical, or academic group may view strict conformity as detrimental to problem solving or creativity. Also, the same person may show conformity to tradition in his work but not in his play. He may conform to most peer standards but still rebel against some past traditions (see Figure 8–1) that are ill suited to the present (e.g., always wear a tie to dinner). "Hippies," for example, are generally regarded as nonconformists, but in their behavior and life-styles they conform to their own group's fairly rigid standards. Social class also relates to the degree of conformity observed within groups, with peer pressure for adherence to group norms very high in the lowest and highest social groups.

Evaluation of conformity in an individual should be related to his personal dispositions and values (whether or not they lead to integrity or unity). A person who is considering conformity in a given situation may raise these questions: Is the conformity slavish and inflexible or is it subject to adaptability? Does it lead to personal growth, creativity, and social contributions? Is this conformity a response to the anxiety which develops in interpersonal situations and, if so, can the anxiety be lowered in some other way?

The above discussion might seem to imply that conformity or nonconformity always occurs as the result of a conscious decision. Yet much conformity occurs without any questioning of the voluntary or nonvoluntary aspect of behavior. One can be caught up in a social situation in a group that demands or that expects certain behaviors of their members. The group may be a social group, a corporation, or a church congregation. If a person in these groups has a need to be liked and accepted by certain people, then he follows their behavior. He observes that most of his chosen group behave in a similar fashion and thus goes along in like fashion in the hope of being more acceptable to them. Similarly one may *identify* with an admired person and imitate that person's behavior. This may lead to *internalizing* (i.e., adopting as one's own) the attitudes and values of the other. Behaving in a manner consistent with these internalized values is itself many times intrinsically rewarding. Internalization is thus the most permanent form of conformity and is not as temporary as mere *compliance* to gain immediate reward or to avoid punishment.

Attempts to understand some of the factors that relate to conformity have led psychologists to create situations in which that particular form of behavior is likely to occur. In an early classic experiment on conformity (Asch, 1956) the subject was asked to judge the length of lines. He was shown a standard straight line, say, 5 inches long, and three other lines: one that measured 4 inches; another, 5 inches; and the third, 6 inches. The subject was to state which of the three was most like the standard—a relatively simple task that usually produced correct answers when subjects performed the task individually. However, in this experiment, the subject made his judgments as one of a group of 7 to 9 people who were coached to give wrong answers. By design, the experimental subject heard most of these wrong answers before he made his own response. The effect of the majority opinion on the subject was quite interesting. The subject tended to conform to the group's judgment and not report what would have been his own, had he been alone. Some of the results showed that if conditions for perceiving the lines were not clear, the experimental subject would be more likely to follow the majority than if there was little doubt about the relative length of the stimuli. If several others also opposed the majority judgment, the number of subjects who yielded to the majority was thereby reduced. Subjects who yielded to the majority early in the experiment later showed greater willingness to conform to group standards on other tasks. Some subjects admitted that they doubted their own judgment; some conformed overtly but when asked later to respond individually it was clear that they had held inwardly to their initial judgment. Similarly, it was found that subjects conformed more often when they made verbal judgments than when they gave their answers privately (Asch, 1956).

POPULARITY

Popularity refers to one's general attractiveness to others and represents another important factor in adolescent socialization. During the teen years, it is important to most people that they see themselves as being popular. Being unpopular can be devastating (see Figure 8–2). Popularity is closely related to, but is not identical with, social prestige. Behavioral scientists have observed that socioeconomic status and such demographic factors as education, occupation, and income are generally found to correlate with popularity as are intelligence, scholastic achievement, and physical and mental health. However, popularity is not solely the result of individual characteristics. It is, in part, related to how much one "conforms" and in this way is also related to the acceptance of values and standards of the group within which one seeks to be popular. Girls, for example, put much emphasis on "feminine" characteristics in evaluating girls; boys, on the other hand, emphasize "masculine" traits such as aggressiveness and assertiveness. Athletes evaluate popularity in terms of their group standard. Individuals from certain ethnic and racial groups are generally popular within their own groups. In sum, popularity is related to attributes that are highly valued by the particular group of which one is a member (McDavid & Harari, 1968).

Popular people sometimes have many admirers but only a few friends (Naegele, 1958), since admiration may isolate a person from close personal relationships. Travelers to other countries have noted the importance and apparent depth of friendship in Oriental and Middle Eastern cultures in comparison to the United States, where more emphasis is placed on easily acquired acquaintances. Friendship necessitates interpersonal relationships that are *interactive* and demands considerable involvement in the life of the other person. Admiration or popularity, by contrast, is an *evaluative* relationship (Blau, 1962). Popularity must be evaluated by the individual who strives for it in terms of his life values

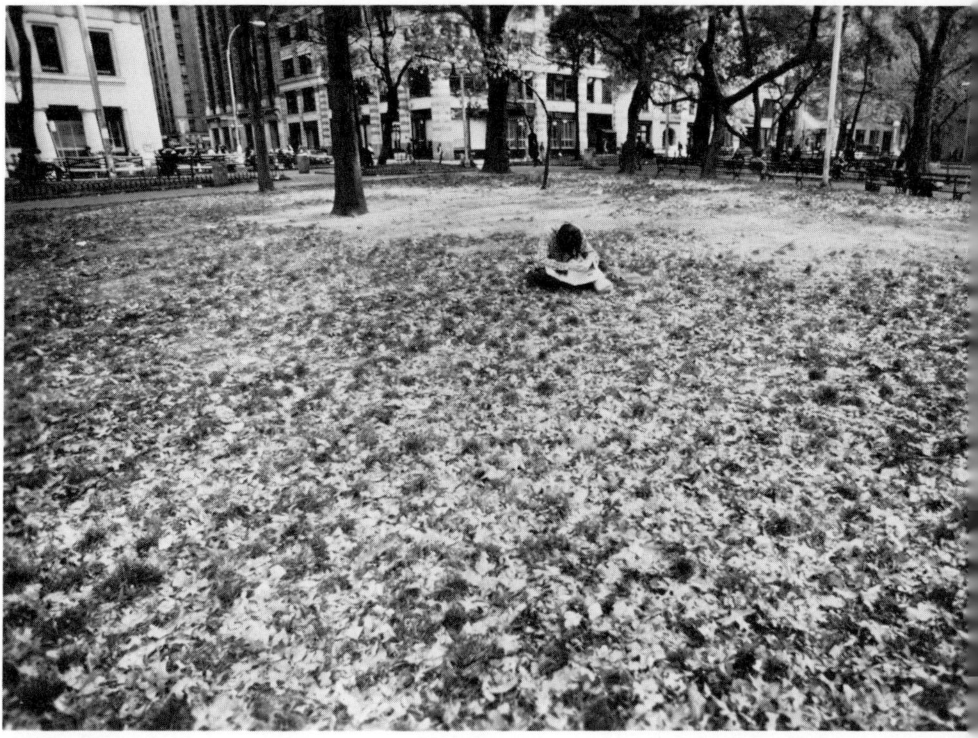

Photo by J. Brian King

Figure 8–2 The Loneliness of the Unpopular.

and his life work; it has benefits in sales work, in the media, and in politics. For the individual whose activities and accomplishments are behind the scenes, for those who seek privacy and deep personal experiences, striving for popularity may defeat their more general life purpose of establishing a few close meaningful relationships.

FRIENDSHIP PATTERNS

Conformity and popularity are important to adolescents because of their relationship to friendship. During adolescence much attention is given to making friends with others. During these years many friendships develop and much time is devoted to maintaining these contacts and attracting new ones. Social scientists such as psychologists and sociologists have attempted to understand more completely how friendships develop.

Persons are drawn together, often, because of *similarity of personality*. They may have similar interests, attitudes, motives, values, and ideals. Hence they are drawn together because they are alike. An example of such a relationship is two men who play on the football team. John and

Bill room together, have classes together, discuss their problems with each other, and even double date on many occasions. They consider themselves close friends; each enjoys the other's company and confidences. Neither of these men has an allowance from home, and both earn or borrow the money for their expenses. They are drawn together by a number of factors common to both of them. Both men enjoy considerable prestige on campus. They share similar hardships and experiences. They know each other's faults and accept them. There is relatively little rivalry between them, so each adds to the other's security. When they are in social groups, John and Bill enjoy the same games, topics of conversation, and interests. They depend on each other for companionship whenever they go places together. Most of all, they appreciate the fact that they can let off steam in each other's presence and even have open conflicts without breaking their essentially warm and stable relationship.

On the other hand, persons may also be drawn together, not because they are so much alike in temperament or personality but, conversely, because they *differ.* Such individuals have *complementary personalities.* Each member of the relationship in some way satisfies the motives of the other. For example, one might have traits the other admires and wishes he might have, but knows he does not possess or cannot acquire. He admires his friend's prestige, possessions, accomplishments, humor, poise, or social competency. Without necessarily knowing it, he may even vicariously live through his friend. He can display strongly desired traits to others by incorporating his friend in his social life and routine. He in turn is able to satisfy needs in the friend and thus bind the relationship. The friend may receive acceptance, sincerity, warmth, or some other satisfaction from him. Typically, this pattern of friendship is likely to become strained if one of the pair becomes too possessive.

Two members of the same sorority who are "devoted" to each other exemplify such a friendship. Linda is pretty, vivacious, and dates frequently. The other girl, Annette, is plain, somewhat shy, yet very unselfish and pleasant. Annette has a large allowance and a car. She feels that her attractive friend, Linda, makes her life more complete and makes her feel more secure. At the same time, the car and the clothes which she lends to Linda add prestige to her attractive friend. They regularly invite each other home. Throughout three years of college they have been inseparable. Each provides the other with what she lacks. The popular girl gets prestige from the money and the name of her less popular friend, whereas she lends some of her popularity to the other. The relationship is thus cemented by the understanding, acceptance, mutual respect, and need that each has for the other.

This type of complementariness is found in some platonic relationships between boys and girls. A girl may need a date upon whom she can depend under all circumstances, even though she may not feel a special affection for him. The boy, on the other hand, may be quite willing to take her out in order to be with her. One may serve the other as a confidant or trusted adviser. Perhaps a boy and a girl will study together. The girl enjoys being with the boy and is able to help him with his work and may even do chores for him. Such relationships are often of the motherly or big-brother type.

Another pattern sometimes cuts across the two already noted. Some people want friends whom they can possess and dominate. They become jealous if they see the friend with another person. Usually such possessive individuals have few friends. They give much but they also expect much. In fact they frequently attempt to obligate the friend through their many services. Often the friend eventually becomes overwhelmed with his debt and the feeling that he must reciprocate. He begins to feel restricted and to sense that the "friendship" simply costs too much. Irritation sets in, and such friendships ultimately end. Some underlying hostility, although unrecognized, may be present in the more possessive of the pair. While he may consciously feel affection for his friend, the possessive friend may also inwardly resent and dislike this person whom he sees as so independent and for whom he must do so much. The overly possessive person may never have been loved, and therefore seeks affection with such vigor that his demands are insatiable. There are, however, persons who want to be possessed, who want to be directed, and, if the friend is such a person, the friendship continues. In these friendships the more aggressive of the pair satisfies the needs of the less aggressive.

The best friendships of adolescence, indeed of any age, allow the mutual satisfaction of most human motives: affection, recognition, security, adventure, and success. Essays on friendship in literature reveal that friends are sources of considerable positive reinforcement. They are described as being deeply understanding and accepting in times of trial or triumph. Friends can share their most intimate thoughts. We see ourselves most openly in the warmth of our friend's acceptance of us, despite our limitations. Friends can do that which we cannot often do for ourselves. They recite our virtues, plead our case, and indirectly help us to see our faults. They furnish companionship and support as we learn to deal with the difficult social and emotional problems of life. They perceive us as doing the same for them. They play an extremely important role in helping us to develop for ourselves an integrated sense of identity.

LONELINESS

One of the most painful experiences for an adolescent is to be without friends, to feel deserted and alone. What are the causes of loneliness?

Why are some individuals devoid of real friendship? In studies of children (Northway, 1944) and in conferences with college students, a number of reasons for the inability to make friends have been observed and are depicted in the following examples.

One student may have grown up in a family that is not socially inclined. His parents have held themselves and him aloof from neighbors and associates. For whatever reason, they themselves have not built friendships. Their children in turn lack the skills for building close relationships.

Another person may be *egocentric* and *narcissistic*. Since early in life he has been given the center of the stage. He has received so much attention as a child that as he enters adolescence and adulthood he expects and demands it. He, therefore, resents any person who receives attention which he believes rightfully should be given him.

A third individual may be lonely because his early experiences have taught him to *enjoy being alone*. He may have grown up on a farm, where he saw few people. As a result, when he first came into contact with others he experienced difficulty in getting along with them. This failure to become socially adept has caused him to prefer solitary tasks and amusements, in which he satisfies most of his motives and finds his greatest pleasures.

Another person does not acquire friends because he is threatened by becoming *too close to others*. He is afraid they will find out too much about him. He does not want them to know his inner life and feelings. He keeps others at a distance and avoids intimacy (see Figure 8–3). He is stiff and formal and can never be "one of the guys." He is oversensitive to their real or imagined gibes and cannot banter with them.

Another student feels that she is not wanted in a group. It is true that she is *different*. She dresses peculiarly, spends many hours alone, and her ideas differ from those of most of her contemporaries. She is bright, but has never learned to socialize, and typically feels inferior and uncomfortable in social situations. She knows that she is not popular, but does not know why. She has never attempted to become acquainted with others, and they make no effort to know her. Therefore, she remains friendless.

Finally, there is the adolescent who was *teased* and persecuted in childhood. As an adolescent he assumes that other people will also be antagonistic toward him. In order to protect himself, he develops a generally negative attitude toward people. He hates and fears them because he thinks they dislike him, and he feels that he is not wanted by any group.

Clearly the opportunity to interact with another is important for the development of friendship. This interaction implies physical proximity to and frequency of association with another person. Once the inter-

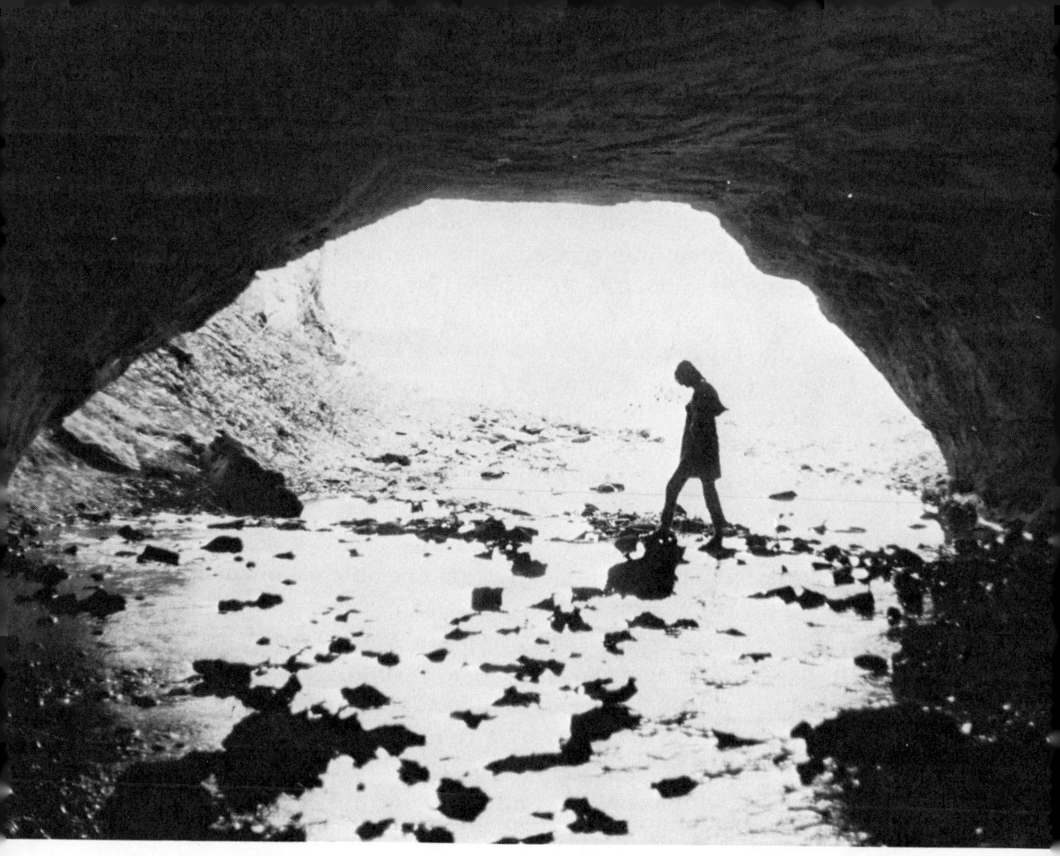

Photo courtesy of *Columbia Missourian*

Figure 8–3 Isolated.

action with the other person is established, mutual attraction develops as each person gradually recognizes similarities of attitudes and interests in the other. Friendships progress in relation to the extent to which the interaction is felt to be rewarding and satisfying to both parties. It is interesting to note that *assumed* similarity (a person thinks his friend is similar) is more crucial in the development of friendship than is real similarity.

The importance of *need complementariness* in friendship (two people who are different satisfying each other's needs because of their differences) is not as clear as similarity of traits. In general, people tend to perceive fairly accurately the extent to which others find them attractive, but unpopular individuals seem more likely to overestimate their attractiveness to others (McDavid & Harari, 1968).

INVOLVEMENT IN PEER ACTIVITIES

A very common way for friendships to begin is in the sharing of interest and activity patterns. Many people move into an activity spontaneously because they had earlier participated in a somewhat similar activity.

There is no assurance, however, that the person who would profit most by participation in a given activity will seek it himself. Social class patterns, for example, influence to some degree an individual's ability and willingness to enter into extracurricular activities on campus. Students in organized groups (e.g., fraternities) participate in more campus activities than students who are not members of such groups—in some cases because they are required by the organization to do so (MacDonald, McGuire, & Havighurst, 1949; Shannon & Kittle, 1947; Williamson, 1948). Another factor that influences participation in activities is personal adjustment: well-adjusted individuals take part in more extracurricular activities than the less well-adjusted (Cavanaugh, 1942; Phillips & Greene, 1939). Some evidence suggests that students most in need of social contacts profit least from the interaction opportunities offered to them (Brown, 1937; Burma, 1947).

Participation in activities such as sports, clubs, church groups, and so forth, has been recommended along with counseling as a positive influence toward personal development. In one study (Aldrich, 1942), students were referred to groups by a counselor after he had held interviews which indicated the extent of their interest in various activities. When compared with a control group, the students who were induced to engage in activities participated in more activities and derived more from them. The girls in this study were judged to have improved in their social adjustment as a result of their new involvements. In another report, a study of teacher trainees indicated that a record of extracurricular participation in college was a good predictor of effective teaching later (Shannon, 1940). A more recent study by Holland and Richards (1965) indicates that academic and extracurricular achievement are independent dimensions of talent—a fact that is certainly known by college instructors! An academically good student may be relatively unknown on the campus by those who are more conspicuous in extracurricular activities and, similarly, a campus leader may be barely passing his courses. We see, then, that not all students voluntarily become involved in extracurricular activities. Unfortunately this often includes those who might benefit greatly by participation and thereby improve their social development.

PLAY IN SOCIAL ADJUSTMENT

Group play has always been regarded by theorists as a great *socializer*, for it brings persons together under pleasant, usually cooperative, circumstances. Ideally, it is a way of gaining facility in interacting with other people besides being enjoyable and relaxing. It allows the player to assume social responsibilities in a less tense and a more pleasant situation than usual and can broaden his interests, offer him additional goals, and keep him from being entirely work oriented. In athletics, individuals must cooperate with or pleasantly oppose one another. The players join purposes as they become absorbed in a common pursuit. Through their games, they can lose self-consciousness, social tensions, and inhibitions.

General lines of evidence indicate that people who have grown up with limited play and companions and little interest in games are less *well adjusted* than if they had experienced a normal play life (Baker & Traphagen, 1935; Cavanaugh, 1942; McKinney, 1939). Play thus has been described as an *integrative* experience. We are completely absorbed in the game when we play it well. Active and satisfying participation provides a sense of wholeness. Every sense organ and muscle work together toward a common goal—improving one's skill and performance.

It should be pointed out that all of the advantages of play do *not* accrue to the limelight athlete, who is under the strict supervision of coaches and whose "play" and mistakes are subject to the scrutiny of thousands (or millions through television). The major goal is no longer the fun of the game, but the need to win "at any cost" in order to maintain a place on the team, with all its extra advantages. His activities quickly begin to take on more of the characteristics of work than of play.

Many of the advantages of athletics apply to other extracurricular activities as well (Arbuckle, 1953; Wrenn, 1951). Since they also are a form of recreation, they serve to integrate, socialize, and satisfy motives that would not otherwise be satisfied. Directors of extracurricular activities in college seek to help students develop skills in socialization, leadership, and discipline (Arbuckle, 1953; Strang, 1946). They also stress the happiness and zest that arise from these activities, the self-confidence they produce, the student's feeling that he has "a place in the sun," and the opportunity students have to lose themselves in causes outside themselves (Hand, 1938; Menninger, 1949).

DRAMATICS

Many of the motives mentioned in connection with atheletics are also satisfied by dramatics. In addition to yielding the prestige that grows from the ability to command the attention of an audience, dramatics may also provide an outlet for dominant traits that cannot be expressed otherwise. When one participates in a play, he lives a role that he may not experience in real life. He can thereby express his inner self. The timid soul may play an outgoing role and glory in the experience. The loud, aggressive blusterer may be told in jest by his friends that if he were really the quiet, mild type of person he played in the dramatic production, he would be more popular. Dramatics may give the participant *perspective* on himself and his role in the group. New roles may suggest new traits and allow him to practice those roles.

One study provides evidence that social changes within the individual grow out of participation in dramatics (Timmons, 1944). Students of psychodrama and play therapy emphasize the value of drama in permitting spontaneity and creativity. Drama offers an opportunity for tensions to be resolved and for new personality patterns to emerge (Axline, 1947; Moreno, 1953).

Dating and Intimacy

The development of friendships individually or through a variety of peer activities reinforces one's social adjustment and provides an essential component to one's sense of self-identity. As mentioned earlier, friendships reflect who we are and how we perceive ourselves. They provide an important element of continuity to our lives and a source of security and support outside one's family. They are also very important in the development of satisfying heterosexual relationships as one moves from friendships in general, to dating, to serious courtship with its possible sexual involvement, to the more mature dyadic relationship which has traditionally been defined as marriage and is presently, in this quickly changing social scene, evolving into a committed sharing of a life-style for two people.

It may be difficult for some to believe that dating, as such, did not exist before the 1920s and that, even today, it is largely an American custom. Currently, dating probably absorbs more of the adolescent's time than any other activity except classwork. Dates devoted to prolonged kissing and varying degrees of sexual intimacy are also relatively recent kinds of behavior in our culture and are seen as occurring as a result of an ongoing social "sexual" revolution. The current dating patterns that extend over the teen years contrast with those of the earlier custom of "courtship"; the older pattern usually carried social obligations and some knowledge or involvement of the pair's parents. American youth now tend to begin to date shortly after puberty, but do not marry, if at all, for many years. This social pattern is less frequent in other societies; in some, the sexes are segregated and chaperoned prior to marriage; in others, the young couple is allowed free personal relations and social taboos upon sexual activity are nonexistent. A major cause of conflict in our society is the intensity with which young people are encouraged to date over a period of years while subjected at the same time to strong social taboos about premarital sexual intimacies. To intensify the conflict further, that dating period occurs at the time in life when the male sexual drive is at its height, and

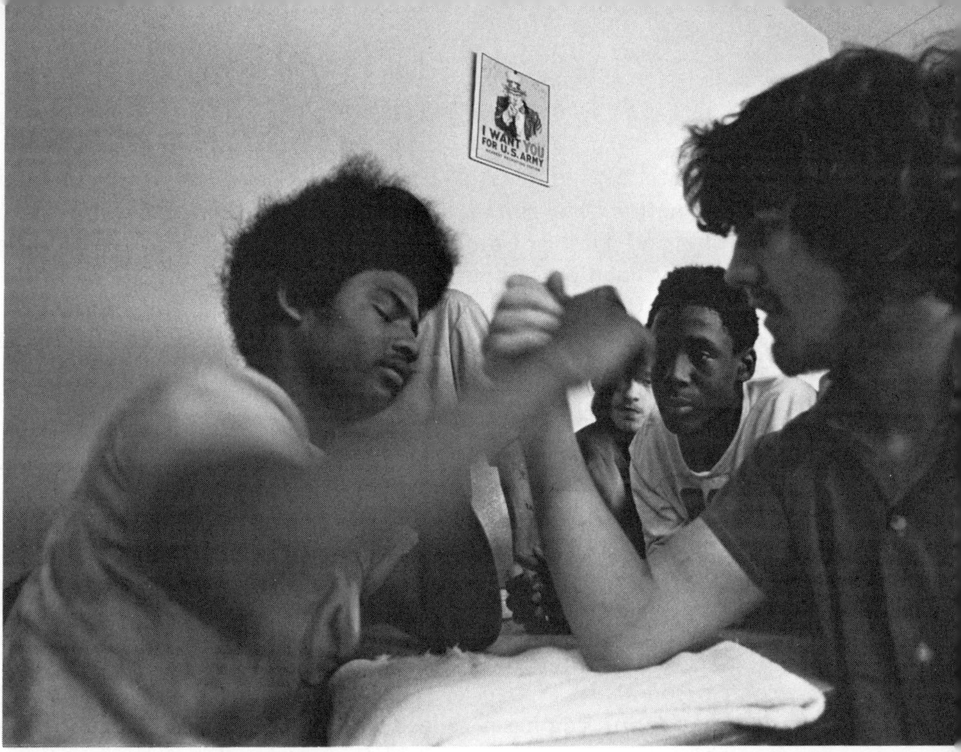

Photo by J. Brian King

Figure 8–4 Adolescent Play as a Means to Social Adjustment.

both sexes are uncertain about how their sexual drives should be integrated into their total personality.

SOCIAL FUNCTIONS OF DATING

Dating has various functions as a social institution, and the relationship that develops during the dating period can affect the personal development of the individual as well as the later relationships between the couple. The boy or girl can come to understand his or her role better and to know what is appropriate in relationships with each other. Dating may reduce the initial awkwardness of interacting with the opposite sex and enhance social maturity. The mere presence of an attractive member of the opposite sex is exhilarating and personally satisfying (see Figure 8–4). If this individual also has prestige and a compatible personality, the pleasure of interaction is even further enhanced. Furthermore dating is an enjoyable source of recreation when members of the pair have similar attitudes, interests, and aspirations. On the other hand, one's experiences on a date can produce strong conflict and anxieties and may so disturb the person's self-esteem that future relationships with the opposite sex are difficult for some time.

Waller (1937), who studied dating on a state university campus in the late thirties, was impressed with its competitive, superficial, and exploitative nature. He summarized his observations under the title "The Rating and Dating Complex." He pointed out the girls' desire to date the "big man on campus" and the boys' preoccupation with the "campus queen," the development of a "line," and the tendency to satisfy one's emotional needs without commitment or involvement. The emphasis in each of these was mainly materialistic, with such factors as fraternity membership, a car, a smooth personality, good looks, and good clothes being important. This study, a later one by Smith (1952), and observation of today's campus reveal that the aims of dating are typically *ego centered* rather than *pair centered.* Still, Smith did report that materialistic factors had lost some of their priority on campus by the fifties, in favor of personality and behavior items such as smoothness, appearance, and ability to dance well. Currently, a sharing of political and philosophical attitudes seems to play a large part in the development of dating relationships on campuses.

A comparison of the Waller (1937) study with the Smith (1952) study suggests that dating emphases reflect the general preoccupations of the culture. This generalization may hold less well today, for one of the most valued goals of youth seems to be the rejection of whatever is regarded as characteristic of their elders. However, it is doubtful whether you can shuck off the parental generation's values as easily as a snake sheds last season's skin. An example is the continuation of the double standard, together with a tendency for young men to reject promiscuous women as potential marital partners. The "new morality" thus encourages sexual freedom at the same time that the vestiges of the older morality penalize those women who practice it.

VARIATION IN DATING PATTERNS

Rogers and Havens (1960) conducted a study at Iowa State College and found prestige to be an important factor in certain stages of the courtship process. Prestige might be found in amount of education, the potential the individual was judged to command, or his probable status in a future vocation. Currently, one could add to these factors involvement in a cause or in protest against some phase of contemporary society. Patterns differ with differences in type of college, region of the country, political and social circumstances, and couples. Probably one can find any type of relationship, based on agreement in any area of life, at a given time on any large campus.

To discover cultural differences, Christensen (1960) compared the degree of premarital intimacy reported by students in Utah, Indiana, and Denmark. The Utah students reflected the influence of the Mormon community, a religious atmosphere that exercises closer social control than is usual in the United States. The Scandinavian students, at the other end of the continuum, reflected a more permissive attitude, but they insisted that a serious psychological relationship should be the basis for physical intimacy—a belief that reduced negative aftereffects.

LeMasters (1957) described several characteristics of the dating system as he found it—again, a study of dating in the fifties that reflects a materialistic youth culture. It was competitive, probably more so for the male than for the female. It was far more youth centered than parent controlled. The double standard of behavior operated, unmodified by growing ideas of more freedom for women. The romantic aspect of dating was stressed, although there were flexibility and variation from age to age and place to place. Dating had become more democratic, with considerable crossing of economic brackets. Continued dating involved progressive commitments on the part of the individuals concerned.

It is clear from the foregoing discussion that patterns of dating behavior differ with conditions like the age of the couple, subculture and peer-group influences on the pair, their personal attitudes and preferences, and the interpersonal relationship they have developed.

Sexual Relationships

Any discussion of sex must take note of its many aspects: the complex matter of self-image; the outlets the person has developed to express the strong physical urge; the feelings of guilt and conflict that can result; the perceived pressures of a peer group to conform to a pattern; the concern about being different from others; the search for romantic love; and the hope, in some people, for a rewarding family life.

None of these problems is new. They have beset young people for many generations, but they seem to be especially acute today. The question of establishing one's own sexual identity complicates relationships with the opposite sex. As one young unmarried male college graduate stated it, "So many young people don't know how they feel about themselves, so how can they know how they feel about a member of the opposite sex?"

In the Western world, sex has meant more than continuation of the family through physical relationship and the extension of the family's social status through marriage. Strong attractions between the sexes under certain conditions have developed into rich, rather stable, long-term love relationships, and out of these relationships have grown intimate and rewarding sentimental values. This romantic aspect of sex in the Western world has been celebrated in much of our literature and arts. True, within most affectional relationships there have been disillusionment, adjustment to different standards of the spouse, arguments, reconciliations, and the eventual development of a way of life (with its satisfactions) that knit the relationship. Under some conditions, difficulties surrounding the expressions of sex have immobilized the individual and destroyed the relationship. We need to recognize that there are few quick, easy, or universal solutions when sexual problems are present. The issues deserve serious thought and effort in the realization that the problem for each individual is unique and that the solution for one person may not serve another.

There is hope for sound solutions to sexual problems in our contemporary culture. Some of this lies in the frankness and openness that allow individuals to discuss the complexities in sexual identity and relationships. Relationships among adolescents are more accessible and varied than when marriages were based on proximity and most young men married the girl on the next farm or down the street. More important, there is a greater acceptance and open discussion of the intimacies involved in marriage. With the readier availability of contraceptives and abortions there is less necessity for bringing into the world an unwanted child and starting, or seriously straining, a marriage as the result of an impulsive sexual encounter. Present-day practices permit more opportunity for premarital discussion and, in some cases, experimentation to test compatibility between partners, based on a larger literature about all aspects of sexual relationships and more accessible professional and nonprofessional counseling. Yet this openness about sex also presents increased temptation to experiment wtih numerous physical relationships a number of which may be self-defeating.

INTIMACY

The earlier taboo against talking about sex is no longer strong; indeed, in many circles broad permissiveness is not only the practice but encouraged as a demonstration of "freedom." Our entertainment, news media, and advertising reveal a considerable preoccupation with, and openness toward, sexual intimacy. Religion, education, and social class continue, however, to affect the individual's response to various levels of intimacy. In the past the middle-class girl was somewhat more sensitive to the risks of petting and more likely to resist sexual advances than were girls from lower-income groups. She was responsive to the standards of her peer group, and concerned about being known as the habitual petter. Men also felt some guilt about petting, especially with girls in whom they were seriously interested. Packard (1968), however, observes a definite tendency for some contemporary students to feel guilty if they *are not* physically intimate with anyone—an interesting reversal of earlier attitudes (see Figure 8–5).

Examining a mass of data, Ehrmann (1959) describes the following trends: The typical heterosexual experience for both man and woman is kissing and caressing, the woman being the primary determiner of the limit of premarital sexual behavior. The "degree of physical intimacy" actually experienced or considered permissible is, among males, *inversely* related and, among females, *directly* related to the intensity of familiarity and affection in the male-female relation. Males often tend to place the beloved female "on a pedestal" (certainly an echo of a Victorian expression). The peer code of both males and females is more liberal than the personal code, since both are more lenient about what is permissible for their companions than about what is permissible for themselves.

Statistical studies of correlates of sexual intimacy do not present the *thoughts* and *feelings* of the two persons. Individuals differ in the motivation that results in the activity, as the preceding discussion indicates. Glassberg (1965), who interviewed young people in his professional

Figure 8–5 Physical Intimacy in Adolescence.

Photo courtesy of *Columbia Missourian*

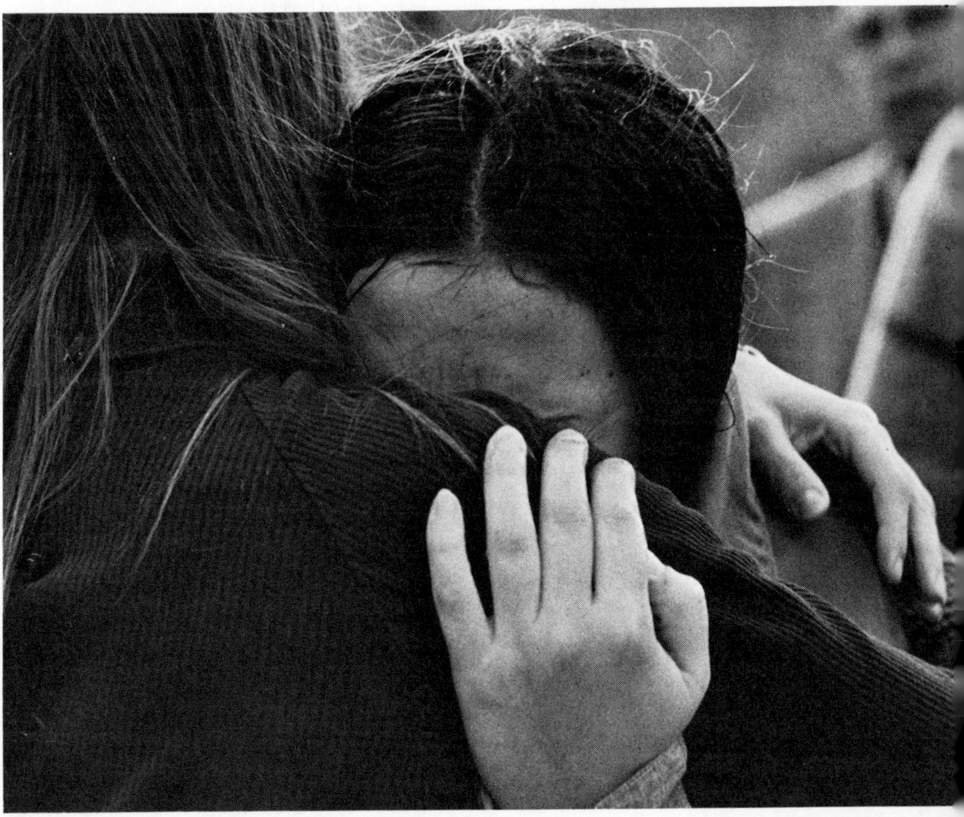

role, describes various individual motivations for heterosexual activity: (1) self-centered needs, such as physical pressures; (2) reassurance of maleness and femaleness; (3) conformity to group norms; (4) compensation for affectional deprivation; (5) "other-person-centered needs" such as the desire to fill the affectional demands of the partner. Individual differences are also found in the personal and social consequences of engaging in sexual behavior. These reactions persist in varying degrees of intensity and character after the incident and will be positive or negative (e.g., guilt, disappointment, anger) depending on the meaning of the act for those involved.

The general effect of premarital sexual relations on marital happiness has not been definitely determined. The entire question is surrounded by value judgments and innumerable positive and negative interpretations (Williamson, 1966). This uncertainty is no doubt due to the fact that the attitude toward premarital intimacy and therefore its effects vary with each individual and across the many subgroups that make up our culture.

DIFFERENCES IN SEXUAL ATTITUDES AND BEHAVIOR

One of the most often quoted results of Kinsey and his co-workers (1948) was their conclusion that no generalized American pattern of sexual behavior exists, but rather that attitudes and practices differ depending on the segment of society sampled. For example, Kinsey used educational level as one measure of class differences. In his survey findings he noted that in total sexual outlet, defined as the number of orgasms one has had, boys who had not completed high school average 20 to 30 percent higher frequencies of orgasm than boys who ultimately go to college. Although we do not know presently the extent to which biological factors separate these two social groups and the extent to which socioeconomic and cultural factors influence them, the latter seem logically more likely to play the greater role in determining sexual practices. Whatever pattern of sexual behavior is established early in life seems highly likely to persist for the balance of the individual's life.

Kinsey also found that attitudes among males about masturbation, premarital and extramarital intercourse, and prostitution are markedly distinct for respondents from different social levels. Members of the lower level perceive masturbation as both unacceptable and unnecessary, are less willing to restrict their sexual behavior to kissing and petting, and find the most satisfactory outlet to be heterosexual intercourse, which they regard as a "natural, inevitable, and desirable thing." On the other hand, the college man in the past, often chose masturbation and petting as a substitute for intercourse because of his social standards. Recent figures clearly suggest that this is changing; that 57 percent of

21-year-old college males have had *some* coital experience (Packard, 1968). Overall, however, it seems reasonable to conclude that significantly more premarital intercourse takes place on the lower than on the higher social level.

In addition to the above-mentioned social-economic differences in sexual attitudes and behavior, those differences found by Kinsey between males and females are worth noting. The reader should, however, recall that these data were obtained nearly two decades ago and therefore do not reflect more recent changes in attitude about sex and womanhood in general that mark the current woman's rights movement discussed in Chapter 6. It is important that social scientists begin to understand such changes systematically so that they may more effectively help both men and women find currently appropriate sexual adjustment.

Kinsey noted that females prefer a considerable amount of *general emotional stimulation* before any specific sexual contact. They are more frequently aroused by love scenes in commercial movies than men, but are less aroused by sexual activities in pornographic movies. They also are more responsive to sexual and romantic literary material, as well as to their own affectional writing than men, who are aroused by pictures of nude females, erotic stories, and other physical stimuli. The *aggressive* component of sex assumes greater importance in the personality of the male than in the female, whereas females are typically aroused more by tender and personal approaches. Females seem more directly and overtly concerned with *romanticism,* whereas males are concerned with *eroticism* (Kinsey, 1953).

Even in dreams, men and women differ; men seem more often than women to be satisfying a need for new experiences in adventure and travel as well as in sex. The most frequent need satisfied for women was the need for affiliation in marriage and the family (Lacrome, 1963).

Thus, it appears, that in the past there were two distinct subcultures—male and female—with respect to sexual attitudes. Within these subcultures individual exceptions occur, of course. Clearly with contemporary social changes women are more open about their sexual desires and experiences. Women can also be more aggressive in expressing their views, wishes, and reactions to sexual situations. Thus there is currently considerably less distinction between the sexual attitudes of the sexes than was evident in the past. Yet even now it appears that adolescent males are typically more sexually experienced than females and usually are the initiators of sexual activities. Their conversation is more open and more centered on sex and they are more sophisticated in their techniques of making sexual advances than are females. The core of interest in sex education for girls lies in the details concerning pregnancy, childbirth, and child rearing, whereas for boys it is sexual techniques and, to some extent, learning the "skills" necessary to maximize the erotic reactions of the female.

Males usually initiate sexual behavior, but females frequently make the first overtures. Furthermore the tendency for them to initiate the behavior increases as they "go steady" and when a love relationship has developed. Males experience orgasm from some source more frequently than females, and cultural standards for their behavior are still somewhat more relaxed.

As One College Woman Sees It

A twenty-one-year-old senior, an attractive young woman, described her impressions of the sexual conflicts among contemporary college students: ". . . most young adults have ignored the existing sexual code and entered into more intimate relationships. It is here that the fact that we are a transitional generation is causing adjustment problems for many individuals. Although we can rationally refute the traditional mores, the fact remains that they were a part of our socialization. Most of us have internalized this code and, combined with religious teachings, it makes it difficult to enter into physical intimacy without a feeling of guilt or wrongdoing. For many these guilt feelings can be rationalized, but they are particularly strong and persistent when it comes to premarital intercourse.

"In weighing the pros and cons of premarital intercourse, psychological factors, then, should be the main consideration. Can you enter into this relationship without feeling guilty? If you do feel guilty, how will this affect your relationship with the partner? How will it affect your self-esteem and sense of integrity? Another consideration is that of a possible break with the sexual partner. Many rationalize premarital relations on the grounds that they will marry eventually. 'Breaking up' is a difficult situation normally but when sexual relations were involved it becomes even more traumatic. It is at this time more than any other that feelings of guilt are hard to avoid. A girl, especially, realizes that she will probably not eventually marry this man, and furthermore that she has to face the problem of her lost virginity in her next relationship with someone else. It is these factors more than any other that point to the need for a new realistic sexual code.

"The present sexual code is negativistic, saying merely that 'nice girls don't. . . .' What is needed is some kind of a new positive definition of what 'nice girls do'—a definition that takes into account that the sexes are mixing at an early age and that sexual experimentation is inevitable, a definition that realizes that couples are being forced to wait for marriage, but most of all a definition that stresses the necessity of responsibility, unselfishness, and deep affection between two people."

INDIVIDUAL DIFFERENCES IN SEXUAL BEHAVIOR

Attitudes and behavior thus differ widely with individuals and are primarily related to the social interrelationships of the couple and to peer and couple codes. Second, personal and social background factors are involved: for the male, heterosexual behavior is associated to an appreciable extent with his attitudes toward sex, adequacy of sex instruction, age, and age at first date; for the female, sexual behavior is associated to a lesser extent with her attitudes toward sex, adjustment to sex, church attendance, and age at first date.

In presenting the above facts, Ehrmann (1959) points out that patterns of heterosexual attitudes, together with behavior and its control, are more sharply defined by *individual sex codes of conduct* and by *intimacy relationship* (being or not being in love) than by any other factors found in his research. Sexual codes include the "single" standard code (the same standards apply equally to males and females) and the "double" standard codes (one standard of conduct for one sex and a different standard for the other). The single standard may be subdivided into liberal and conservative, with the conservative prohibiting premarital coitus for both sexes and the liberal either advocating it or allowing individuals the right to make individual decisions about their sexual behavior.

Anyone who wants to build satisfying relations with the opposite sex makes choices regarding his partner and the general nature of the date on the basis of his own attitudes and values. He tries to leave open the possibility of developing an enduring relationship with his partner. We will consider the implications of establishing an intimate relationship more fully in the following chapter. First, however, it is appropriate to review some of the sexual problems faced by adolescents as they struggle to integrate their sexuality into a meaningful identity.

Sexual Problems in Adolescence

MASTURBATION

Few habits have caused more personal unhappiness and concern than masturbation. In fact the practice itself causes neither mental nor physical problems; rather it is the *attitude* held by people toward masturbation that is the major cause of the emotional difficulties which sometimes accompany masturbation (Kinsey, 1948).

The term "masturbation" includes a variety of self-induced sexual activities involving genital stimulation. Many animals masturbate. Masturbation occurs almost universally in small children. Parental censorship usually terminates the practice at this time, but it is rediscovered in adolescence. This discovery is made either accidentally or through another child or adult. The sensations that accompany masturbation change with adolescent physical development. Originally, it provided primarily a pleasant physical sensation. With increasing age, it becomes more intense and vivid and in both males and females, may now lead to orgasm.

Masturbation therefore is a typical experience of many persons at different times in their lives. The highest frequencies occur in those men who reach adolescence early. Frequencies are somewhat lower for boys raised in rural areas and for the devoutly religious. The reaction to and duration of the habit vary greatly, depending upon the individual's emotional background. Questionnaires answered by various groups of men and women in college and elsewhere indicate that 62 to 98 percent of men and 40 to 64 percent of women have masturbated at some time in their lives (Ramsey, 1943). While the frequency decreases at college age, it does not do so as greatly for this educational group as for those of less schooling. Generally, females masturbate less frequently than males; in females its frequency has no apparent relationship to age of onset of adolescence (Kinsey, 1953). The above percentages are given because often those who continue to masturbate in college believe their behavior makes them abnormal. This view is erroneous. Statistically, the practice occurs in a large proportion of young adults.

Several generations ago it was believed that masturbation caused insanity, sterility, feeblemindedness, "loss of manhood," ill health, acne, physical weakness, and other dire consequences. Often, children were assured that those who practiced this evil behavior were scarred for life. The young adolescent still picks up beliefs of this type, and in some instances he retains them and broods over them. Even if he later learns that these beliefs are false, he may continue to be influenced subconsciously by them.

Examples of the manner in which the habit of masturbation influences the individual in his teens and early maturity are numerous. Some young people wrongly believe that certain "telltale" characteristics indicate to the world that they have been or are guilty of the practice. Different individuals isolate aspects of their physical makeup as "giving them away," such as the expression of their eyes or a facial blemish or peculiarity. One college coed feared she would become epileptic in class—a fear that was caused by a childhood belief that masturbation causes epilepsy.

Guilt and anxiety reactions to masturbation are similar to responses to other sex practices that are regarded as wrong. Frequently bodily sensations occur after an orgasm, and some persons center their attention on these sensations. They continue to be anxious about them that day or the next. The quiet, introverted, reclusive young person may become so emotionally upset over the effect of masturbation on his health that he mistakes for illness the natural changes that occur during the occurrence of sexual sensations.

The eradication of masturbation, as with other forbidden sex practices, is a goal that sometimes assumes prime importance in the individual's existence. The end of the behavior becomes an all-consuming goal that demands all of the person's energies and interest. At the other end of the continuum of attitudes toward masturbation are those people who regard the practice as an enjoyable and convenient way to obtain sexual release to be used whenever interpersonal sexual contacts are unavailable or undesirable. Most people probably have some residual guilt about masturbating, as we might infer from the fact that most continue to be quite uncomfortable in openly discussing their masturbating practices. Nevertheless people are becoming more accepting of the practice and more willing to discuss it objectively and realistically with their children.

Masturbation is one of several sexual outlets that might occur in any individual under strong sex stimulation when other sexual outlets are not acceptable or possible. Its physical consequences are negligible. It varies in frequency, depending on many factors. It seems that when the individual who has a conflict about masturbation is engaged in other absorbing, satisfying activities, masturbation is a minor concern to him. The false and frightening beliefs that float around in folklore complicate the problem rather than reduce it and themselves produce the more serious consequences of self-derogation and disintegrating guilt. From a strictly behavioral point of view, if this form of sexual behavior conflicts with a strong negative attitude, the individual has the choice of finding another outlet or of seeking to change his attitude, possibly through counseling.

BISEXUALITY

In his classic work on the topic, Kinsey (1948) points out that there are several possible outlets for the sex drive in human beings. Among these are dreams (e.g., nocturnal emissions in the male), homosexual contacts, and heterosexual contacts including petting, premarital, marital, and extramarital coitus. An individual may have experienced several of these outlets in his life span and then limited himself to one, or he may struggle with the need to express his sexual impulses in several directions. He may find that, whereas one inclination or outlet is strong or has been reinforced by his past experiences, behavior through other outlets may occur occasionally. For example, an otherwise heterosexual adult may revert to masturbation as a supplementary outlet when he is unable to have sex with his usual partner. An individual who has a heterosexual preference may also have infrequent homosexual contacts. Kinsey regards the use of the term *bisexual* as unfortunate because of the difficulty of defining it. Persons who have histories of both heterosexual and homosexual physical relationships differ widely from each other as total persons. They differ in terms of the frequency of homosexual and heterosexual behavior; in terms of the time of life when such contacts were made; and the circumstances under which either behavior has occurred. Kinsey suggests that it would be more accurate to discriminate between persons in terms of the frequency of each behavior. He uses the concept of *homosexual-heterosexual balance* to discuss the sexual preference of both males and females. Thus the balance for a given person would tip in one or the other direction as a function of the greater frequency of either same- or opposite-sex contacts. For people in general, there is a wide continuum of balance patterns, ranging from persons who have had exclusively heterosexual experiences at one end of the continuum to those who have had exclusively homosexual experiences at the other end.

HOMOSEXUALITY

Even in this era of sexual freedom and of the Gay Liberation movement, discussion of any homosexual inclination in an individual typically produces anxiety in our culture. This anxiety usually leads to various defense mechanisms. For example, many people with homosexual inclinations simply repress those impulses and never permit their expression. When one hears about the famous men in history who have been homosexual, it is often quickly pointed out that they weren't *really* homosexual, or that they had no other available outlets, or that "everybody did it then." Each of these rebuttals provides a good example of the use of rationalization. In reality many famous historical figures were acknowledged homosexuals and their sexual preferences had little relevance to their intellectual or humanitarian contributions. Nevertheless the overt declaration of "atypical" sexual inclinations (which, by definition, are those *not* practiced by the majority) commonly carries with it major threats to one's social and economic standing. It is therefore very difficult for an individual (particularly for a male in our culture) to be honest with himself and admit homosexual incidents in his history. Often a youth or adult who does become aware of the underlying cause of his anxieties may defensively fight any incidents of homosexuality in society or he may engage in a variety of compensatory activities (e.g., weight lifting, participating in dangerous events, even have a number of heterosexual affairs) to prove his own masculinity.

In our culture, homosexuality is not the accepted means of expressing one's sexual urges. Whereas normal-developing individuals idealize members of their own sex and are often attracted to share many activities with them, only a small percentage of either sex seeks to satisfy its sexual urges in physical relationships with members of their own sex. As noted before, it is, therefore, necessary to distinguish between those who are mainly or exclusively homosexual and those who at some time in their lives have engaged in homosexual activities. Kinsey (1948) reported that 36 percent of American males at some time during their lives exhibit some kind of homosexual behavior. However, only 4 percent of all men were exclusively homosexual. Some males have an extremely athletic, masculine appearance in their public life, and yet distinctly prefer members of their own sex in physical relations. Conversely, there are blatantly effeminate men who may enjoy shocking others with their exhibitionistic, atypical mannerisms and yet have never had a homosexual contact. Other men and women are openly attracted to members of their own sex. They usually live in a society of their peers and frequent places where they can meet fellow homosexuals. A distinction between homosexuals is sometimes made on the basis of the copulatory role they assume. Those who assume the female role are called *passive;* those who assume the male role, *active.*

HOMOSEXUALITY AND PERSONAL ADJUSTMENT

Ellis (1966) reminds us that the homosexual may be classified in various categories. Some have overwhelming interest in assuming the normal role of members of the other sex, to the point of wearing clothes and accessories that are more appropriate for the other sex. Often, transsexuals (i.e., people who are physically members of one sex but feel psychologically that they belong to the other sex) will participate in "homosexual" contacts because in that way they feel *psychologically* as if they are engaging in heterosexual contacts. Thus a man who perceives himself as a woman will attempt to express his feminine sexual needs by relating sexually with a man. Some homosexuals actually have a *phobia* for members of the opposite sex that prevents their having satisfactory relations with them. Still others have a sexual *fixation* for members of their own sex that they cannot escape. The existence of these obsessions, phobias, and fixations suggest that the exclusively homosexual individual is emotionally disturbed, at least to some degree. This condition is understandable in terms of their upbringing (discussed below) and because many have experienced feelings of inferiority and rejection during their developmental years. Furthermore they must face, even with the more permissive attitudes of today, a society that is essentially hostile to their way of life. The recent "Gay Liberation" movement has attempted to counter these beliefs by claiming that their sexual tendencies do not, in fact, reflect their emotional disturbance but rather, their ability to accept and adjust to their own perceived needs and drives. Given the anthropological fact that homosexuality has existed in a wide variety of cultures and is found in otherwise well-adjusted individuals, the "Gay Liberation's" position should, in fact, be given very serious consideration. The central questions that must be answered are whether the behavior causes the maladjustment, whether the maladjustment causes the behavior, or whether the *reaction* to the behavior causes the difficulty.

The public in general associates the word *homosexual* with very negative stereotypes of one who is weak, perverted, makes lewd public advances to members of his or her own sex, and seduces children. It is easy to see how a homosexual individual of either sex in a rejecting environment can come to perceive himself in negative terms, to feel unworthy, and to anticipate complete rejection from others. Such an individual finds it very difficult to accept his more intimate experiences and internal impulses, which further undermines his self-esteem. The rejection of one's inner self certainly militates against positive self-esteem and as a result creates new and more serious problems. Doidge and Holtzman (1960) found that certain homosexual young men can show relatively pervasive and severe emotional disorder on various tests of adjustment as a function of their sexual inclination. Despite these findings on a given group of homosexuals, we are unable to say that all homosexuals have emotional disorders. In fact the American Psychiatric Society recently approved a change in its official manual of psychiatric disorders. Homosexuality when considered by a psychiatrist [1] is no longer officially regarded as "a psychiatric disorder" but labeled as a "sexual orientation disturbance." Some persons who are exclusively homosexual might well seek professional assistance, to aid them either to accept their decision to remain homosexual or, if they so desire, to work toward developing heterosexual interests. The decision to seek much help, however, should always be made by the person himself rather than by "interested" others who seek to force him into accepting their way of life.

SEX DIFFERENCES IN HOMOSEXUAL FREQUENCY

Kinsey (1953) reports some sex differences among homosexuals. As contrasted to the 50 percent cumulative incidence of all homosexual contacts of the male population, the percentage for females was 28 percent. The percentage of males who have had overt homosexual contact to the point of orgasm was 37 percent and for the females only 13 percent. Furthermore, the women had engaged in homosexual contact for shorter periods of time and were less promiscuous, having only one or two partners—far fewer than men. The statistics reveal too a class difference. It appears that more lower- than middle-class males have had

[1] Concerning the status of Homosexuality among psychiatrists, see a debate between two psychiatrists, Dr. Robert L. Spitzer and Dr. Irving Bieber, in the *New York Times*, Sunday supplement, December 23, 1973.

homosexual experience, whereas in the case of females the opposite is true.

Antecedents of Homosexuality

Some of the developmental antecedents of homosexuality known today have been gleaned through clinical and developmental studies. Parental attitudes toward the child may be a factor. Parents who dress and treat the child as though he were a member of the opposite sex can shape him in this direction. Extensive identification with the opposite-sexed parent may also be a factor. This is an especially potent possibility when the same-sex parent is cold, rejecting, and arouses fear or hostility. An incestuous-like attachment to the opposite-sexed parent which results in guilt may later affect possible sexual relationships with members of the opposite sex. Other developmental attitudes produced as parents instill their values in the child may make the individual unsure of his own sexual role and (as often happens) produce fear or guilt about heterosexual attachments. In such a case the only legitimate sexual expression becomes a homosexual one.

Physical factors may prevent the individual, either in his own mind or in reality, from being an eligible heterosexual partner. Not all youths meet the cultural ideal of physical attractiveness appropriate to their sex. The person may feel that he is too large or too small or be overly conscious of some other atypical physical feature that he perceives makes him unattractive to members of the opposite sex.

Certain attitudes may also develop from environmental factors, such as isolation from the opposite sex or being exposed to derogatory attitudes about them. If conditions that produce love, approval, or sexual outlets from members of his own sex are coupled with such factors, and he or she finds success with the opposite sex difficult, the result may be a definite movement toward homosexuality (Ellis, 1966).

It should be clear from this discussion that a major factor in homosexuality is *developmental,* and that conditions in one's sex typing and attitudinal growth operate to produce tendencies toward both homosexuality and heterosexuality. Since homosexuality in our culture has such negative connotations, the experience of anxiety and all its ill effects add to the person's confusion and render more difficult his developing an identity.

THE INDIVIDUAL AND SEXUAL BEHAVIOR

The findings we have been discussing speak for categories of individuals and are only generally relevant to the individual person whose problem appears to him to be unique. As indicated above, many factors combine to produce a given pattern of attitudes and behavioral tendencies. In addition the contemporary youth in the United States grows up in a social climate of peculiar ambivalence toward sex. Studies not many years ago revealed that some high school and college students rated sexual irregularities among the primary crimes and sins, and considered certain sexual offenses more serious than jeopardy to human life (Pressey, 1946). A large segment of our culture continues in this strong defense of the conservative code. On the other hand, the mass media like movies, magazines, fiction, and television programs furnish songs, jokes, and other presentations that provide constant stimulation, and some endorse free sexual experiences with no insistence on entangling alliances, as in *Playboy*.

Ellis (1966, p. 253) has documented this ambivalence and states that the mass media "voice the view that sex is nasty and tasty, a vicious and delicious business." In consequence, the average American is consciously almost completely muddled and confused in his sex view, feelings, and acts. It is to be expected that some young people may be unclear as to their own identity with respect to sex and also as to the behavior expected of them or permitted toward members of the opposite sex. Unfortunately the phrase "making love" has become synonymous with sexual intercourse, no matter how brief or brutal the encounter may be. There are individuals, however, who constantly give priority to a love relationship that points to a satisfying permanent family relationship, rather than to promiscuous experimentation with sex.

On the other end of the continuum, the individual who holds chastity as an ideal and who searches for love and romance will find others who have similar values. Love is a more complex and less impulsive experience than lust. It involves sentiments, tends to be more selective, and has elements of unselfishness that lust lacks. It is a fusion of physical attraction, ideals, and sentiments; as such, it has been the source of great art. Love involves the enrichment of the physical relationship, especially when it is enhanced by the reciprocal emotions of the beloved. Some college students recognize these characteristics and, as the above-quoted studies indicate, regulate their relationships with the opposite sex by this code. Self-respect and responsibility to one's self and one's partner are vital items in this code, and the physical relationship with the selected lover is usually related to a broader life of commitment and ideals.

CONCLUSION

If the youth is able to achieve satisfaction in his interpersonal contacts and in his more intimate personal relationships, he is well on his way to establishing a meaningful self-identity. The well-adjusted adolescent enters adulthood with a generalized sense of who he is and how he fits into the environment of which he is a part. That is not to say that all of his actions and decisions will necessarily be the mature, correct ones. Adjustment does not imply perfection. Rather, it implies the ability to recognize the realistic options that are available and to select among them. If the decision is correct, the adjusted person learns from that experience. If the decision is in error, the adjusted person accepts that fact and is able to cope with the negative consequences of his mistake and programs the experience into future behaviors. So it is for the adolescent whose sense of personal role has become defined through the social and sexual demands of youth. He can now confidently carry into adulthood the identity he has developed and put it to the test of the new developmental conflicts that await him. As he encounters and deals with those conflicts, his sense of who he is is further refined and he becomes more capable of adjusting to the daily happenings he must face throughout his life.

Summary

1. Adolescence is a critical developmental period in which the healthy person must establish his own *identity* and thereby become increasingly independent in determining his life.
2. During adolescence one experiences not only significant psychological pressure but also important physical changes that accompany puberty and the maturation of reproductive organs.
3. Social adjustment is very important during this period. Peer pressure for the establishment of relationships and conformity to group norms is typically quite intense on high school and college campuses.
4. One reaction to peer pressure is to conform to the demands and standards established by a person's reference group in order to be popular. At times such conformity is quite conscious, but often it occurs through unconscious psychological mechanisms such as identification.
5. A number of factors determine with whom one establishes friendships including similarity of interests, attitudes, values, and ideals. Additionally, some persons become friends because their personalities complement each other. Friendship during adolescence provides many positive benefits and helps the person develop his sense of identity.
6. A common pathway to establishing friendships is through involvement in a variety of peer activities. The present chaper discusses a number of extracurricular programs available to high school and college students.

7. Eventually friendships and involvement with peers lead to dating and increasingly more intimate relationships. Dating enables adolescents to become comfortable in heterosexual situations and to adjust to their evolving sexuality.
8. Dating patterns vary with one's socioeconomic and familial background and appear to be a more well-established middle- and upper-class phenomenon than a lower-class one.
9. An important component of the adolescent's developing identity is his evolving sexuality. Changing social customs are permitting more open discussion of these feelings and also encouraging somewhat more experimentation of practice.
10. Important male and female and social class differences have been observed in sexual attitudes and practices. These changes appear to be in keeping with the contemporary recognition of "woman's rights."
11. Adolescents also must learn to deal effectively with a variety of sexual problems that accompany maturation. These include myths and concerns about masturbation, bisexuality, and homosexual impulses.
12. The well-adjusted adolescent has successfully coped and profited from the demands that accompany the integration of the social, personal, and physical demands of maturation into a satisfying identity. He is then ready to face the tasks of adulthood.

Words to Remember

Bisexuality
Egocentrism
Fixation
Heterosexuality
Homosexuality
Identification
Internalization
Masturbation
Menarche
Narcissism
Phobia
Puberty

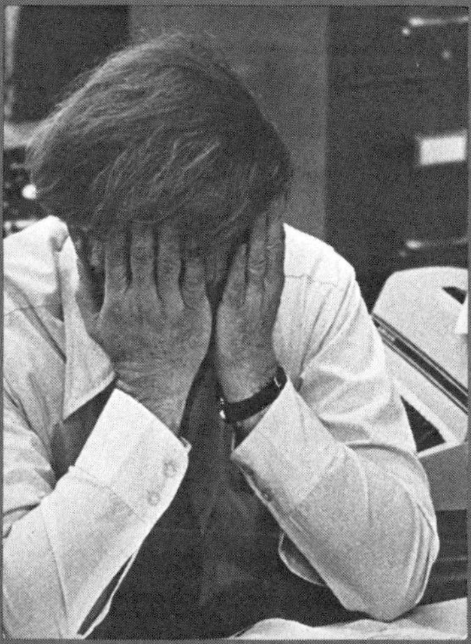

9. Adjustment to Adulthood

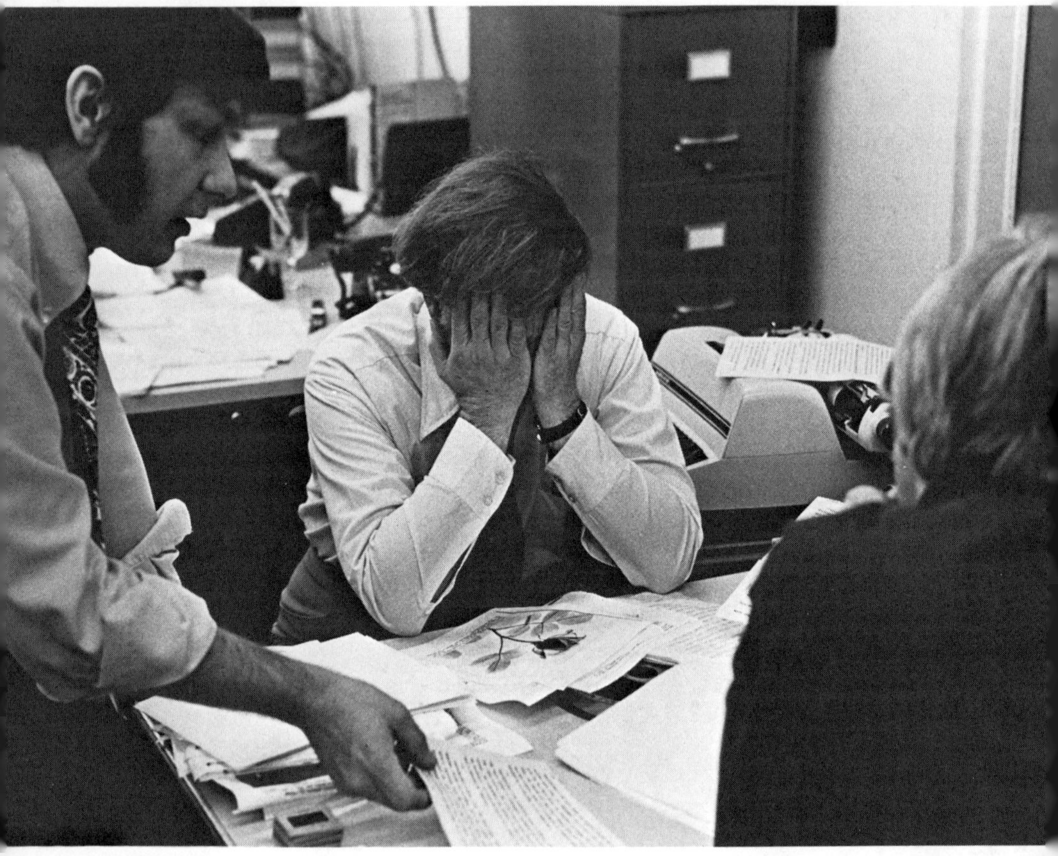

Photo by Chris T. Quillen

Objectives

After studying this chapter the reader should be able to:

1. List Erikson's developmental tasks for this stage of life.
2. Discuss the factors in career choice that lead to adjustment of individual needs.
3. Identify the important factors in marital adjustment.
4. Discuss parenthood in terms of Erikson's developmental tasks.

From Erikson's point of view (Erikson, 1963), the well-adjusted young person enters adulthood after having mastered the conflicts involving identity and role confusion; he is then prepared to embark on some of the very important business of adult life. This sense of identity is tested in adulthood, however, by two new conflicts that must be mastered. The first has to do with his capacity to achieve *intimacy* against the alternative of remaining an *isolated* individual. The second has to do with the basic human need to pass something of oneself on to later generations—in Erikson's terms, *generativity*—rather than to suffer *stagnation*.

It is paradoxical that after struggling to establish his self-identity, the young adult feels called upon to share that identity by fusing it with that of another. Intimacy involves the capacity to become committed to deeply meaningful interpersonal relationships. This process requires a certain amount of sacrifice and demands a willingness to make many compromises within the structure of the identity that emerged during adolescence. To become a close friend, a truly committed spouse, or a deeply feeling person in general, one must be willing to share something of himself. To achieve the ultimate in a sexual relationship, he must be able to abandon controls temporarily and to give in entirely to feelings. Such requirements, therefore, test the achievements of the adolescent period.

If one cannot give enough of himself to achieve intimacy, he remains psychologically distant from others. Preserving one's integrity by refusing to give up any aspect of one's individuality must be paid for by remaining apart from other people who might threaten this individuality. This isolation can lead some individuals into an existence quite apart from other people, but allow them to meet their needs and satisfy their motivations. The activities required on the job should be compatible with one's attitudes, habits, and personality traits. Considering that the average person will spend approximately one-third or more of his life's hours (between ages 23 and 65) in his vocation, the need for satisfactions through work is apparent. The influence of occupation extends beyond the working hours. It determines social status, style of living, neighborhood and, to some extent, leisure activities. The occupation is not only an extension of life's choices, but it may actually determine them, as when it dictates dress, life-style, and general behavior.

The selection of a vocation is not usually an automatic movement from talents and interests into a field of work. It is, more typically, a synthesis of wishes and reality and a compromise choice from among interests in many areas, each offering different satisfactions and disadvantages. Much that follows will imply that the choice of vocation is a *process* associated with one's own personal growth. To demand, as our society often does, that a choice be made early may well present serious problems for a given individual. This will certainly be the case if he feels himself locked into a situation in which he is unhappy but which he does not feel he can easily escape.

Vocational Selection and Adjustment

How does our discussion of vocational selection relate to the broader problems of adjustment? Vocational adjustment, because it affects such a wide segment of an individual's life, is an important basis for the development of one's self-concept. Working by plan toward a life endeavor helps one to discover who he is and what he might become—that is, his identity. A vocation (or a job and an active avocation) is a major source of *satisfaction of basic needs* or personal motivation. Usually the behavior that will satisfy these needs must be learned through the development of appropriate skills and attitudes. These learned skills are developed best when based on interests (another form of motivation) and adequate aptitudes. One aspect of personality is of vital importance in finding a vocation—one's basic values. What we want to do with our lives depends primarily on what we believe about how a person finds meaning in his life. This is one reason why the individual himself must discover his vocation.

NATURE OF A CAREER

Although *occupation, career,* and *vocation* are often used synonymously, they differ in precise meaning. *Occupation* means employed activity in which the tasks are similar from situation to situation. *Career* is broader in meaning; it includes activities outside the job and denotes a general life pattern. *Vocation* also reflects a life pattern. Both suggest a deeper motivation, a meaning in life, and possibly dedication to socially valuable ends. A vocation typically includes activities both during and outside working hours.

A career suggests (1) working with *purpose;* (2) *growth* in a vocational field, planning, and using imagination; (3) making a game out of work; being *creative,* using work as a creative outlet for self-fulfillment; and it involves interesting experimentation and exploration.

A man or a woman may teach English in a high school or do bookkeeping for a firm and be forced to go through the same prescribed duties year after year. In such a situation the person may feel that he is in a rut and needs to turn elsewhere for the satisfaction of dominant motives, even if it is toward excessive drinking or other dubious means of adding interest to life. Another may teach English in a high school and see promise of larger satisfactions within the limits of the position. He may write; he may see the young personalities before him as characters in a novel; he may see his students' separate needs and help them to meet them; he may experiment in methods of teaching and publish the results in scholarly journals; he may devise a textbook that suits the needs of his students; he may continually reorganize his course so that it meets the needs and growth potentials of more students; or he may furnish professional leadership on the staff or in organizations of teachers. In short, he can grow personally and professionally in his vocation. In a similar fashion the accountant can escape the bounds of his immediate job. He may see the figures on his ledgers as having meaning, as an index to trends in customers' behavior, and as signs of future events—a basis for changing policies in the firm; he may devise more efficient procedures and records for his office. He too may make his work creative and grow personally in what seems to others to be a routine job.

JOB SATISFACTION

Studies have been made of job satisfaction. In one widely circulated questionnaire, 25 percent of college graduates apparently do not find job satisfaction and wish they had prepared for some other occupation in college (Havemann & West, 1952). Obviously these findings suggest that large numbers of people do not find fulfillment or opportunity for personal development through their work, so careful and informed choice of vocation is important as a source of personal identity and growth.

Job satisfaction is related to fulfilling one's important *personal needs.* Schaffer (1953) discovered a substantial relationship here. Men in professional and semiprofessional positions answered a questionnaire designed to assess the strength of 12 needs, such as recognition, achievement, self-expression, economic security, independence. They also rated their general job satisfaction and the degree to which their specialty allowed for satisfaction of each of the 12 needs. A significant relationship was found between job satisfaction and the extent to which the individual satisfied his two strongest needs through his job.

Brophy (1959) had nurses express their concepts of their actual and ideal occupational roles, their self-concepts, and their vocational satisfactions. The larger the discrepancy between self-concept and the perceived occupational role, the lower the vocational satisfaction. Also, the discrepancy between actual and ideal occupational role was correlated negatively with vocational satisfaction.

Brophy's study introduces an issue related to alienated youth. These are young people who cannot accept much of what the materialistic culture offers, who see the usual occupations as devoid of personal meaning. In an occupation, they feel, they will lose their autonomy or they will find no personal relationship to the occupation. To them, the vocations are monotonous and actually degrading. This condition of alienation occurs more frequently now, either because today's youth expect more of life or because they are more conscious than earlier generations of the dehumanizing factors in commerce and industry (Goodman, 1956; Josephson & Josephson, 1962).

The implications of several job satisfaction studies (Crites, 1961; Jurgensen, 1949) have relevance for the college student. Individuals differ in their needs (security, affiliation, achievement, etc.) and in the roles they prefer to play. These needs and roles relate better to certain vocations and jobs than to others. Some people prefer free-lance work, in which they can plan their own schedules and procedures, rather than a more secure job in which the planning is done for them and they work on schedule.

We can best see the whole process of vocational adjustment through the review of a case of someone who has been searching for the right kind of job.

The Case of Donald

Donald S. was a clerk in a shoe store in a small Kentucky town. He had taken the job two years previously at the end of his formal education. Because of his dissatisfaction with it he visited a vocational counselor. He confided that he was not interested in his work; he had liked the job when he first took it, his salary was satisfactory, but he was tired of fitting people's feet. Still, no other occupation seemed to interest him. He felt that he should be working in a stimulating calling; the shoe business failed to provide the stimulation he needed, but he couldn't think of a job that would.

The counselor explained that in order to become interested in a field one must obtain information about it. He recommended that Donald read up on the history of shoes: learn from books in the library or from an encyclopedia that shoes probably started as a crude sandal and evolved through many variations throughout history. He suggested that Donald examine one of the shoes he showed customers daily and see therein structures that have been carried over or have evolved from the styles of other centuries and other peoples. This information should hold interest for a salesman of shoes, as well as being practical. It should make him style-conscious and alert to niceties in design. Tracing the manufacture of shoes from the artisan shoemaker to the present-day factory process would offer enjoyment, and a visit at a large modern bootery on his next vacation would allow him to point out the intricacies of manufacture to his customers. By this time the zest of discovery would lead him on to new aspects of the study of shoes.

Donald readily accepted these suggestions. He became a voracious reader, quizzed traveling men from wholesale shoe houses about styles and construction. One of these sales representatives, the sales manager of a large manufacturing company, was struck by the fund of solid information the boy possessed, as well as by his urge to learn more. He offered Donald a position that doubled his salary. Donald has since been promoted to the position of assistant sales manager of this company.

It so happened that Donald, who disparaged his job because he saw nothing in it but daily routine, had the needs and potential to which his counselor could appeal. After his reading and discussion with salesmen, shoes became more than something he put on the feet of his customers; they became an expression of man's history. His interest in them and their significance grew until he became an authority on shoes. He obtained for himself the sort of education that a specialist in any given field might gain from a series of courses.

VOCATIONAL COUNSELING

Many young people are aware that counseling is available for help with educational and vocational decisions. The professional counselor indicates to the client that vocational planning involves more than one decision and that at various points in his development he must make decisions that to a certain extent will influence the direction he will take. At the high school level he must choose between types of schools and curricula. At this time too the counselor attempts to guide the client toward self-knowledge as well as to inform him about the world of work. He may also try to communicate to the client something about the decision-making process and involve him in it. As Super (1957) points out, occupational choice is a synthesis between wishes and reality occurring over a period of time, during which the individual tests his personal needs, aptitudes, and personality traits against the demands and resources of society. This process may involve tryout jobs, reading, discussions with people in the occupation, and extracurricular activities that are related to the occupation.

Bordin (1946) has classified under five diagnostic constructs the problems considered by counselors as they deal with students who seek vocational counseling and who have some behavioral difficulties. Pepinsky (1948) tested Bordin's categories and modified them to produce this generalization: The categories that consistently identify the cause of students' problems in vocational choice are *lack of assurance, lack of information, self conflict* because of the views and pressures of other people, and *self conflict within the individual.* After he reaches this kind of diagnosis, the counselor can more easily structure remaining interviews.

PERSPECTIVES IN PLANNING

A growing number of young people select and plan thoughtfully for their careers with a view to the wide variety of occupational specialties, but some analyze occupations as superficially as Lewis:

> Now, I don't think I would like medicine; I never did care to be near sick people or to visit hospitals, or to go to our doctor's or dentist's offices. Law doesn't interest me; I am not a good speaker, and a lawyer should be able to sway a jury. I am not mechanically inclined, so that eliminates engineering. I know I would never make a good minister, and I would not want to be a teacher all my life. I can't write, although journalism ought to be interesting because I'd get to interview famous people. Well, what is left to choose from? Business. Yes, business—I'll register in the business school at the university.

Planning is helpful for satisfactory vocational selection. Studies of groups of students show that for many their aspirations extended far beyond their later achievements (Miller & Form, 1951). Had their goals been set on the basis of informed and practical choices, fewer failures might have occurred.

Many people enter college with the idea of entering a profession, but professional colleges usually have more applicants than they can accept. Counselors and testing bureaus can assist students in this regard, for they can inform the aspiring student of his chances of being considered by various professional colleges in view of his ability test scores and grades. Disappointment and unhappiness may be prevented by a judicious adjustment of the student's aims in keeping with his interests and abilities to make it possible for him to attain satisfactions, community respect, and whatever else he seeks through his vocation. The store manager should not be discontented because he is not a lawyer; rather, he should be content to see his business grow.

CLASS FACTORS

We must face the reality that despite our open educational system and the strong emphasis in our culture on upward social mobility (the attitude that every person should try to better his position in life), not everyone having ability can utilize it, and not every person of limited ability remains at the level predicted for him. American society is stratified, with social and economic conditions operating to keep the disadvantaged in low-rated vocations (see Figure 9–1) and to elevate the

Figure 9–1 A Class-Related Vocation.

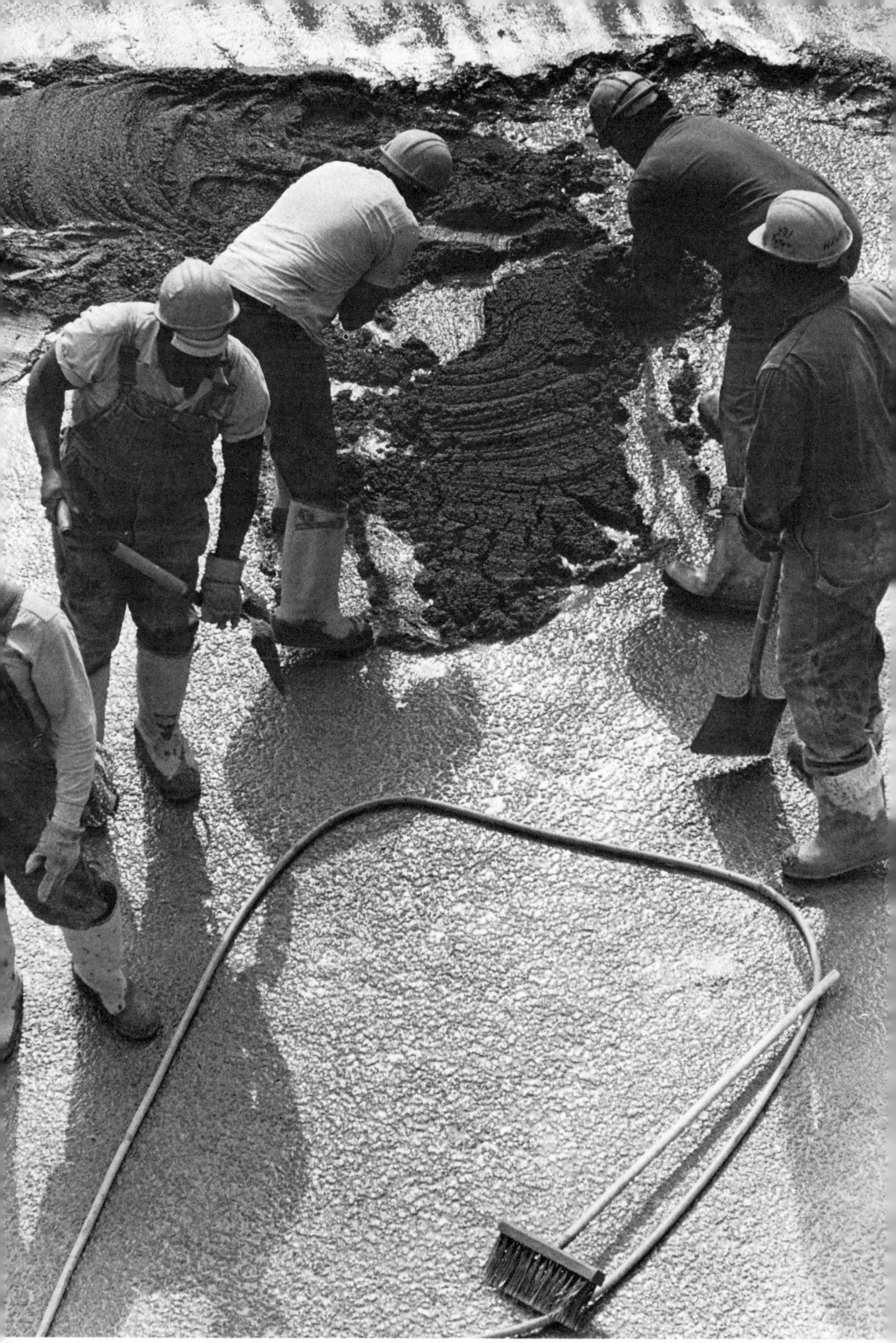

Photo by J. Brian King

advantaged to the most desirable ones. Consequently many individuals feel considerable frustration and vocational maladjustment, and society suffers the waste of good manpower (Super, 1957). Because of these conditions, efforts are being made to correct the effects of cultural deprivation on academic achievement and test scores and, thereby, to open doors for the disadvantaged to vocations that have heretofore been closed. Special attempts are being made by both private and governmental agencies to recruit the culturally handicapped who show promise for positions in higher education and industry.

VOCATIONS AND PERSONAL DEVELOPMENT

Basically, in planning for a vocation one is seeking a source of personal growth that will be integrating and realistic in terms of one's aptitudes, interest, and self-concept. This growth ideally will allow both satisfaction of deep personal needs and a means of contributing to society. Planning for a vocation usually involves a prolonged trial-and-error process of testing one's aspirations with the realities within oneself and the world in which one lives.

One of the standard plots for stories of personal tragedy is based on the parent who projects his unrealized vocational desires upon his child. This situation requires, from the young person, understanding of the parent's viewpoint along with recognition that it is he—not the parent—who must be satisfied in his chosen career.

One writer about vocations advises young people not to expect to find a "perfect niche," or to be naively deluded by the "attractiveness of the remote" or by the "glorification of the unusual." Briefly stated, one should be practical. Nor should the old idea that through hard work and proper living, any position can be reached by any person, regardless of ability or opportunity, be perpetuated. This has been called the "fallacy of perfectibility." One must learn to regard the occupational world realistically.

PREPARATION DOES NOT BEGIN OR END AT SOME DEFINITE TIME

The prelaw program is just as much a preparation for practicing law as courses in contracts or evidence. An advertising writer once confessed that a course in classical mythology was the most useful he had taken for furnishing ideas in his daily work. Of the hundreds of lawyers in every large city, how many have taken three or four years of chemistry as prelaw students to prepare them to handle effectively cases that involve such chemical processes as those used in the manufacture of dyes, foods, or explosives? Just as all preprofessional schoolwork is preparatory for a profession, so are early practical experiences preparatory for later success.

MAN CAN ELEVATE CAREERS AS WELL AS BEING ELEVATED BY THEM

Suggest to a college student that the position of a detective is open to him, and he will reply that one does not need a college education for such a position. By the same token, one need not have a degree to preach or to practice law, but how many noted lawyers are without college backgrounds? At one time medicine could be entered without a college degree. As the number of men who had been formally trained in reputable institutions increased, those who lacked such training found themselves of inferior standing in their profession. Many pursuits traditionally devoid of college men may be elevated to the status of a profession by superior preparation. A few examples are private secretaries of executives, camp directors, fine-gift merchants, and managers of employment bureaus or travel agencies.

TIME OF CHOICE

There is some debate concerning the merits of early career choice. An inappropriate rigid choice, made early, would obviously seem undesirable, especially if it involves vocational training that precludes a broad educational background. A 10-year follow-up of college men shows, however, that early vocational decisions made in line with family tradition and boyhood hobbies tend to be stable (Dyer, 1939). Investigation of another facet of vocational choice reveals that a good percentage of college graduates do not enter fields closely related to their college training, yet they consider their college training valuable (Hawley, 1938).

VOCATIONAL DECISIONS

The decisions reached at each stage of vocational development are inevitably a compromise. Individuals usually begin with broad areas. Numerous pros and cons are considered as each aspect of the various vocations is surveyed. The upshot of all these rational processes is a decision for a given time period. A temporary decision is desirable because, with industrial and social changes, the demand and supply for certain kinds of personnel fluctuates. For example, from 1920 to 1930 the number of insurance agents, stockbrokers, college professors, and electrical engineers increased greatly, while the number of untrained nurses, stenographers, typists, and street railroad conductors decreased (see Figure 9–2). The post–World War II era opened new fields such as electronics

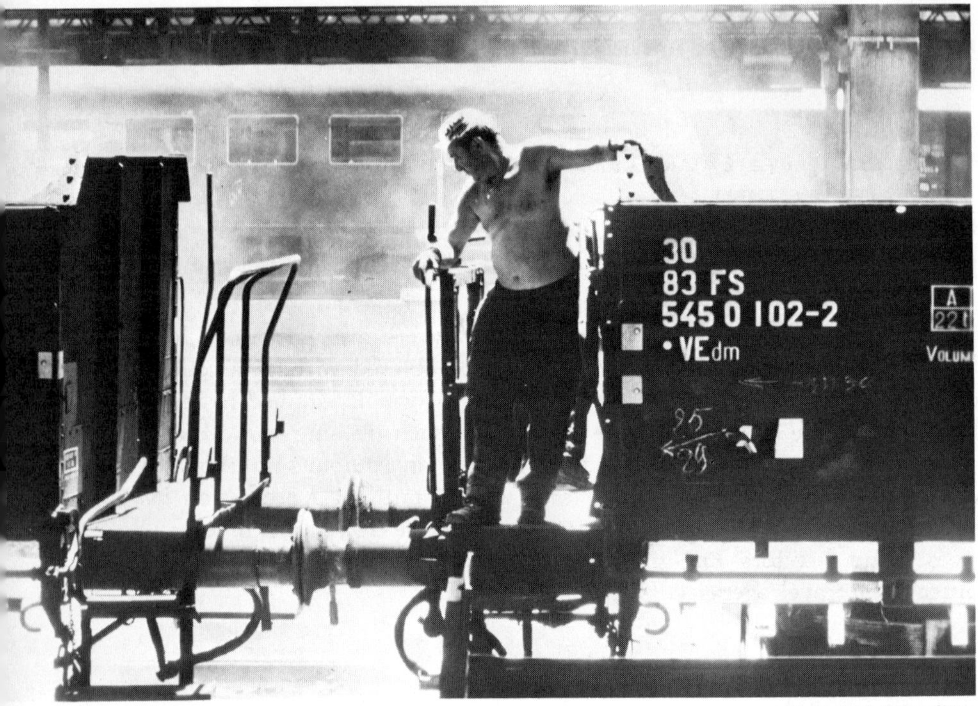

Photo by J. Brian King

Figure 9–2 A Dying Vocation.

and plastics. Such changes are continuing, to the extent that vocational publications emphasize their information on trends and new careers. Information of this type should be utilized in making vocational decisions.

Psychologists have recently become interested in studying scientifically the nature of decision making and have developed a "decision theory." Anastasi (1964) has simplified decision making in vocations into these aspects: (1) predicted possibility of the outcomes of our different choices, (2) estimates of the risks involved or seriousness of failure in choices, and (3) consideration of the relative value or importance of different goals. Today, with accumulated data on ability, interest, personality, and previous achievements, the counselor can inform the client on the predicted possibility of his completing certain curricula and of gaining vocational satisfaction. He and the client can also appraise the risks and consequences of failure. Together they can weigh the importance of goals and of taking risks in terms of the client's values. Some of this information can now be presented in numerical probabilities, and such estimates will become increasingly available in the future.

The client's values and life goals, some of which are shown in the tests he will take, may overshadow other factors in his selection of a field.

How he defines success also carries much weight. His definition may involve inner satisfaction, monetary gain, compliance with family tradition, satisfaction of social needs, creativity, immediate results versus later status, or growth as a person.

AVOCATIONS AND LEISURE

Because of circumstances beyond their control, many individuals make a compromise in their choice of a vocation and thereby leave some strong motives unsatisfied and some aptitudes unutilized. For such people—and there are many—avocations, hobbies, or strong interests can fulfill the personal needs that are not met adequately in their vocation. Avocations are becoming more important because with the specialization and mechanization of industry work hours are being shortened and free time increased. However, idle time is not synonymous with leisure; it may indeed lead to boredom. *Leisure* means freedom from time-consuming duties and responsibilities, but it also means freedom to explore, to develop, and to recreate in personally rewarding directions. Further, stereotype is encroaching on even the more complex vocational fields, and this mechanization and computerization reduces the worker's opportunities for creative expression. Avocations, therefore, are becoming essential as avenues for satisfaction of urges to create (Super, 1940).

DEEPENING OF INTERESTS

Natural growth toward maturity promotes a deepening of interests (White, 1966), a progressive mastery of knowledge, and skill in a sphere of interest. By the same process, interests grow broader as well as deeper. Anyone who is intensely interested in an occupation can spend hours in a state of absorption. Reward for such a person comes from doing something for its own sake. The deepening of interest is important in personal effectiveness and happiness in one's vocation and avocations.

The distinctive factor in professional and creative workers like artists, physicians, and biologists is that they become interested quite early in life in the subject matter they pursue as a vocation (Roe, 1953). This interest deepens cumulatively; it guides their careers and to a large extent determines their success (see Figure 9–3). These professionals may be contrasted with workers who do not find deep satisfaction in their work, who see only monotony and relative meaninglessness in the roles they have to perform, and who have—if they are wise—turned to projects outside the vocation in order to satisfy important needs and express their values.

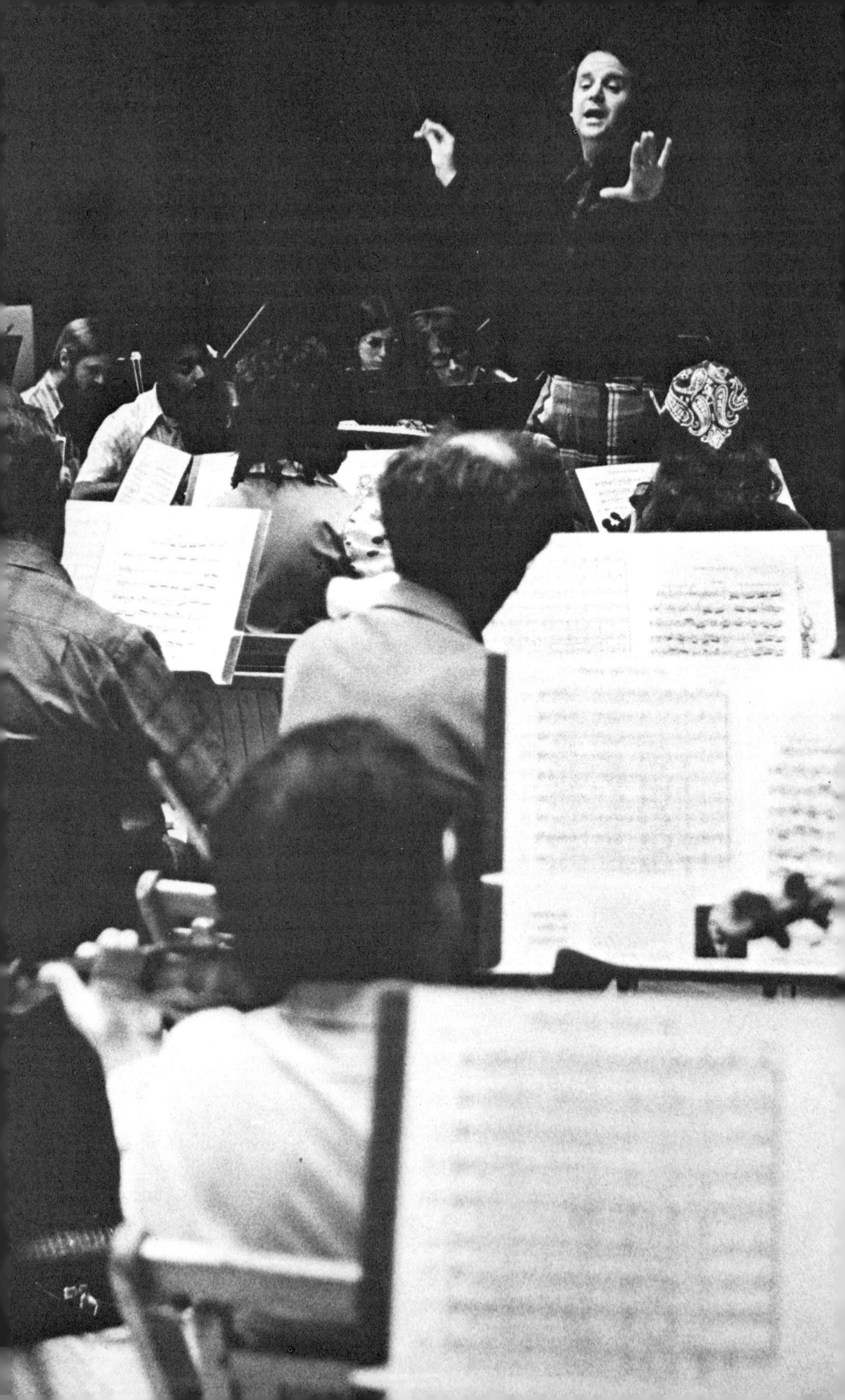

Marriage

Marriage has different meanings for different individuals and different societies. A majority of people in our culture idealize marriage as an end-point in personal-social development. Despite this, we find many married people who show no great compatibility of feelings, attitudes, or motives; presently one out of every three marriages ends in divorce. In a recent interview, Mead (1968) speculated that marriages that last a lifetime will become less frequent as life expectancy increases, and people become less willing to tolerate indefinitely an unsatisfactory marriage. Indeed, studies show that many marriages do decline in satisfaction and happiness as the years accumulate (Blood & Wolfe, 1960; Pineo, 1961).

Marriage in our middle-class culture usually is the culmination of romantic love and courtship (see Figure 9–4). It is a fusion of the relationships existing in friendship, companionship, and sexual attraction. Ideally it occurs after numerous friendships with the opposite sex and after a courtship that has tested the social and temperamental compatibility of the pair. It is a public declaration of affection and fidelity and usually has the approval of one's immediate social group.

UNMARRIED INDIVIDUALS

A certain percentage of our population, either through choice or circumstance, do not marry. Another percentage will marry and then appropriately decide that they prefer to live as a single person. Many such unmarried individuals in our society live relatively full lives, rewarding to themselves and to their fellows.

Some of the circumstances leading to the single state include the fact that in this country more women than men of marriageable age want to marry. It is estimated that there are 6 million females in the United States over 14 years of age, many of whom would choose to marry but who will not do so for many reasons (Adams, 1951). Let us consider just a few of the factors: women in certain vocations and in certain geographic areas have more opportunities to marry than others; for example, teachers and city-dwelling women meet fewer acceptable men than do women in business or in rural areas. Also, the more educated the woman, the less likely she is to marry. Seventy-two percent of college women marry, compared to 90 percent of the population as a whole. A study by Baker (1968) compared 38 women who had never married with married mothers. He found that they manifested equiva-

Figure 9–3 A Profession Requiring Years of Preparation.

Photo courtesy of *Columbia Missourian*

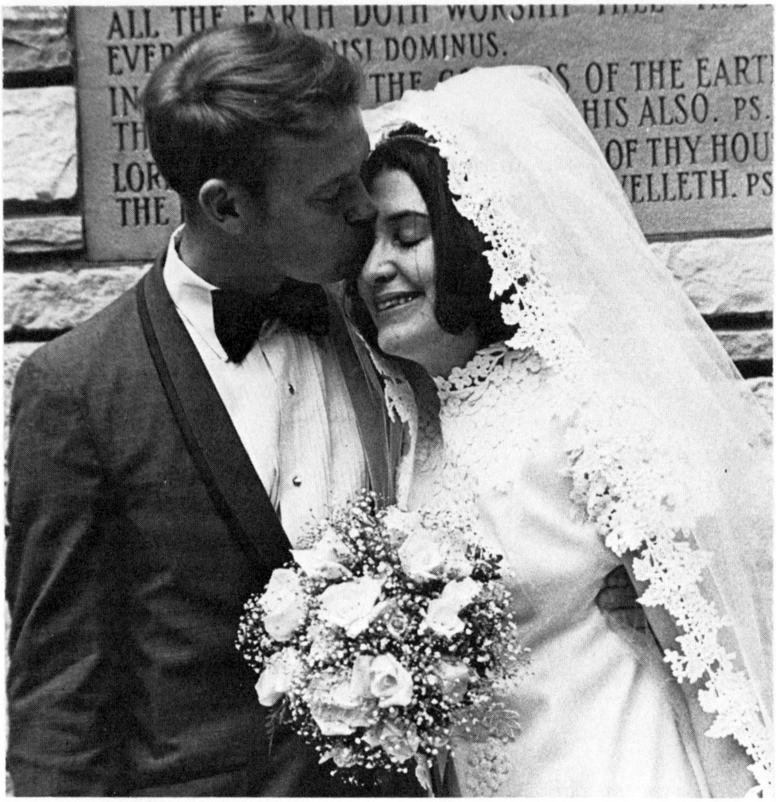

Photo by Chris T. Quillen

Figure 9–4 A Typical Marriage.

lent adjustments and that the never-marrieds may achieve self-fulfillment without husband or children.

The unmarried obviously have to resolve the problem of satisfying their sexual needs. Five percent of women and 8 percent of men between the ages of 35 and 44 never married (U.S. Bureau of the Census, 1964). Even though unmarried people may find mates through computer-dating services, clubs for singles, or other agencies, the mathematics of the situation are such that many women will not find husbands as long as our society is monogamous. Those who are unmarried must go through life without the "accepted" type of regular sex partner. Hence, four choices seem to be open to them: (1) total abstinence, (2) masturbation, (3) homosexual relationships, or (4) extramarital sexual relationships.

Choosing between these alternatives will presumably be determined by several considerations; for example, homosexual relationships may not be appealing or inflict too great a social stigma; extramarital sex may not be available or may be too fraught with potential guilt and other problems (the man may be married and his wife one's best friend);

masturbation may be too deeply disturbing to be a satisfactory solution; and abstinence, no matter how frustrating, may be the only answer.

FACTORS IN MARITAL ADJUSTMENT

As in all complex social relationships, many factors produce a desirable marital equilibrium. Not all these factors need be present to produce a satisfactory happy marriage. One or two conditions may be so important that their presence will be more significant than a combination of six or eight other factors.

FAMILY BACKGROUND

Studies on marital happiness began in the early 1930s in the Los Angeles and Chicago areas (Terman & Buttenwieser, 1935; Burgess & Cottrell, 1939). Other studies have added information since then (Burgess & Wallin, 1953; Locke, 1951; Landis & Landis, 1963). One outstanding factor found in these studies was the importance of a happy family background for both the married persons. Kirkpatrick (1963), in listing factors roughly in order of importance, places happiness of parents' marriage first on his list. Pond, Ryle, & Hamilton (1963) found that the best single predictor of happiness in marriage was happiness in childhood; emotional disturbances in childhood tended to be correlated with unsatisfactory marital adjustment. Among other items listed are approval of marriage by parents and others, harmonious affection and lack of conflict with parents during childhood, and personal happiness in childhood. Other important factors in the family background are presence of siblings, higher socioeconomic status of parents, a religious atmosphere in the home, and conditions leading to appropriate sex roles (Terman, 1938).

The relationship with parents is important in marriage, for sometimes, when conflict arises between parents one of them will turn to a child for the response that is lacking in the other partner. This creates a real problem for the child's future relationships. An example of such a problem is provided by the case of Margot who, upon marrying, endowed her husband with qualities that neither he nor any other man has ever possessed. When the husband turned out to be an ordinary man, she was disappointed and no longer found him attractive. Still, she maintained hope in their marriage, since they had a son, Cyril, whom she could attempt to turn into the perfect man, the type of man she thought she had married. Margot worked at this, and at 20 years of age the boy seemed nearly perfect in her eyes, but was actually neither attractive to nor attracted by girls of his own age. His mother loved him dearly, and his whole life was shaped around her life. He viewed his father critically, never regarding him as a person to emulate or with whom he could identify. Unless an entire reeducation takes place over a period of time, Cyril will have difficulty adjusting as a husband or may never desire to marry. If the change does occur, his mother will have difficulty adjusting to his marriage—a real threat to the happiness of the new family.

SIMILAR INTERESTS

Practically all studies on marriage and friendship support the generalization that those with similar interests and attitudes have mutual appeal, tending to disprove the saying that "opposites attract." The specific areas explored in which agreement was greater among happy couples in contrast to unhappy ones include recreation, religion, table manners, conventionality, philosophy of life, friends, care of children, and family finances. The climate of cooperation and agreement on certain matters is more important than the *number* of mutual interests. Men have different interests than women, and this difference is accepted in an essentially happy marriage. However, mutual interest in the home, the children, in religion, and in demonstration of affection is important (Benson, 1955; Frumkin, 1954).

Not all personal characteristics need be similar in order for the marriage to be happy. A difference in age between the partners is typically not a highly important factor affecting the happiness of the partners. There is no evidence that the husband must be older than the wife for an effective adjustment (Terman & Buttenwieser, 1935) or that marriages in which the husband is considerably older than the wife are likely to fail.

EDUCATIONAL, CULTURAL, AND ENVIRONMENTAL FACTORS

Nationality and *religious differences* likewise tend to be minimal in happy marriages. A study by Burgess and Cottrell (1939) failed to show that religious preference made much difference, but the author indicates that many of the individuals studied were emancipated from religious controls. Sometimes couples themselves may feel that a marriage is workable despite their cultural background differences. Their friends and parents, however, may view the marriage differently and through their interference cause unhappiness (Bossard & Ball, 1957). The wealthy girl, for example, who has married an unconventional, lower-middle-class man may later find herself unwilling to lose former friends and be unable to endure the snubs of her acquaintances. Social class differences between spouses are strongly related to later difficulties in marital adjustment (Roth & Peck, 1951).

To be sure, trends do not show the facts found in individual cases, but if we look at most of the data available, as did Landis and Landis (1963), we would have to point out that Catholic-Protestant marriages, especially before the institutional changes suggested by Vatican II, presented special difficulties. Prior to these changes, the non-Catholic had to agree to raise all offspring as Catholics. This often became a very controversial issue for the couple when the children arrived or reached their adolescence and wanted to adopt the religion of the non-Catholic. These marriages were more likely to lead to a break than homogamous Catholic or Protestant marriages.

When these background cultural factors run deep into the personality of the individual, similarity of attitudes in the mate is important. Sometimes persons of two different religions are more similar in attitude than are two persons of the same religion. A nonorthodox Jew and a liberal Protestant may be much more similar attitudinally than an orthodox and a nonorthodox Jew, especially if all the cultural attitudes of Judaism have not been emphasized in the development of the nonorthodox Jew. On the other hand, it is hard to see how a literal-minded Roman Catholic and a Baptist fundamentalist could be happily married. Usually, however, the couple discover important discrepancies in attitudes if the courtship is long enough and if these matters are frankly discussed (Marcson, 1953).

ATTITUDES TOWARD FINANCES

Indebtedness and unemployment are among the factors associated with marital difficulties (Williamson, 1952). Economic conflicts often arise because of *dissimilar attitudes* on the part of husband and wife regarding the use of income. Further conflict arises when previous standards of living conflict with present income (Terman, 1938). Apparently, if couples try to fuse their aims in the spending of money, the marriage runs smoother. If, instead, they become competitors in the use of their resources, friction results. Engaged couples might well work out individual budgets as well as a family budget for their future home. They might save and buy home furnishings together and then after marriage make an active attempt to live within the family budget. Security and stability, shown in regularity and steadiness of employment rather than in *income level,* are important in marital happiness (Burgess & Cottrell, 1939).

REWARD BY CONSENSUAL VALIDATION

The psychological reason why common attitudes and interests lead to more happy marriages is that both partners have common goals and do things that lead to mutual satisfaction. Knowing that one's mate agrees with one has been called *reward by consensual validation* (Byrne & Blaylock, 1963). The accumulation of satisfactions in a marital situation results in both spouses evaluating the marriage as a happy one. The more emotionally mature individual makes a greater effort to bring about events that are satisfying to his partner. He readily rewards or compliments his partner's activities. Psychology is replete with studies showing that rewarded behavior is repeated and leads to human satisfaction.

Some conflicts about the best ways to spend time and money may be inevitable, and the resolution of these conflicts will sometimes require great tolerance and ability to compromise. Ideally each partner should probably encourage the other to continue independent interests if the two cannot agree on mutual participation. Such encouragement will be more likely to lead to more positive interactions than would complaints and frustration of each other's activities. It is difficult to find a marriage free of disagreements. These inevitable disagreements may stimulate fairly good-humored interchanges of information, in which both partners avoid destroying each other while gaining their points. In such cases, grouchy, semihumorous banter provides a vehicle for voicing complaints without threat to either ego. On the other hand, one partner may become very hostile or extremely sensitive, and a "good fight" will turn into a "bad fight," in which the participants are hurt rather than informed. Two people are not likely to go through marriage without quarreling. They would be unwise to transfer from courtship to marriage without testing out this area of adjustment—not intentionally, but incidentally to knowing each other well enough so that a situation of conflict arises. One part of knowing each other well will be a growing awareness of the other person's areas of sensitivity. This is one aspect of a necessary, absolute, mutual respect for the integrity of the marriage partner. If one or both partners start chipping away at the ego of the other, a happy marriage cannot survive.

Since marriage involves cooperation, communication, and learning to make adjustments, the engagement period is a good time to ascertain the extent to which these processes can take place between the pair. The greater the congruence between the roles the couples manifest, the greater the likelihood of marital satisfaction (Tharp, 1963). They can begin by testing their potential for significant communication and by making compromises in arriving at mutually satisfying solutions to everyday problems.

Happier marriages, studies show, are based on longer periods of acquaintance and engagement as contrasted with a brief acquaintance of a few months (Terman, 1938; Burgess & Cottrell, 1939). Divorce data substantiate the finding that *length of engagement* is related to satisfactory marriages. This factor may be a reflection of other more important factors such as class, or education, or emotional instability. The longer the couple had known each other, the longer the marriage lasted. In 71 percent of the divorces, this period was shorter than six months, and in 19 percent there was practically no engagement period (Goode, 1956). A marriage that is contracted too early or too impulsively, as many war marriages were, does not allow a sufficient period for work and play together. Because it is not clear how much and which couples change after marriage, as indicated by Stagner (1965), the testing of interactions before marriage becomes highly important for marital success.

EARLY MARRIAGES

There is considerable evidence that marriage contracted between very young people—usually under 20—is a poor risk (Kephart, 1961; Burgess & Cottrell, 1939; Terman, 1938). Yet maturity rather than chronological age is the critical measure of readiness for marriage. Indeed, some 20-year-olds are more mature than their parents.

Some very young people marry early to escape an unhappy home situation or parental domination, or because their contemporaries are marrying. They do not perceive clearly what marriage entails in the way of responsibilities. The person who chooses marriage as a solution to personal problems without attempting to cope directly with these problems is a poor risk. Childish habits are found in many unhappy spouses. Some spouses expect to be indulged and anticipate being treated by their partner as their parents treated them. Members of this group are often irritable or hurt when the spouse expects them to assume their adult responsibilities.

An overoptimistic young man (or young woman) may recognize the incompatibilities existing between him and his fiancée but may still plan to marry the person with whom he has had numerous quarrels. The rationalization he uses is, "It will change after marriage." What do the studies show? There seems to be little tendency for either of the spouses to change their interests and traits toward those of the other after marriage (Kelly, 1955).

Premarital background predicts marital success accurately both for those married more than fifteen years or for less than five years. This suggests that change in personality is not great. If personality changed drastically over the years, the accuracy of prediction for the early-married and late-married should not be the same (Stroup, 1953). The consistency of partners is also reflected in the finding that marital tensions in the first three years of marriage give a good prediction of tensions after fourteen years.

SEX IN MARRIAGE

Happiness in marriage in general is related to the spouses' total personalities, and not to single factors including the one that is greatly emphasized in our culture—sex. Terman (1938) found that fear of pregnancy, pain during first coitus, a history of "sex shock" in the wife, her rhythm of desire, and the particular method of making love were not related to happiness in marriage. A somewhat related fact is that a newly married husband who is experienced with promiscuous women is *not* necessarily well prepared to initiate an inexperienced bride (Stroup, 1966). Stroup points out (p. 224) that these men often lack the patience, understanding, tact, and foresight necessary to lead their wives toward mutually satisfactory sexual interaction. Terman (1938) also found some indication that sex habits inconsistent with marital fidelity affected the happiness of the marriage.

MUTUAL SEX SATISFACTION

Since sexual gratification is today a major expectancy in marriage, sex frustration can become an important factor in individual marriages. Indeed several decades ago, Terman (1938) showed that happiness in marriage is related to the wife's ability to achieve an orgasm. Thomason (1955) repeated Terman's early studies and also found the wife's capacity to reach an orgasm important. He concludes that the total marriage is happier if intercourse was by mutual desire and the mates were willing and able to have intercourse as often as they wished.

Studies of sex attitudes and roles indicate that some *adaptation in attitudes* of the man and woman during marriage must take place. Men and women in our culture differ in the stimuli that are most effective in arousing them sexually. Men have a history of easy arousal to sex thoughts and impulses prior to marriage through various stimuli that refer to the physical aspect of the woman and sex activity. Women often have aversions to the "crudities" of physical approaches and reflect a life history of inhibition; they reach a stage of readiness through a tender, personal, love attitude (Kinsey, Pomeroy, & Martin, 1948). With frankness, understanding, patience, and time, partners make a more effective mutual affectional adjustment (Ort, 1950).

In reviewing studies of marriage, Bakan (1966) observed that the more successful marriages have a balance within the spouses of the traits of *agency* (self-protection, assertion, self-expansion, mastery) and *communion* (openness, human contact, and union of feelings). He points out that men tend more to overemphasize the agency aspect in their lives, and he suggests that this emphasis affects the happiness of both spouses. Often marital partners expect these intimate relationships to be natural and not subject to a learning process. The resulting early frustrations and disappointments lead to self-recrimination or recrimination of their spouse, or of both. Studies show these adjustments do improve over a period of time (Duvall & Hill, 1945).

RELIEF OF SEXUAL DYSFUNCTION

After their research on the physiological aspects of the sexual response in humans, Masters and Johnson (1966; 1970) reported the results of counseling sexually incompatible marriage partners troubled by frigidity, impotence, or lack of satisfaction. Their technique involves working with both members of the marriage, in addition to direct therapy for the sexually inadequate partner. They were most optimistic about therapeutic gains when they were able to enlist the complete cooperation of the adequate spouse—the husband of the frigid woman or the wife of the impotent man. Their therapeutic approach also aided the partners to communicate with each other (often for the first time) highly personal feelings about their sexual needs and fears. In this way the married couple began to work together in solving a very personal problem.

Some psychologists believe that a good sexual adjustment in any context depends on self-confidence and mutual acceptance by the participants. In the atmosphere provided by such acceptance, almost any problem can be solved, and the partners feel a freedom to do whatever is natural to them without any thought of rejection. In such a situation, and perhaps in any successful sexual relationship, a peculiar paradox occurs: (1) the most selfish thing to do is to be unselfish, and (2) the most unselfish thing to do is to be selfish. The paradox is resolved if the extreme mutuality of successful sex is understood. Statement (1) is true in the sense that it guarantees satisfaction of the partner and thus one's own maximum enjoyment. Statement (2) is true because one's partner will derive maximum satisfaction if he or she feels that you are doing whatever is most enjoyable for you.

Sex and the other factors considered are interrelated. It has been said that the extent of sexual adjustment is a good index of the marriage as a whole. If, for example, the wife or husband respects the spouse because of education, athletic, or economic accomplishments, it will be easier to adjust sexually than if these attitudes are negative. If one spouse is irritated with the other's performance as a parent or in domestic matters (breadwinner, housekeeper), he will be less solicitous of the other's sexual desires. Conversely, if the spouse is entirely satisfying as a sexual partner, the other roles will seem satisfactory even though they do not conform to original preferences. We discussed a similar phenomenon earlier as the "halo effect." Basically, in a happy marriage each partner is constantly working to satisfy the spouse's needs in ways that can also satisfy his or her own. When necessary, both are willing to compromise to find a mutually acceptable solution.

Process of Adjustment in Marriage

COMMUNICATION BETWEEN COUPLES

Married people are *always* communicating in some way or other. Even when they refuse to talk to each other, they are communicating rejection or hostility. Communication goes far beyond the spoken word. We communicate nonverbally through gestures, facial expressions, timing of our responses, and tone of voice. It is not always clear to us what we are communicating to the other person; even though he may receive our deeper intentions accurately. For example, a husband may constantly communicate to a wife that he regards her as incompetent and inferior to himself without being conscious that he has revealed this judgment so clearly.

In many marriages, communication is far from a complete interchange of all attitudes and feelings. One of the partners may not dare say exactly what he or she feels until anger forces hidden feelings and attitudes to the surface. Then the negative information cannot be used effectively by the spouse because hostile overtones produce defensiveness. In some marital relationships and in some subcultures in the United States verbal or deep communication is not the usual pattern. In other marriages the personality of one or both of the partners is such that most of the communication has the nature of a contest, each partner competing with the other to satisfy his or her own needs and perpetuate his or her own attitudes and habits.

Disclosure of one's feelings to a spouse is correlated positively with general marital satisfaction. Also, as one partner shows disclosure the other partner tends to follow (Levinger & Senn, 1967). Another study of happily married couples revealed that sensitivity to the needs of the spouse and ability to communicate one's feelings and emotions to the partner were important to the success of the marriage (Mudd, Mitchell, & Taubin, 1965).

Several other investigations empirically emphasize the importance of communication in marriage. Communication patterns are found to differ for happily and unhappily married couples. Happily married couples talk to each other a great deal and indicate that they understand what is said and felt. They tend to keep avenues of verbal and nonverbal communication open (Navran, 1967).

Inadequate Communication: Virginia and Oliver

Oliver and Virginia were attending college together, particularly enjoying their courses in the Humanities. Both had strong interests in literature and the arts, and had a pleasurable year amid atrocious housekeeping conditions in two substandard rooms. Although they had grown up in the same neighborhood, each had dated others and discovered only when Oliver returned from military service how much they had in common and how much they enjoyed each other's companionship.

Virginia's relationship to her father was ambivalent. They loved each other, but they quarreled bitterly when she failed to meet his expectations. Oliver's father had died young, and Oliver had become a father to his younger siblings. He reared them, and when he entered the Army he became the parent-substitute sergeant for a number of immature rookies. He is a massive and calm, but colorful, individual, his liberality representing an almost bohemian veneer over his stable traits. Virginia is bright but submissive and nervous, with a strong need for someone on whom she can lean. Unlike her father, Oliver is understanding, tolerant, and helpful. Their particular personal styles appeared to mesh quite well and their marriage seemed to be happy.

They came to the counselor after a hysterical evening when Oliver had an unprecedented verbal battle with a friend of his. This brought back to Virginia's mind the parental scenes, and she went to bed trembling and sobbing. She feared that Oliver might some day show similar aggression toward her.

Virginia had not shared with Oliver her feelings about the hostile interchange she witnessed between Oliver and his good friend, nor had Oliver communicated his concern over Virginia's unprovoked "going to pieces." In the relative calm of the counselor's office the next day, Virginia could own up to her fears that her loved husband might become like her father, and Oliver could admit the implications to him of Virginia's apparent loss of emotional control. With this block removed they could express their love for each other.

The Problem-Solving Approach

Despite similar interests and attitudes and mutual love, disagreements and overt conflict arise in marriages. It is best that they be anticipated before and during marriage as much as possible and that methods be devised for coping with them. The more objectively problems can be viewed and verbalized so various solutions can be worked out, the greater the marital satisfaction. Ort (1950), for example, found that happily married couples resolve conflicts by discussing them, whereas the unhappily married use aggression and avoidance of the issue. Diane and Joe represent one couple who were committed to a problem-solving approach. They are not the typical couple, so some readers may not agree with the solutions they reached. The important point here is not the solutions, which are a personal matter, but the process of problem solving.

Case of Diane and Joe[1]

Older than Joe, Diane has been providing the larger share of support for the family unit while Joe works on an advanced degree. This arrangement could be a source of friction, since both are stepping out of the usual culturally defined roles. Yet they share convictions and a realistic problem-solving attitude that has so far guaranteed the success of their marriage.

Diane, the daughter of a Midwestern psychiatrist, and Joe, a southerner, met as students at a Southern university. Diane, eight years older than Joe, had been married and divorced. Nevertheless, Joe found himself tremendously attracted to her. Diane felt similarly but rejected the thought of marriage because of the difference in their ages. She had nearly finished her work for a Ph.D. while he was still an undergraduate.

When Diane got her degree and accepted a job at a Midwestern university, Joe transferred to her new school as a graduate student in order to remain close to her. They continued to see one another, and after a two-year courtship, his continuing affection and persistence overcame all obstacles, and they were married.

They shared a deeply held belief in a systematic approach to the study and understanding of behavior and applied this view, derived from their professional work and training, to their marriage. Consequently, they recorded frequency of intercourse, quarrels, and social engagements both in and out of their home systematically. In addition, Joe periodically recorded his current evaluation of the success of the marriage.

They found from their records that they never had intercourse during menstruation, but never missed having intercourse the day before menstruation began. This general pattern is often reported, but is far from universal. One of their purposes in keeping records was to determine whether a relationship existed between frequency of intercourse and frequency of arguments. They found no evidence of such a relationship suggesting that, whether or not love really conquers all, intercourse does.

In addition to recording intercourse and arguments, they established certain rules that regulated their behavior in each part of their apartment. For example, no arguments were permitted in the bedroom (arguments were regarded as being inconsistent with the proper use of a bedroom). Many arguments did, however, occur in other places. An argument was defined as an unpleasant interaction in which at least one of the pair became uncooperative. They did not count as arguments the "good fights" in which some couples deliberately indulge as an enjoyable game. To reduce the number of arguments they worked out a signal which could be used by either partner as an indication that he wanted hostilities to cease. A bean bag, to be used for no other purpose, was arbitrarily chosen as a

[1] The authors are indebted to W. A. Hillix for this case.

means of providing the signal; when it was thrown into the middle of the floor, the uncooperative partner had to stop arguing. Their graphs showed that the bean-bag signal worked beautifully; the number of arguments steadily declined over a period of months.

Then an unexpected problem arose. The birth of a baby boy (Scott) resulted in disagreement on methods of handling the child. Joe wanted to make observations on Scott's learning abilities, but Diane's "maternal instincts" prompted her to protest. The number of arguments shot up until Joe convinced her that his procedures would be harmless. They began simply to require Scott to push a panel with his foot in order to "earn" the milk from his bottle. This settlement reduced the number of arguments and produced one of the earliest instances of systematic operant training in a human infant. In this case, as in others that could be cited, Joe's was the dominant view. They had decided mutually at the outset that, despite the reversal of the usual pattern of relative age and status, Joe would be the dominant figure.

Diane is able to continue her teaching partly because of the purchase of two infant living chambers in which Scott can be placed—one at home, the other in her office. These chambers are thermostatically controlled in temperature, and fresh filtered air is continually circulated by motors whose quiet hum helps to mask external noises.

Scott is thriving in his thermostatically controlled "home away from home" and in the loving atmosphere provided by his stable mated parents. Joe has won a national prize for research design and has finished his work for the Ph.D. At this writing, they would seem to constitute a living testimonial for a systematic, problem-solving approach to marriage.

Parenthood

Having achieved *intimacy*, the mature adult begins to experience a desire to leave something of himself, to achieve some form of immortality, however small. Thus, as his career, trade, or occupation becomes established, he finds increasing satisfaction in sharing his experiences with younger men. When a vocation does not permit sufficient opportunity to feel productive and creative, many men try to give expression to this need through hobbies. The form of the activity does not matter, but it must provide a sense of doing something worthwhile. Thus some men, such as architects, can find their satisfaction in the structures they design; doctors, in the patients they help; teachers, in the students they educate. Others such as laborers and unskilled workers take similar pride in their efforts. A truck driver, for example, may find considerable satisfaction in his ability to handle skillfully a 40-foot trailer through narrow streets and heavy traffic. Those who do not find complete fulfillment of this need for *generativity* in their work may invest considerable effort on their home, their lawn, their automobile, even their putting stroke. Without such satisfaction, Erikson reminds us, we would *stagnate* and lead dull, empty lives. Without achievement of some kind, our daily, weekly, yearly efforts become routine and mechanized. We become unable and unwilling to go beyond ourselves at all, and tend, in fact, to lose ourselves and thereby, ultimately, to lose the very intimacy we struggled to maintain. The following chapter will consider at some length the consequences of stagnation for the middle and later years.

Just as the adolescent developed an *identity* that was to be tested by the demands for *intimacy* accompanying young adulthood, so the adult must test the solidity of this *intimacy* by going beyond it in his drive toward generativity. As Erikson (1963) himself noted: "the strength acquired at any stage is tested by the necessity to transcend it in such a way that the individual can take chances with what was most vulnerably precious in the previous one" (p. 263). In addition to the various ways in which the adult does so through his occupation and hobbies, the primary means for testing the intimate relationship of a marriage is through parenthood in which both partners must now share their emotional ties with one or more offspring.

BECOMING A PARENT

During the past two decades, much about parenthood has changed. Previously, marriage and children were almost synonymous and generally in that order. The appearance of children was typically determined as much by nature as by man, since the only absolutely effective birth control procedure was sexual abstinence (a technique which, to this day, has never been very popular). In those instances in which no offspring were produced, there was usually a reproductive dysfunction in one or both partners. Children, therefore, were conceived and born whether or not the family was emotionally and financially prepared for them. Families tended to be larger than the modal two children of today's standards and, often, family resources were carefully budgeted in order to meet basic needs.

While this description continues to apply to many low-income families, middle- and upper-income families are increasingly planning the occurrence and frequency of children in their families. As communication and social services increase for the poor, they also demonstrate a strong desire to limit the size of their families. As one parent noted: "It's not that I don't love each and every one of my five children, only if I hadn't had so many I could provide much more to them. I also would have been able to really begin to know my husband and develop a better understanding of him as a person had I not had the children so quickly after we were married."

Thus significant medical advances in birth control methods have had major social and psychological consequences for marriages and parenthood. Husband and wife can now opt to delay having children for a time, indeed forever. In some instances, both partners achieve sufficient satisfaction from their occupations, interests, and relationship that they feel neither a need, nor a desire, for children. Changing social mores also are reducing the number of times they must hear in whatever form, the oft-repeated question: "When are you going to have children?" As noted in an earlier chapter, the prevailing movement to break down established stereotypes of women as housewives and mothers provides further support for those who choose not to bear children. Still another source of encouragement of childless marriages is the growing social concern for the possibility of overpopulation and its attendant problems. Thus zero-population growth is an ideal for many young couples that prompts them to limit sharply family size.

The decision to remain childless throughout life cannot be made by either partner individually. It is a choice that in the later years will be irreversible and unless carefully made can lead to much bitterness and anger between the partners.

As a relationship develops and approaches marriage, each person should seriously consider his or her attitudes toward parenthood. Both partners should discuss their positive and negative feelings openly, and not only listen to the words of the other but also attend to the more subtle indications of the person's desires as expressed by his or her reactions to children, in general, and to close family members' children in particular. This does not imply that adults who don't have children must hate kids, but only that at times, for the sake of maintaining a relationship, one person may deny his true desire to have children.

It is important to identify each partner's real feelings about having children so that the couple can arrive at some mutually satisfying decision around the issue of parenthood. If there is any doubt in either partner's mind prior to the marriage, he or she must consider carefully the implications of choosing a partner who is unalterably opposed to children. The well-adjusted person's options in such an instance are few and include (a) delaying the marriage until a greater degree of certainty is achieved; (b) terminating the relationship as unworkable; (c) openly sharing with the partner one's ambivalence and perhaps agreeing to marry with the understanding that parenthood will be delayed for some specific length of time and then carefully reconsidered. The last-mentioned solution, though perhaps the easiest to accept, carries with it a certain potential for placing the marital relationship in jeopardy at some later date and should only be selected after much careful discussion. Those readers who find themselves in the dilemma of having to choose between a partner and the chance to have children should seek out help in making the decision through clergy, a close friend, or the school counselor. An objective sensitive listener can often help one learn what he or she really wants.

Parenthood, therefore, has become a real choice for adults. Those who genuinely feel unable or unwilling to accept the responsibility of children can now decide not to do so with decreasing social pressure. Those who are unsure can delay the decision until they feel more able to commit themselves one way or the other. Couples who fall in either category should realize that a decision made in the early twenties or during the first hectic year of marriage may seem less satisfactory once they have done many of the things they wanted to do, and grown together in their relationship. For this reason, in selecting among birth control procedures, it's typically best not to begin with the more permanent measures such as sterilization. As the years pass and the couple's decision becomes clear, open discussions with one's physician can lead to the most satisfactory solution.

The majority of marriages will, however, produce some offspring. In some cases, the child will have already been conceived at the time of marriage and its imminent arrival has hastened, if not in fact motivated the marriage. Unfortunately this situation often occurs with very young adults in their mid or late teens and results in considerable strain on what would have been a rather tenuous relationship in any case. The potential for the success of such marriages is relatively low, and often a hastily arranged marriage harms rather than protects the resultant offspring. Such marriages frequently end in divorce and produce many difficult adjustment problems for both spouses, and especially for the children. While it is not easy to consider objectively the consequences of an unexpected pregnancy and forced marriage in the middle of such a crisis, it is important that all involved—both the couple and their parents—carefully weigh the available options. The stronger, more mature the relationship between the two parties the better the chance that the marriage may succeed. If the relationship is remote or tenuous, it is unrealistic to assume that a good one will develop simply because the couple marries and shares parental responsibilities. In such cases both partners and potential offspring may fare best if the marriage is not forced and the child released for adoption at birth. While this is certainly a very difficult (and often unpopular) decision, it is often the most sensible. Once again, perhaps the wisest move to make in such a situation is to seek counsel from a trusted, mature outside party such as a counselor or clergyman.

In most cases, conception follows marriage and the couple then decides mutually when and how many children to have. An important determinant of their decision will be their religious beliefs. Additionally, their own positive experiences as children and the happiness of their early family life also relate to the probability of their wanting children. Those couples who do plan their families usually consider a number of factors in spacing their children. First, many couples use their first married year or two to learn to know each other well both as individuals and as marital partners. They seek to understand and adjust to the personal, emotional, and sexual characteristics of each other and thereby, hopefully solidify their relationship. Given this base, the couple assumes that they can securely share their mutual affections with children. Thus in delaying, their goal is to provide the child with a stable family setting.

Many other couples opt to postpone having children during their first years of marriage in order to solidify their family's financial base. Without children, both partners can work full-time and the innumerable initial expenses of setting up a home and saving for the medical and related expenses of childbirth can be handled. Such couples assume that they will be much better able to deal with the interpersonal complexities of having a child if they are free of financial pressures. An important caution they must recognize is that it becomes increasingly tempting to put off the birth of a child until "the car is paid for" or "the down payment for the house is put away" and thus each financial goal is followed by another. In such a situation, when a child does arrive, the couple may overindulge him after having waited for so long or may (contrary to their original intentions) feel that his presence denies them of yet another material possession.

No specific guidelines exist to help one decide when "the right time" has arrived. The development of effective and efficient birth control procedures provides married couples (and unmarried ones, as well) with an option previously not available. It does not, however, necessitate that each couple exercise that option. A man and woman must choose for themselves whether or not they are able to accept the responsibilities of parenthood. If they are and can maturely integrate the new child into their relationship, financial concerns may be relatively unimportant to them. They may simply accept the reality that having a child now rather than later entails certain financial sacrifices. They may decide that material security can be delayed but children cannot. The important thing is that at this time, as never before, parents can control whether or not they will be parents.

The reader should be well aware that there is no evidence that the addition of a child can save a "rocky" marriage. Occasionally, the added responsibility successfully motivates a man or woman to accept their role in the marriage. More often, the added demands made by the child will strain the already frail relationship and if not hasten its termination, increase the discontent and hostility between the partners.

Thus, if a couple is having difficulty in their marriage, they are well advised to seek a solution to their problems before having a child. Ultimately, they will be better off without children if the marriage must end and, if it succeeds, to bring their children up in a more secure relationship.

THE DEMANDS OF PARENTHOOD

The birth of a child is a very significant event in a marital relationship. The "couple" now becomes a "family" and assumes responsibility for the health and welfare of their offspring. Suddenly, decisions about how and where they will live, how to spend their time, and how to manage their finances must all be made with the new family member in mind. The *intimacy* achieved earlier in their relationship is clearly tested as the child demands and receives a significant portion of each parent's, especially the mother's, time. As each succeeding child enters the family even more sharing and understanding is necessary from the parents. For those relationships in which either or both partners were already insecure, the arrival of a child may be a very threatening event.

The infant requires much nurturance and attention and may therefore be perceived by the father as monopolizing the mother's feelings or by the mother as an obstacle to being close to the father. When either partner feels that his or her affections are not returned in kind and amount by the other, they may transfer those feelings onto the new child and thereby actively displease the other in the relationship. The consequences of such distorted parent-child relationships are often observed only much later in the child's life as he attempts to relate to peers and other adults. The child may then be highly dependent and constantly demand attention or he may be very reluctant to form any attachments in order to avoid the hostility and resulting sense of guilt that have accompanied his earlier relationships. In most cases, however, the new parents are genuinely pleased with the arrival of a child and are able to maturely integrate it into their relationship. Although adjustments will be necessary and the problems and demands of parenthood recognized, most adults cope adequately with the realities of having a child. Through their efforts, they gradually discover that in working together and in sharing each other with their child, their relationship gains rather than loses.

As noted, parenthood is not an easy lot. Indeed, it is a complex and often frustrating role in which one is never certain that decisions made today will prove to be the "right ones," ten, twenty, or thirty years in the future. We are all in some way affected by techniques of parenting and, yet, surprisingly, no formal training for the task is available. Although some consideration is currently being given to the required preparation of all expectant parents in child-rearing techniques, it seems unlikely that in the foreseeable future a person will be required to pass a test before becoming a licensed parent. An important reason for this is that while there are numerous "experts" on the topic (both professionals and, even more abundantly, family, friends, and mild acquaintances) there is no single appropriate technique that well suits all parents and all children. Numerous books, articles, and syndicated columnists debate the pros and cons of every aspect of child rearing from demand versus schedule feeding to the potential harm or benefits of spanking a child. While they do not typically agree on specific recommendations, it does seem fair to summarize their positions by suggesting that common sense and respect for the child as a person should be the main ingredients in any parenting approach. Needless to say a spanking is not a beating and under no circumstances is physically injuring or endangering a child a responsible disciplinary measure.

The primary task of a parent is to support and facilitate the maturation of a child's physical, emotional, interpersonal, and cognitive potential. In essence, that implies aiding the child to deal successfully with each of the developmental crises through which the adult himself has already passed. It is in this sense that parenthood truly enables one to share actively in the responsibility for coming generations. As we proceed through each of the developmental stages considered in the preceding chapters, we gain experiences from our own behavior and from what we learn from our parents on how to resolve the conflicts which arise. As parents, we pass that part of ourselves on to our children and, ideally, enable them to benefit from the mistakes and successes we have already had. Additionally, as parents we shape the attitudes, goals, and behaviors of the succeeding generation and, in this way, achieve some portion of the sense of immortality which characterizes Erikson's concept of generativity.

GINOTT'S CONCEPT OF PARENTHOOD

As noted earlier, the present volume cannot provide a comprehensive treatment of child and developmental psychology. Rather, the authors hope to present an overview of some of the relevant issues at each maturational stage and thereby stimulate the interested reader to delve further into the primary source material referenced throughout the book. Those readers concerned with approaches to parenting are therefore encouraged to review at some length the more extensive coverage of this topic provided by Wolf (1951), Arnstein (1964), and Halpern (1963). Among the more recent and widely acclaimed works of this type is Dr. Haim G. Ginott's (1965) *Between Parent and Child,* which emphasizes clear communication between family members as the key to an effective parent-child relationship.

Basic to Dr. Ginott's approach is the establishment of a clear distinction in a parent's mind between the recognition and behavioral expression of feelings. Emotional reactions, whether positive or negative, occur automatically in response to internal and external situations. An individual can neither control nor choose what feelings will be elicited in him. He can, however, determine the form in which his affect will be expressed. For example, when he is angry he may engage in destructive acts against his environment, direct verbal and/or physical abuse against those with whom he is interacting, march off abruptly to be by himself, or through repression, denial, or another of the defense mechanisms (discussed earlier) attempt to avoid direct expression and recognition of these feelings. The last-mentioned solution is most likely when the person has learned from childhood that certain feelings (once again be they positive or negative) are unacceptable and "bad." Hence, allowing such feelings to surface can only lead, in this person's mind, to further guilt and rejection. Unfortunately, denying a feeling means denying a very real part of oneself and thereby can eventually lead to a constantly troubling sense of incompleteness. The consequences of this state and recent innovative ways of dealing with it will be discussed at some length in Chapter 14.

Dr. Ginott assumes that a parent's responsibility is to facilitate a child's recognition and acceptance of all feelings be they positive or negative. This can be accomplished through a communicative process in which the parent encourages verbal expression of feelings and their meaning. Children gradually learn that *all* feelings are appropriate and acceptable because the parent does not reprimand a child for *feeling* but only for inappropriately expressing the feeling. Thus an angry child begins to accept his anger and to communicate it to others in a socially approved way. In doing so, his anger, sadness, hatred, or discouragement can be shared with others without being negatively reinforced. Dr. Ginott's approach to communication between parents and their children is based upon the maintenance of *mutual respect* between both parties and upon the parent's expression of *understanding* of the child's perspective and experience prior to providing advice or instruction. It also assumes the child's right to his feelings and discourages a parent's attempts to deny their existence. Consider, for example, the following excerpts from Dr. Ginott's book: [2]

[2] From *Between Parent and Child: New Solutions to Old Problems* by Dr. Haim G. Ginott. New York: Macmillan Publishing Co., Inc., 1965. Reprinted by permission of the publisher and Dr. Alice Ginott, Executor of Dr. Haim G. Ginott's Estate.

Son: I am stupid.
Father: You are not stupid.
Son: Yes, I am.
Father: You are not. Remember how smart you were at camp? The counselor thought you were one of the brightest.
Son: How do you know what he thought?
Father: He told me so.
Son: Yeah, how come he called me stupe all the time?
Father: He was just kidding.
Son: I am stupid, and I know it. Look at my grades in school.
Father: You just have to work harder.
Son: I already work harder and it doesn't help. I have no brains.
Father: You are smart, I know.
Son: I am stupid, I know.
Father (loudly): You are not stupid!
Son: Yes I am!
Father: You are not stupid, Stupid! (pp. 29–30)

Dr. Ginott suggests the following approach as a growth-producing response to a child's negative self-perception:

Son: I am stupid.
Father (seriously): You really feel that way, don't you? You don't think of yourself as smart?
Son: No.
Father: Then you suffer inside quite a lot?
Son: Yeah.
Father: In school, you must be afraid a great deal of the time
. . . afraid you'll fail.
. . . afraid you'll get low marks.
When the teacher calls on you, you get confused. Even when you know the answer, it doesn't come out right.
You are afraid that your words will sound ridiculous.
. . . and that the teacher will criticize you.
. . . and that the children will laugh at you.
So, many times you prefer to say nothing. I guess you can remember times when you said something and they laughed at you. It made you feel stupid in your own eyes. Hurt and angry, too. (Here, the child may tell you of some of his experiences).
Father: Look son! In my eyes you are a fine person. But you have a different opinion of yourself (pp. 30–31).

The first child is called upon to defend his feelings and the father finds himself debating an issue against which he can never raise irrefutable evidence. Most important, the father misses the point of the child's problem; that is, he *feels* stupid. That is a reality and may very well be unrelated to the validity of the feeling. The second child discovers that father accepts and understands what he is feeling and is given an opportunity to vent some of these feelings. Later, both father and son may consider the facts of the matter, for thus far in the conversation father has neither agreed nor disagreed. Instead, father has communicated to his son that it is acceptable to feel negatively about oneself. For Dr. Ginott, that is the essence of good parent-child communication and forms a solid base for healthy development.

Through the medium of conversation according to Dr. Ginott, parents can enable their children to develop self-respect, a sense of identity, and perhaps most important, a sense of responsibility for their behavior and its consequences. This is most clearly demonstrated in his discussion of disciplining children through the clear specification of what are the acceptable limits to behavior. Essentially, this technique refers to providing a child with accurate feedback about the acceptability of certain behaviors and the inappropriateness of others. The consequences of such is made clear to the child, for example, "if you throw the toy again, I will have to put it away." The child must then assume responsibility for his action. If he throws the toy, *he* causes it to be put away. If he plays with it as he should, *he* decides to do so. A parent, then, need not argue or constantly issue increasingly serious threats if he simply follows through on his earlier warning. The child learns that parents mean what they say and can be trusted. The child further learns that he can be assured that when he senses that his feelings are overwhelming and uncontrollable, his parents have the strength to ensure that his impulses will be controlled.

The central theme in Dr. Ginott's work and in the writings of others involved in parent counseling is the importance of providing the child with a sense of self-respect and self-worth. With this, the child can gradually become increasingly independent and develop a secure sense of his ability to select among alternative courses of action. Dr. Ginott sums up this goal in this manner:

> The essence of permissiveness is the acceptance of children as persons who have a constitutional right to have all kinds of feelings and wishes. The freedom to wish is absolute and unrestricted; all feelings and fantasies, all thoughts and wishes, all dreams and desires, regardless of content, are accepted, respected, and may be permitted expression through appropriate symbolic means. . . . Overpermissiveness is the allowing of undesirable acts. Permissiveness brings confidence and an increasing capacity to express feelings and thoughts. Overpermissiveness brings anxiety and increasing demands for privileges that cannot be granted (pp. 110–111).

Summary

1. The major conflicts of adulthood as described by Erikson involve *intimacy vs. isolation* and *generativity vs. stagnation.*
2. Mastering these conflicts is illustrated in the process involved in establishing a career, marrying, and becoming a parent.
3. One's occupation is an essential, time-consuming aspect of life that requires a compromise between one's wishes and the circumstances of reality.
4. Many workers are dissatisfied with their jobs. In large measure, job satisfaction is related to the degree to which one's occupation fulfills important personal needs.
5. Vocational counseling is a process through which the client is guided to self-knowledge and is informed about the world of work.
6. Social class has been a factor that has enhanced or limited vocational opportunities.
7. Vocational choices as compromises virtually always leave some powerful motives unsatisfied. Avocations or hobbies are, therefore, utilized to fulfill personal needs that are unmet through a vocation.
8. To see marriage in perspective, it is well to observe it in different cultures as well as in the American middle-class subculture. There are, however, several possible models within these subcultures.
9. Among the factors leading to good marital adjustment one of the outstanding is family background and relationship with parents. Similar or homogamous interests, attitudes, background, and values of the spouses are also very important factors in marital happiness. Furthermore, courtship is a means of testing compatibility, and data show longer engagements are related to more satisfactory marriages.
10. Many specific aspects of sexual relationships do not seem to be related to marital happiness, but the wife's ability to achieve an orgasm does relate to marital adjustment. Methods are available today for the relief of frigidity and impotence.
11. Marriage always involves problems and conflicts and open communication of feelings and attitudes between the husband and wife helps to meet them. Also a problem-solving approach to differences that allows discussion is highly important.
12. Parenthood is related to the need for generativity as described by Erikson.
13. Improved birth control methods and increased concern about overpopulation have led to a tendency to limit the sizes of families on the part of many couples.
14. It is essential that a couple contemplating marriage be fully candid about their attitudes concerning having children.

15. When a marriage is entered into primarily because a child is on the way, its chances for success are generally not good. Unless the couple has a strong, mature relationship they are best advised to avoid marriage.
16. Many couples who plan for their children elect to wait until they have been married for a year or two before having children in order to adjust to each other before taking on the added burden of offspring. Others postpone children to solidify their financial base. No formula is available to guide couples in the determination of the best time for children.
17. Having a child makes numerous demands on a couple. No formal training can prepare a couple to deal best with these demands and no single technique will well suit all parents.
18. The primary task of parenthood is to prepare the child to deal successfully with the various developmental crises lying before him.
19. Ginott stresses the need for parents to recognize and accept all that a child feels and to help him to find appropriate ways to express these feelings. This stance is seen to lead the child to a good sense of identity and personal responsibility for his behavior.

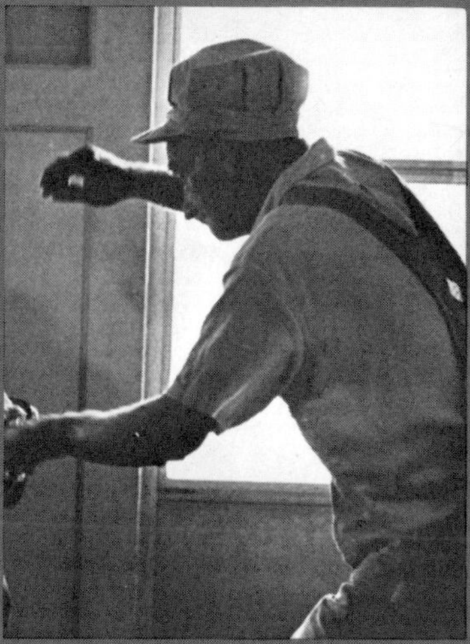

10. Adjustment to Middle Age and the Later Years

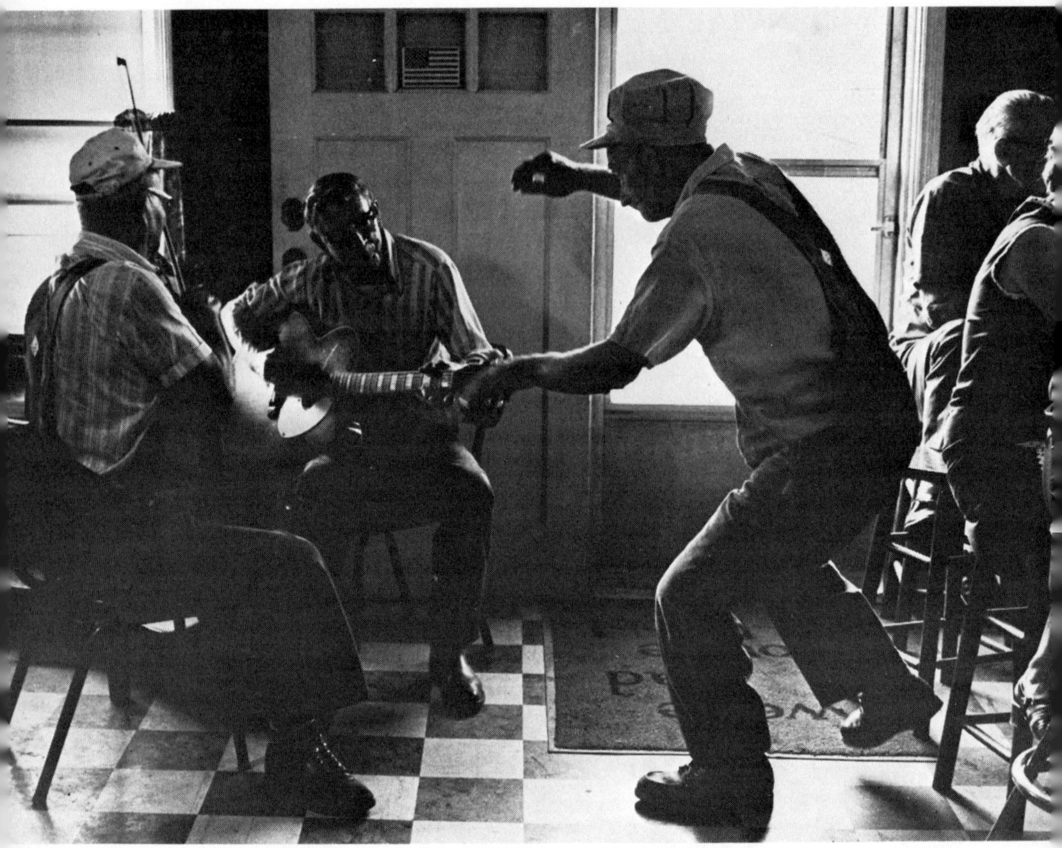

Photo courtesy of *Columbia Missourian*

Objectives

After studying this chapter the reader should be able to:

1. Describe Erikson's developmental task for this stage.
2. Identify the factor of *loss* in adjustment problems faced by the older adult.
3. Compare and contrast the *activity* theory with the disengagement theory in explaining adaptation to old age.
4. Discuss society's view of the elderly and identify some of the potential adjustment problems that this situation presents.

In the various ages of man described by Erikson (1963) the conflict that best typifies what people in their middle and later years face is one described as involving *ego integrity versus despair.* For Erikson the person who achieves ego integrity has the sense that he has taken care of things and people in his lifetime and has managed to adapt to the various successes and failures that characterize anyone's life. Such a person accepts his own life cycle as something that had to be the way it was and faces its end with a sense of completeness and satisfaction. For such an individual, death is confronted as a natural conclusion to what has been a reasonably satisfying process.

The person who fails to achieve ego integration fears death desperately. He has not been able to accept his life cycle and perceives what he has done and been as inadequate and unfinished. He is filled with despair that time has run out on him and much that he would have liked to accomplish will never be achieved. He feels that he has lost his only chance in life and must depart as an unsuccessful and unhappy man. It is helpful for the reader to hold Erikson's characterizations of the basic conflict of later life in mind, as he looks at some of the specific problems faced by man upon reaching middle age and the later years.

Middle Age

Reaching the middle years of life can produce a vast array of problems for people depending on the nature of their earlier adjustment and their particular life circumstances. Clearly one of the problems that occurs during that time of life is the growing awareness that one is getting older and is approaching the last stages of life. Often, this feeling is accompanied by a sense that unachieved ambitions are no longer likely to be accomplished. In one's earlier years, a person is full of dreams about what he wants from life, the kind of successes he hopes to achieve, and the type of family life and community status that he expects to win. For most of us, these dreams are not fully realized. Yet as long as we remain young we can hang onto our dreams and feel secure in the belief that some day they might come true. When a person reaches middle age, he must now begin to face and accept the reality that if youthful ambitions have not yet been accomplished, they are probably not likely to be.

The meaning of this realization in a person's life is likely to vary from individual to individual. A great deal depends on what early goals a person has set for himself and the areas in which his ambitions reside. For example, if he has been striving for abundant material success and professional accomplishment, middle age may be extraordinarily stressful for the person who has not yet reached the top in an occupation where age becomes a penalizing factor. For example, the salesman whose success requires much physical vigor and drive to keep up with the times and to present a good personal front may well find middle age to be a serious problem. He must now fight to overcome his normal tendency to slow down physically. He finds it increasingly difficult to remain current in a fast-changing scene. Most of all, he becomes ever more aware of the pressure of younger colleagues who have the drive he used to have, and who now challenge his hard-won position. Such a person may see his earlier successes fading away, may be frustrated in his efforts to compete with younger men, and may find himself working harder and harder only to fall more and more behind.

In certain occupations people reach their peak effectiveness fairly early in life and then find the decline of the middle years to be extraordinarily stressful. The professional athlete, for example, suffers considerable strain as he grows older when he must give up the fame, material success, and satisfaction of the status brought him by his profession. Many such individuals experience a psychological decline similar to that seen in middle age, only several years before actually becoming middle aged chronologically. Similarly the nuclear physicist ambitious to produce the kind of research that will win him Nobel prize honors may find upon reaching the mid to late thirties that he cannot easily accept the idea that he's not likely to achieve the kind of success that he had hoped for, since a large percentage of physicists who perform work of the highest caliber do so while still in their twenties.

On the other hand, many people work at occupations in which experience allows them to accumulate knowledge that steadily increases their job success and makes them progressively more valuable to employers. For such individuals, middle age is less likely to be threatening unless their ambitions are unrealistically high. The university professor, for example, who, during his long years of experience, accumulates more and more knowledge and an even greater perspective on the important issues in his field, gradually comes to achieve the honors and status of an "elder statesman" and is not seriously penalized by reaching middle age. Likewise, the business executive whose background and experience enhance his value to his firm may accomplish his greatest managerial triumphs during the middle years.

A second problem that arises for most individuals during middle age has to do with events that are beginning to occur within the family circle. As we noted in Chapter 8, late adolescence brings to most people a need to develop an identity of their own and to establish oneself as a mature adult. For most people who marry in their twenties, middle age coincides with the time when their children are beginning to seek such independence. Parents who have devoted a considerable part of their life and energy to generativity begin to find themselves less necessary to their children than they once were. Their need to be needed is no longer being met. This can create serious adjustment problems, particularly for mothers.

Typically the mother in the family has most of her status invested in the role that she plays with her children. In essence, as long as the children are young she is an executive in a very active business which demands considerable time, energy, ingenuity, and attention. Much gratification comes to many women from this role they play with their children. As the youngsters grow older, and begin to leave the family, parents come to feel less significant in their youngsters' lives and lose an important purpose in their own lives. If such a purpose has been paramount for them, considerable psychological reorganization must take place. The difficulty for many women in easily accomplishing the necessary role shifts when parental duties decrease has been one of the underlying stimulants to the current "woman's rights" movements. By providing women with meaningful roles (other than mother) early in their lives, it is felt that the transition that often occurs at middle age will be much easier.

Still another source of stress for the middle-aged person is the fact that his physical powers are beginning to wane and, in many cases, physical attractiveness is also fading. Those who have set great store by their youthful physical manner and their appearance find this fact of middle age particularly difficult to accept. Women, particularly, in our culture often perceive their physical appearance as an extraordinarily important asset in their interpersonal relations. No longer being slim and youthful and the development of facial wrinkles—all of these normal signs of aging may pose a very serious threat. Furthermore, it is at this time of life that women encounter menopause. In addition to feeling that they are becoming less attractive physically, women are also confronted with the loss of their reproductive powers. Whether they wish to have more children or not, this too is extraordinarily threatening, for their personal sense of themselves as women must now be redefined.

While the decline of physical attractiveness and the problem of menopause are particularly acute for many women, men too may experience considerable threat during middle age because of their changing physical state. The professional athlete was mentioned earlier as one who finds his life disrupted to a marked degree because physical changes make him unable to maintain the skills that brought considerable honor and acclaim. Many men who do not aspire to professional athletics, however, also lay great store by their physical youthfulness and ability to compete with younger men on that plane. For such men the middle years are very threatening. On the sexual side, it is not uncommon for men who have been uncertain of their sexual adequacy earlier in life to find the advancing years extraordinarily threatening. They accept the myth that sexual potency decreases with age and begin to assume that they can no longer function adequately in sexual situations. Recent studies by Masters and Johnson (1968), among others, has demonstrated the error of this assumption.

Finally, all who reach the middle years inevitably face a growing awareness that the peak in life is past and that death must ultimately be faced. As Erikson has pointed out, for the individual who has been dissatisfied with the life he has lived, who feels that its direction has not gratified his ambitions and hopes, the prospect of death is very threatening. At some point, the person becomes aware that time is running out and that he has lost his only chance to accomplish the great dreams of youth. For some, this can be overwhelming and lead to serious feelings of sadness and failure.

SERIOUS MALADJUSTMENT TO MIDDLE AGE

Considering the nature of the pressures of the middle years of life, it should not be surprising that many who have serious emotional problems at this time suffer from *depression* (Figure 10–1). This tends to be a time of life characterized by serious losses: one's hopes and dreams; the feeling of being needed by dear ones; and cherished physical powers. Along with this, inevitably, is a loss of self-esteem. It hardly is surprising, therefore, that many who cannot manage to adapt unscathed during middle age become depressed, downhearted, discouraged. Characteristically the depression felt at this time of life is often accompanied by much anxiety associated with anger held fairly close to the surface. Along with feeling downcast such individuals feel resentful at what is happening to them. They feel deserted by a family to which they have devoted themselves. They feel unappreciated by employers for whom they have

Figure 10–1 Middle-Age Depression

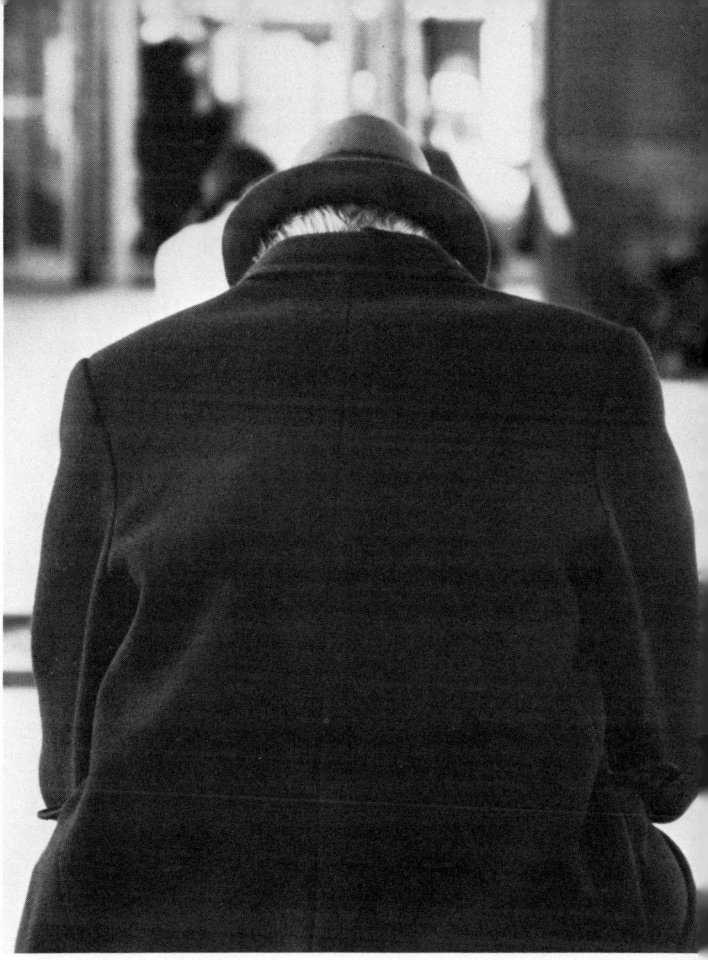

Photo by J. Brian King

worked hard, and they fear rejection by an unfeeling society. The mixture of anger and depression results in agitation, a tendency to be jittery, hyperactive, and tense. This is an extraordinarily uncomfortable state and one in which the danger of suicide is very serious. The sense of loss and powerlessness can be overwhelming, and some people in their attempts to strike back and assert themselves "for one last time," choose to do so through some self-destructive action. Fortunately many such attempts are unsuccessful and do cause important others in the person's life to intensify their contacts and thereby replace some of that which the person senses has been lost.

Also common during middle age is a disturbance characterized by *paranoid* symptoms. In such cases, the individual blames his problems on others whom he sees as the cause of his difficulties. Thus children are accused of having deserted him; fellow workers are accused of plotting against him and thereby causing his work effectiveness to decrease; at times, even the decline in physical powers may be blamed on the food he's eating. As in the case of the person whose disturbance takes a depressed form, much resentment lies quite close to the surface. Both individuals will require some form of professional assistance to aid them to accept their changing role and to express their anger and resentment in more adaptive fashion (Figure 10–2).

MAXIMIZING ADJUSTMENT TO MIDDLE AGE

Clinical experience demonstrates that those who are most susceptible to serious adjustment problems during the middle years have typically lived a relatively narrow life up to that time. Characteristically the woman who develops serious problems has been singlemindedly devoted to her home and family. She had relatively few activities that took her outside of the home and never had a wide circle of friends. The man who finds it most difficult to adjust to the stresses of middle age was, typically, very much tied to his work. He belonged to relatively few organizations or groups and had a narrow social life. For such individuals the many losses associated with middle age are, of course, particularly stressful. In effect, such singlemindedly devoted people tend to lose or are threatened by the loss of everything that they know how to do that provides them with a feeling of worth.

Those who are best able to adapt to the changes experienced during the middle years have had broad interests and are into a variety of activities. Such individuals are assured of self-esteem from many sources and thus can withstand far better the losses associated with the changing physical and social conditions of middle age. Maximizing adaptation to middle age, therefore, requires the early development of a broad spectrum of interests and the willingness to engage in a variety of activities particularly as one grows older. It would preclude investing overly heavily in any involvements that would obviously have to be given up as old age approaches. Parents must anticipate their children's growing independence, and as it emerges they should be acquiring their own interests which give satisfaction and relieve their children of the burden of parents who must dote on them long after they feel the need for it. For many women middle age is an ideal time either to begin a career or to pick up the pieces of what had been a career prior to marriage. Many activities that may have been deferred earlier in life because of the presence of children, insufficient finances, or simply the unwillingness to take the time for them can be successfully carried out by the middle aged. Travel, for example, can be a source of great satisfaction to many who always wanted to do it but never felt that it was a practical thing for a family person.

In summary, the major problem of middle age is withstanding the serious losses experienced in a variety of realms. An adaptive solution

TWO EXAMPLES OF SERIOUS MALADJUSTMENT IN MIDDLE AGE

Karl T., a fifty-six-year-old druggist, voluntarily entered a private mental institution in a large city in the South. Married, and the father of three teen-age children, he had recently retired to live, in upper-middle-class circumstances, off income from investments.

He was born in a small southern town, the sixth in a family of nine children born to German immigrants. His father, an extremely hard-working man, had developed a successful hardware business, and he was described as a very ethical person who made many friends and gained a respected position in the town. Because he spent so much time in his business and because there were so many children in the family, the patient rarely got individual attention from him. Nevertheless, he felt closer to his father than to his mother, whom he described as a frugal, exacting person who worried constantly lest her children fall in with bad company. Although she was a devoted person who cared for the physical needs of her children, she was not warm, and her efforts to divide her attention among the several children resulted in many of the siblings feeling emotionally distant from her. She died about fifteen years before the patient's hospitalization, after a lingering illness. His father, who had remarried, died ten years later.

After high school Karl attended a pharmacy school on the advice of a cousin who pointed out that one could support oneself while attending such a school. After he received his degree he was employed as a druggist in a local store. At the age of thirty-three he married, eventually having three teen-age children. He continued to work for others until the age of forty-two, when he opened his own store and made a great success of the business. His daily routine called for him to work twelve hours a day seven days a week. His only interest other than the store was athletics, and he frequently exercised in the local Y.M.C.A. gymnasium. There he became proficient at squash and was proud of his ability to beat much younger men at this vigorous sport.

Even though Karl was successful in business, and wise in his financial investments, he saw himself as a dependent, insecure person who had always been apprehensive about the future. Perhaps as a result of his insecurity he never felt satisfied if he merely met the requirements of a job, and felt that he must do more than just what was expected of him. He was very reluctant to accept responsibility, and considered it a great accomplishment when he was able to operate his own business so successfully.

About two years before his hospitalization he suffered a fall in which he tore some of the cartilage in his leg, and was then forced to abandon his athletic activities. Eight months before his hospital admission he impulsively sold the pharmacy in order to have more time to relax. Although he still received an adequate income from property investments, Karl found that he was unhappy without his accustomed routine. Symp-

Figure 10–2 From M. Zax and G. Stricker, *Patterns of Psychopathology.* New York: Macmillan Publishing Co., Inc., 1963. Reprinted by permission.

Figure 10–2—continued

toms developed five months before admission to the hospital, when he began to brood over having sold the business. This feeling gradually became more intense, and was accompanied by feelings of guilt. In an effort to dispel these he tried working for others, but this only intensified the depression. He began to have difficulty falling asleep and would awaken at four or five in the morning and pace up and down. His interest in his surroundings waned, and having no appetite, he suffered some loss of weight.

Karl was constantly preoccupied with having sold his store, and he began to feel that he had let his family down and "killed his future." He felt guilty over not having spent more time with his family and accused himself of being impulsive and childish. He refused to dine out with his wife because he felt too inferior to be seen in public. He gave up the hope that he would ever do anything worthwhile again, and his concern lest something happen to his family grew because he felt that he could no longer care for them. When a well-to-do businessman of his acquaintance committed suicide Karl was quite shaken and feared that he might do the same. At this point he saw his family doctor, who recommended hospitalization.

When interviewed after his admission to the hospital Karl presented the picture of a well-developed, neat man who looked younger than his stated age. He was anxious and restless as he talked and intermittently ran his hands through his hair, walked around, sat down, wrung his hands, and twiddled his thumbs. His mood was clearly depressed, and tears came to his eyes as he discussed his mother's death. He was generally friendly and cooperative and well able to reason logically. Orientation, attention, memory, and his grasp of general information were all good. He admitted to sexual impotence, which upset him a great deal during the previous four months, and caused him to worry that he would never be well again. He regretted not having been more attentive to his parents when they were old and alone and worried about the stigma his emotional illness might place on his family.

Karl was hospitalized for approximately one month, during which time he was treated with five electroconvulsive shocks. After the third he was free of all symptoms, but on discharge he was advised to continue psychiatric treatment in order to consolidate the gains made during hospitalization.

Ella D., a fifty-two-year-old woman, was committed to a state mental institution after an attempt at suicide while a patient in a general hospital. She was married but childless, and had never been hospitalized before for any mental disturbance. Her education was limited to grade school, which she completed while in her late teens, indicating that her progress there was slow. After working for several years as a semi-skilled factory worker she married her present husband, at the age of thirty-five. He owned a small business and economically they were of middle-class standing, living in a medium-sized midwestern city.

Figure 10–2—continued

Ella was born in a large midwestern city, the youngest of four children, two of whom had died before she was hospitalized. The only remaining sibling was an older sister. Her mother died when the patient was five and the responsibility for raising the family fell to the father, an immigrant to this country, who had recently died of old age. Raised as a Catholic, Ella lost interest in the Church as an adult, and was married in the Protestant church of her husband. She had always been a seclusive person with a pessimistic outlook on life. She tended to be moody and never had many friends. Her interests seemed centered about sewing and housework. Ella was never interested in raising a family, and it was presumably by choice that she remained childless.

Her symptoms became noticeable about six months after going through menopause and about six to nine months prior to her first hospitalization. At this time Ella became irritable and discontented, expressing the desire to leave the apartment where she was living with her husband, because she feared "things" would be done to her and to her husband. She began to suspect her neighbors and storekeepers and felt they were pointing at her and poking fun at her behind her back. These symptoms subsided briefly but then she began losing interest in her daily activities, neglected household chores and threatened suicide. Shortly before her hospitalization she wandered away from her home and was found by police six hours later wandering the streets of a suburban community. At that time she was confused, disoriented, and expressionless. Her explanation for leaving home was that someone had told her that her husband had left for the army (World War II had just begun) and that she had to get out of her house. She was placed in a general hospital for a few days, and during this time thought and activity were slowed and she seemed to be in a "mental fog." After a few days she tried to strangle herself with a wash cloth, subsequently explaining, "I tried to kill myself to learn when I was born." Shortly thereafter she was committed to the state institution.

Upon examination in that institution Ella was oriented for time and place and both recent and remote memory were good. Despite this she remained somewhat confused and delusional and threatened suicide. She felt people were talking about her and accusing her of having stolen things. She wept frequently and proclaimed that her husband was a wonderful person from whom she wouldn't be parted for the world. Ella made a point of spontaneously denying that she had ever been married or that she had any vile disease. On the ward she was very restless, shouting to an imaginary self and to others through open windows, and obviously misinterpreted occurrences around her. She refused to eat and was negativistic and grossly resistive to ward routine. Ella expressed fear that she would be electrocuted, that people would bury her or that they would put her in a penitentiary. At times she expressed fear that her sister wanted to do away with her and her husband in order to get their property. She insisted that no one could prove such things against

Figure 10–2—continued

her as illegally signing checks. She developed the delusion that a man came into her room one night and that she subsequently heard that same man's name mentioned on the radio.

During a six months' stay in the hospital she gradually became less restless and aggressive, became neat and began to comply with ward routine. At the end of this period she was described as friendly, but not sociable. She was able to recall that she had been very ill and had felt responsible for all of the world's ills at one time. Placed on convalescent care in the custody of her husband, she made a good adjustment for a short while. However, she became actively psychotic once more, and it was necessary that she be returned to the hospital nine months later. During the next fourteen years she was in and out of the hospital three times, managing to maintain herself outside of an institution for only a few months at a time before her earlier symptoms recurred. Eventually she was discharged and to date, three years since, has not returned.

to this problem is to minimize these losses by living a broad life full of satisfactions from a variety of sources. In such cases the losses that are inevitable represent only a minor portion of the total life satisfactions and are unlikely to damage the personality seriously.

The Later Years and Retirement

As pointed out, middle age is a time in life when most men and women become aware of a discrepancy between what they felt they wanted out of life and the way in which they are living (Figure 10–3). This represents a crisis in which the individual in a sense must decide whether to stagnate or to grow. He has two alternatives: he can try to continue his customary life style by reinterpreting his goals; or he can change his behavior in an effort to accomplish his earlier-held aims. The manner in which he deals with this mid-life crisis is looked upon by some (Lowenthal, 1972) as a significant sign of how he will deal with the adaptations required still later in his life when retirement and the inevitable physical decline associated with aging must be faced. At such a time, many forces over which the individual has no control require a reorientation of life's goals.

BIOLOGICAL AND SOCIAL FACTORS ASSOCIATED WITH AGING

All living species go through a somewhat similar biological cycle. At birth an era of growth and development of physical abilities begins that culminates in a period of maturation when one is at one's peak followed by a stable plateaulike period in which decline is relatively slight.

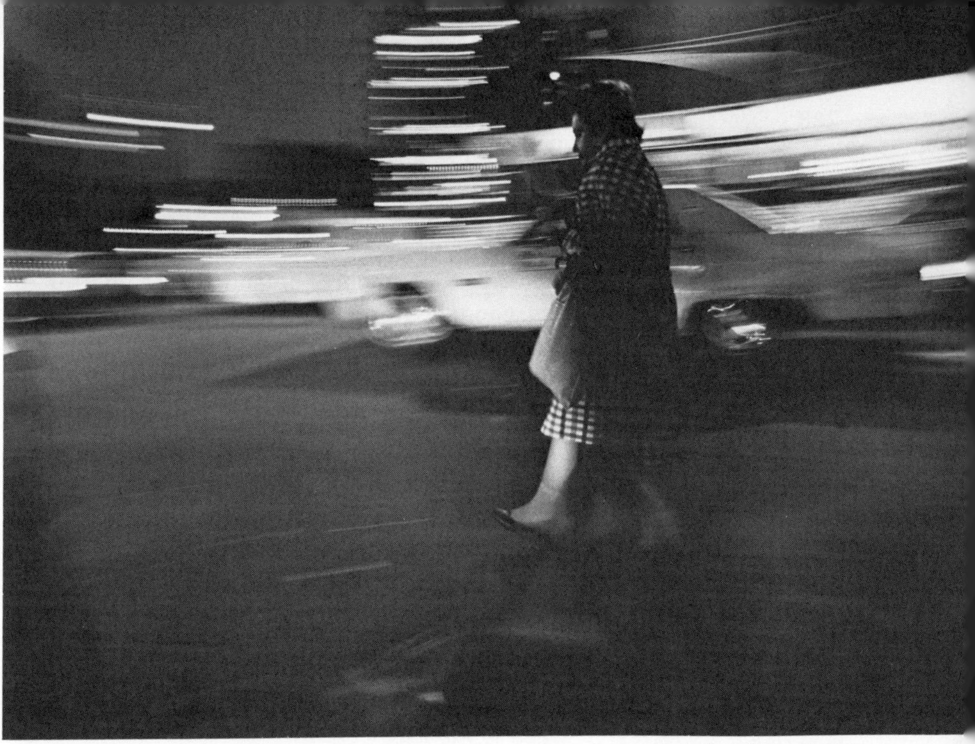

Photo by J. Brian King

Figure 10–3 A Busy World Passing By.

Decline gradually accelerates and eventually death occurs. Variations occur between species with respect to the exact shape of the curve of rise, peak, and decline, and for humans the plateau period has probably been greatly extended during the past 50 years due to an increase in knowledge about man's physiology and the accompanying advances in the medical sciences.

Man's physiological decline results in the reduction of many of his physical capacities. Advancing old age is associated with a slowing of reaction time, impairment of memory, particularly for recent events, and increased difficulty in learning new material. Many of these decrements are associated with subtle changes taking place in brain functioning. These changes can involve the collection of deposits in blood vessels which impede the efficient flow of blood or they may involve the actual atrophy of brain tissue. While cells in most parts of the body are constantly regenerating, brain cells do not do so, thus those lost during life are gone forever. Only later in life do losses associated with aging affect behavior. In extreme cases the elderly may become senile and are very confused and incapable of caring for themselves.

In many respects society creates institutions in accord with man's biological cycle. For example, children and adolescents are protected during the years of growth and development, when they have not yet reached their full productive capacity, in order that they may maximize their potential upon reaching maturity. Thus we have laws regulating child labor, and requiring minimal amounts of schooling. Retirement is another social institution developed to protect society and to ensure maximum output from its members. Retirement is intended to allow for the replacement of workers by younger workers who are functioning at the peak of their efficiency in a way which minimally disrupts the productive process as a result of the growing infirmity of older workers. Cost factors are also very important here. As the worker grows older, he is more subject to disruptive illness and potential accidents. Thus, taken from the viewpoint of the overall functioning of a society, mandatory retirement at a particular time in life seems to be an efficient procedure to ensure the society's smooth and effective functioning.

On the other hand, what seems like a sensible and necessary process of worker replacement turns out to be far from an efficient one because men vary so widely with respect to where they are in the biological cycle. Retirement at a particular time in life would be most efficient if all men were to decline at a particular age and would decline at the same rate. This is very far from the truth and, as a result, enforced retirement can lead to the waste of extraordinary talent as well as the creation of costly social problems with respect to many retirees. Further complicating the issue is the fact that people in different occupations reach their peaks at different times in life. Mathematicians and physicists are thought to reach their peak while in their 20's; musicians are thought to be at their best in their late 20's and early 30's; behavioral scientists and architects are thought to function at their zenith while in their late 40's. In many occupations the accumulation of experience over a period of many years may well help one to approach the peak of his productive powers relatively late in his life.

THE MEANING OF RETIREMENT

The term "retirement" may be used in a number of different ways. One of the more common ways of using it refers to a man's economic condition. From this viewpoint, the person who is retired has been removed from the labor force or works so few hours per week that his contributions are negligible. The term also refers to an event—that period in life when one leaves behind him the responsibilities of work. The psychologist sees this particular event as one that ushers in a very critical life period, one in which a crisis is experienced and where some special kind of adjustment is required. Sussman (1972) points out that retirement, the act of removing a person from society's work system, takes away from the individual a number of the roles that he had served and reduces his status in many others. For example, the income reduction requires that he live in a different way from what he could afford earlier. On the other hand, retirement can carry with it the connotation that many roles in life sectors outside the work system are continued. This is an important point, since retirement may well feel like an anticlimax for a person who has been an active, useful, productive citizen, and the retiree may well see himself as consigned to the anteroom of death's chamber.

PROBLEMS BROUGHT ON BY RETIREMENT

One of the most obvious problems introduced by retirement is an economic one. In giving up work the retiree must depend on his income from some source other than the job that has supported him for much of his life. In effect, there are a limited number of such sources. The family of the retiree is one possibility. The federal government, through social security is another, along with whatever retirement income the individual may have been able to develop through personal savings or contributions to some pension plan. Another potential source of income is through what the retiree may be able to earn in various part-time jobs. In their survey, Havighurst and Albrecht (1953) indicate that families are the least reliable income source for retirees and that personal earnings was the largest single source of income for the older people they surveyed. More recent studies may show that pension plans and government support programs for the elderly prevail to a greater degree than was the case in the early fifties, but the economic problem remains a serious one for the retiree. Pensions may suffice in a stable economy but become totally inadequate in an economy that is showing a great deal of inflation. Furthermore medical costs have risen dramatically and can be extraordinarily damaging to the economics of an older person who is more likely to need considerable medical care at that time in his life than during his younger years.

The economic problems of retirement are, of course, more serious for those in the lower socioeconomic classes. Medical costs for the lower classes are likely to be no less than for the very wealthy, and similarly the upper and lower classes will pay the same for the necessities of life. On the other hand, the low socioeconomic classes are likely to be living on relatively low pensions involving fixed incomes whose value shrinks in an inflationary economy. Furthermore, Belbin (1972) points out that retirement rates are inversely related to occupational status. Thus, the occupational groups having the lowest retirement rates include professionals, managers, and farmers. The occupational groups with the highest retirement rates are service workers, craftsmen, and foremen. Apparently those in high-status occupations are in a position to control when they will enter retirement and often choose to delay. Those in low-status occupations are more likely to have retirement forced upon them.

The economic handicaps of living as a retiree are, therefore, most severe for the groups that are most likely to have the least to say about the timing of their own retirement.

Modern society affords man a vast array of options concerning how he will live his life. He has wide choice with respect to his participation in political and social activities. There are a variety of organizations he can choose to belong to or avoid. He can become a part of a vast array of reference groups. For most people such options are limited only by their social position and their own psychological and personality attributes. Different options are open to different subgroups within the society and to some extent certain groups, defined by racial and ethnic factors, may suffer greater limitations than other members of society. Within these constraints, however, man can choose the role that he'll play in a variety of life sectors.

When a person retires, he is challenged to retain as many options as possible and to resist the tendency to drift back into a social role resembling that of a child. Several factors can play a significant role in determining how well he resists this regression. The physical losses that characterize aging certainly is one of these factors. Inevitably as one becomes older and grows disabled, his options in life are reduced. A previously used example of the professional football player who is forced to retire while only 30 or 35 is a good example of one whose options are constricted as the result of biological changes. In the elderly the physical changes are more profound and impose far more dramatic limitations on the individual. In the extreme case of the senile individual, virtually all options are closed off and there is no choice but to revert to the dependency of childhood.

A second factor that places limits on life's options is the geographical location of the individual. Climate, the availability of needed services such as places to shop, and places where medical care can be provided are related to the place where one lives. Furthermore opportunities for access to religious, recreational, social, and welfare facilities also fall into this category.

A third factor that relates to the degree to which the retiree, and particularly the elderly, remain in a position to choose among life's options is the government under which he lives. Inevitably many retirees must depend on government assistance to look after their most fundamental needs. When this is done, the elderly have available more options than in cases where they are not properly cared for by society. When a man is secure in his income, and his expectation that his health needs will be cared for, he has considerable freedom to exercise a variety of options. Clearly the trend in modern society has been toward erecting society-wide economic supports for the elderly.

Finally, a fourth and most significant factor related to the degree to which the retiree maintains options concerning his life are the values and expectations of society concerning what his role ought to be. Such values exercise a broad influence over the individual. They guide him in directions he thinks he ought to take and prevent him from taking directions he might otherwise take. Those who willingly accept such value orientations try to harmonize their behavior in keeping with them, and behavior ultimately depends on their perception of these values. These values are found with respect to a variety of life sectors. With respect to work, the retiree is expected to be a good sport and not to resist giving up his job. He is expected to stop being a producer and to become a consumer exclusively. This message is contradicted by values in other areas which suggest that the retiree ought to "do his own thing" independent of family, friends, and other of society's groups.

Another important human need that is threatened by retirement is the feeling of self-respect that assures one he has worth as a person. It is also important for most people to feel that they have some social responsibility. The anticlimactic nature of retirement and the not uncommonly negative attitudes that people have about the role the retiree should play tend to shunt the older person aside and rob him of a sense of self-worth and make him feel that he is no longer needed by his society. Having accumulated a lifetime of experience, most men would like to feel that his fellows respect what he has accomplished and perhaps even need to communicate with him in order to benefit from his background. This feeling does not diminish when a man retires. Yet when the society in which a man lives no longer sees him as being potentially useful, he suffers serious damage to his self respect.

Belbin (1972) has pointed out that intellectual and other abilities decline with age and to some degree are associated with physiological changes. However, the decline in abilities does not proceed at the same time rate as the decline in physiological functions. Decline in abilities is often offset by various compensatory mechanisms and the transfer of skills from some physiological systems to others. What is noticeable, however, is that decline in functional ability is closely related to the roles assigned to the aged in a particular society and the attitudes of its members toward the retired. In those societies where retirement takes place fairly early in life and where the aged are pushed aside and expected to stay clearly out of the mainstream of the society's functioning, the aged display more extreme characteristics of aging than is the case in societies where retirement occurs later in life. Thus, even the reaction to physiological changes which are common to all who become older is in great measure determined by the roles assigned to the retiree and by the attitudes of members of society toward them.

Another problem confronting the older person is that often he experiences a gradual decline with respect to his sexual activity. Because the elderly expect or are led to expect this decline to take place, many become "sexual dropouts" long before it is physiologically necessary that this must occur. For many the loss of this aspect of their functioning becomes a source of unhappiness. Again, it should be underscored that this decline is less the result of the physical aging process than it is a set of attitudes pervading society which leads the elderly to expect that sexual behavior will simply no longer be part of their later life.

While certain regularities exist with respect to the physiological changes that occur among aging men and women, the effects of such changes on the sexual responsiveness of the aged are by no means entirely a function of physiology. For example, Masters and Johnson (1968, p. 269) point out with respect to the menopausal woman that "endocrine starvation has an indirect influence upon, but certainly not absolute control over, female sexual capacity or performance. Steroid starvation also has an indirect influence upon the female sex drive. However, sex drive is but one in the total of physical and psychosocial factors influenced by the aging process." These researchers indicate that if endocrine changes were alone responsible for the character of the sexual behavior of the woman who has passed through the menopause, all women should respond in much the same way to the gradual diminution of sex hormones. Such regularity of response among different women is not found. In fact, within the same individual, differences in total response are found as a function of life experience.

Among men, Masters and Johnson (1968) indicate that there is little question but that some waning of sexual responsiveness occurs with age. However, they question again whether this diminished responsiveness is solely a function of physiological factors. The aging male cannot run or walk as fast as he could when he was 20 or 30 years younger. He cannot lift and carry as heavy a weight as he was once capable of. In the same respect, the aging process does have some limiting effects on his sexual capacity. It tends to take the older man more time to acquire an erection and to reach a climax. His ejaculation is more sparse and he experiences fewer genital spasms. Before he can have another erection, it takes a longer time than was the case when he was younger. While such changes are common to most men as they grow older, they do not invariably detract from the pleasure that the aging male experiences from intercourse.

It seems that the sexual behavior and responsiveness of the older person is heavily related in important ways to a variety of psychological and environmental factors. The psychological factors include, quite prominently, the attitudes that the individual has had concerning sex throughout his lifetime. For example, the person who has always questioned his or her adequacy in this area probably looks to the menopause or the climacteric as an excuse for giving up an activity with which he or she has never been comfortable. Another psychological factor related to the sexual activity of the older person would be the set of expectations that he or she builds up with respect to what their sexual behavior ought to be as they grow older. Our society, for example, tends to show relatively little acceptance of the notion that an older person should have a full, active sexual life. In essence, despite the openness about sex with respect to younger people, a Victorian prudishness characterizes attitudes toward the sexual side of the aging person's life. To be a "dirty young man" is a mark of some distinction, whereas to be a "dirty old man" is reason for disapproval. As a society we simply tend to believe that as people grow older their sexual functions should be given up. The combination of such a set of expectations plus the physiological slowing that takes place with aging in both men and women is often sufficient cause for a reduction in sexual activities and at times for giving them up completely.

Among the environmental factors that have bearing on the sexual responsiveness of the aging person is, most prominently, simply the matter of opportunity for continuous sexual contact. When an older woman is widowed, she often finds little opportunity for acquiring another partner with whom to share her sexual life. Usually the problem is somewhat less acute for the aging male because he can be more active in seeking out partners and because younger women are frequently more willing to engage in sexual behavior with an older man, whereas the reverse is less often the case.

In still other ways our society's puritanical attitude toward sexuality among the aged inhibits sexual functioning among older people. Homes for the aged, for example, as well as nursing homes, provide little opportunity for aging men and women to be together privately. Living arrangements provided for older people in such institutions assume that a sexual life will no longer be part of the older person's functioning. Not uncommonly when evidence of such a drive manifests itself in the aged, it is regarded as a sign of aberration. A recent article on sex and the senior citizen (Lobsenz, 1974) points out that in some institutions men and women are forbidden to watch television together in the late evening, and such rules apply even to married couples who happen to be living in the same institution.

Despite the social and psychological barriers to a rich and continuing sexual life among the aged, the few surveys that have been done to assess the nature of the sexual activity of older people indicate that a significant percentage both remain interested in a sex life and manage to maintain one. Kinsey, for example, found that 4 out of 5 men above the age of 60 were capable of intercourse and that women displayed no evidence of a sexual decline until much later than that age. One study has provided evidence that 15 percent of men and women showed an increasing rate of sexual interest as they got older. Lobsenz (1974) summarizes the findings of a long-range study of sexuality among the aged done at Duke University to indicate that 2 out of 3 men beyond the age of 65 remain sexually active and that one out of 5 is still active while in his 80's. Even in cases where activity has declined, interest remains, as evidenced by the fact that half of the 80- and 90-year-olds in this study indicated a moderate degree of interest in sex. For women, the frequency of sexual contact during the later years is lower than for men. While in their 60's about 1 in 3 indicate sexual interest and only 1 in 5 are actually having sexual contacts. Among older women, however, the interest rates and the activity rates do not decline as age increases. Apparently the lower activity rate for women in this age group is accounted for by the lack of an available partner, or at least a partner who would be acceptable to women who may be relucant to engage in nonmarital sex.

Masters and Johnson conclude from their studies and from their review of other studies of sex among the aged that there is no physiological reason why the rate of sexual contact for the young woman should not be maintained in the postmenopausal years so long as the individual remains healthy, active, and well adjusted. For the aging male, Masters and Johnson feel that the single most important factor in determining whether effective sexual expression will remain is the consistency of an active sex life. Those men who have been stimulated to a high degree of sexual activity when they were in their formative years and have carried this through middle age seem consistently to maintain their high level of sexual functioning as they grow older. This applies no matter what manner of sexual expression has been followed. Furthermore, Masters and Johnson feel that the aging male who has developed a sense of sexual inadequacy in the later years need not resign himself to a sexless existence. They feel that the male over 50 years of age can be treated successfully in a high percentage of cases to revive a dormant sex life. They also conclude that if a man is in reasonably good health he can maintain an adequate sexual performance well into the 70's or 80's.

Adjustment to Retirement

Two prominent theories have been advanced with respect to the issue of how one adapts optimally to aging (Havighurst, Neugarten, & Tobin, 1968). These theories are based on the observation that as people move from middle age to old age they become less active and they interact less with other individuals. The two theories for explaining these behavioral changes may be called the *activity theory* and the *disengagement theory.*

Basic to the notion of activity theory is the idea that the psychological and social needs of the older person are much the same as those of the middle-aged individual. The reason his interaction with others tends to diminish as he grows older is because society withdraws from him, for the most part against his wishes. To adjust optimally to this situation, the person must resist the loss of social ties that he once had by remaining active as he grows older (Figure 10–4). This is managed by maintaining the activities that were typical of his middle-age life as long as possible and by finding substitutes for these activities when he is absolutely forced to give them up. When retirement is imposed on him, he must find substitutes to replace the work activity he was engaged in. When friends and loved ones die, he must find other people to replace them. Thus, from this point of view, maximum adjustment is achieved in old age by actively resisting the loss of important social and psychological ties that had been held earlier in life.

Disengagement theory, on the other hand, holds that the observed decrease in social interaction is a mutual process in which society and the aging individual withdraw from each other with the older person ac-

Figure 10–4 Maintaining Social Ties.

Photo by J. Brian King

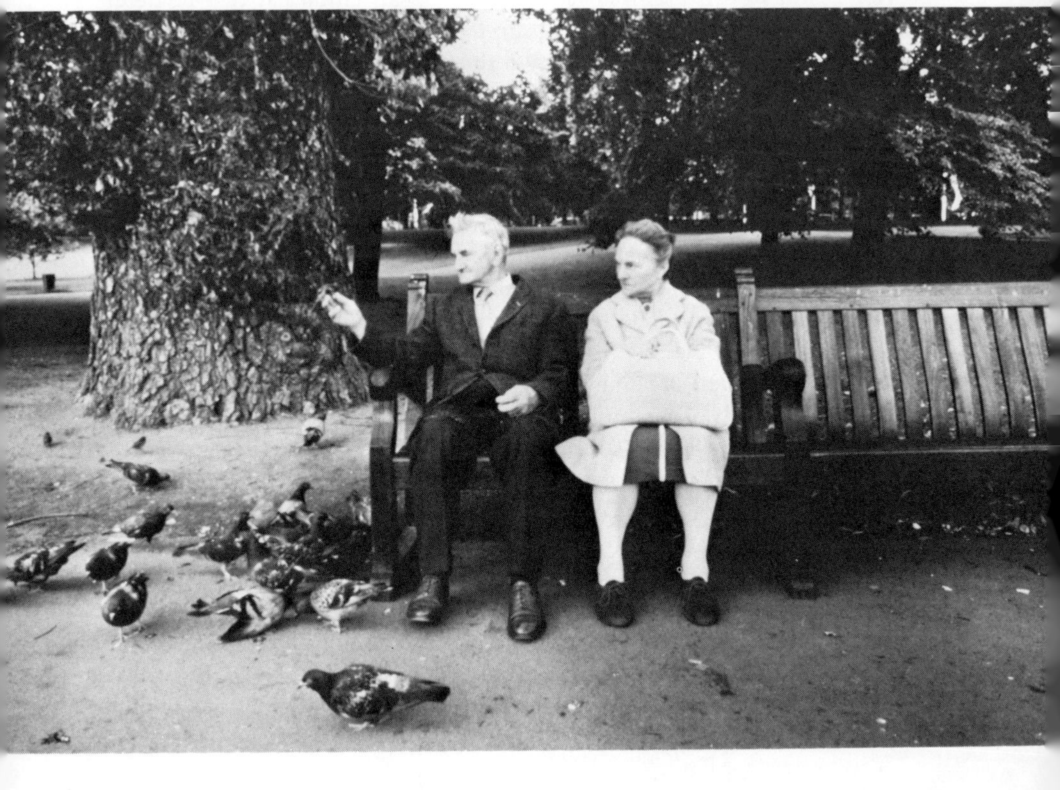

cepting this decrease in contact willingly. For the most part the decrease is even thought to be desirable for the aging individual. Social withdrawal from this point of view occurs along with or may even be preceded by a tendency to become self-preoccupied and to invest less intensely in the people and the objects that had once been important. Thus disengagement is simply part of a natural process that all people experience as they grow older. From this point of view, maximal adjustment is achieved by the individual who manages a psychological equilibrium characterized by different kinds of relationships from those that he knew when he was younger and ones that involve more psychological distance and greater insularity than was characteristic in the earlier part of his life.

As Havighurst, Neugarten, and Tobin (1968) point out, both of these theories imply certain basic values. Activity theory assumes that, at least in our society, activity is preferable to inactivity and maintaining a life-style that characterizes middle age is superior to adopting a new way of life in old age. Disengagement theory assumes that one is better off living in a state of equilibrium rather than disequilibrium and bowing gracefully to a process that is considered "natural."

Since there is a fairly clear-cut contradiction between these two points of view, it has been possible to put them to an empirical test to determine which is more valid. Havighurst et al. (1968) have done such a study and found that each of the two theories seems to have some merit. The longitudinal data of these authors indicate that a process of disengagement does indeed occur. Over a five-year period, the age groups studied showed a decline in ego energy and in various measures of role activity. It was also found that the psychological process of disengagement tended to precede the decrease in social role activity by about 10 years. Thus subjects in their 50's showed a high degree of psychological disengagement, whereas those in their 60's and 70's were high in social disengagement theory. The fact that the disengagement does occur supports the theory. The fact that psychological disengagement precedes social disengagement is somewhat contradictory, since the theory would imply that the two occur mutually.

A second finding lends support to the activity theory. This was the indication that a measure of satisfaction with life actually increased as their subjects grew older. Furthermore those who were engaged in the greatest amount of activity reflected the highest degree of life's satisfaction. In addition, however, these findings seem to be in part related to the personality characteristics of subjects. Those individuals who have well-integrated personalities showed a great deal of satisfaction in life whether or not they were active, whereas those who were poorly integrated tended to be low on the measure of life's satisfaction whether they were active or not.

The upshot of these findings seems to be that neither of these two theories can successfully explain good adjustment among the aged in the absence of some consideration of personality styles. For some, the business of remaining active and substituting new roles for old ones that must be abandoned seems the most feasible response to aging (Figure 10–5). For others, there may well be a mutuality in the process of disengagement.

In a recent book Kimmel (1974) has pointed to another significant variable with respect to adjustment to aging. This involves the importance of having a "confidant." Kimmel points out that a recent study has found that it is particularly important for the older person to have an intimate relationship with someone in whom one can confide problems. Such a confidant serves as a "buffer" against the losses that are inevitably experienced by the older person. As a result, those having such a stable intimate relationship were found to be less likely to become depressed at the fact that they are interacting with fewer people as they grow older and that they are losing considerable status. Even significant losses such as being widowed and having to retire seem more bearable for those who have such an intimate relationship.

The individual character of the various types of adjustment to old age which are suggested by the theories and experiments cited above is elaborated on by Lowenthal (1972). She points out that the process of adaptation to retirement is a relatively easy one for those working people whose life goals and behavior have been heavily invested in nonwork activities. When retirement does come, such individuals can look toward the period that follows as a better opportunity to fulfill what have always been important goals, since they are at last freed of the burden of a job. For such individuals work has been necessary only to provide their basic livelihood needs. It has not been a primary aim in and of itself. Thus retirement is a blessing rather than a burden.

On the other hand, the person who has derived most of his important pleasure and feelings of success and status in life from his work will be enormously threatened by the prospect of retirement. It may not be possible for such a person to elevate nonwork goals to the same level of importance as his work had held. He may not be able to alter the behavioral style that suited his job very well but is not particularly adaptive to other kinds of activities. For such a person the process of adapting to retirement is extraordinarily difficult and when retirement is forced upon him he may suffer physical illness or clinical depression. Likewise, a person who has used his work as a means of protecting himself from becoming close to other people may find retirement a serious trauma if it should expose him to close relationships with others. Some individuals whose important goals have been work oriented may function in a profession in which full retirement is not required and thereby may find it

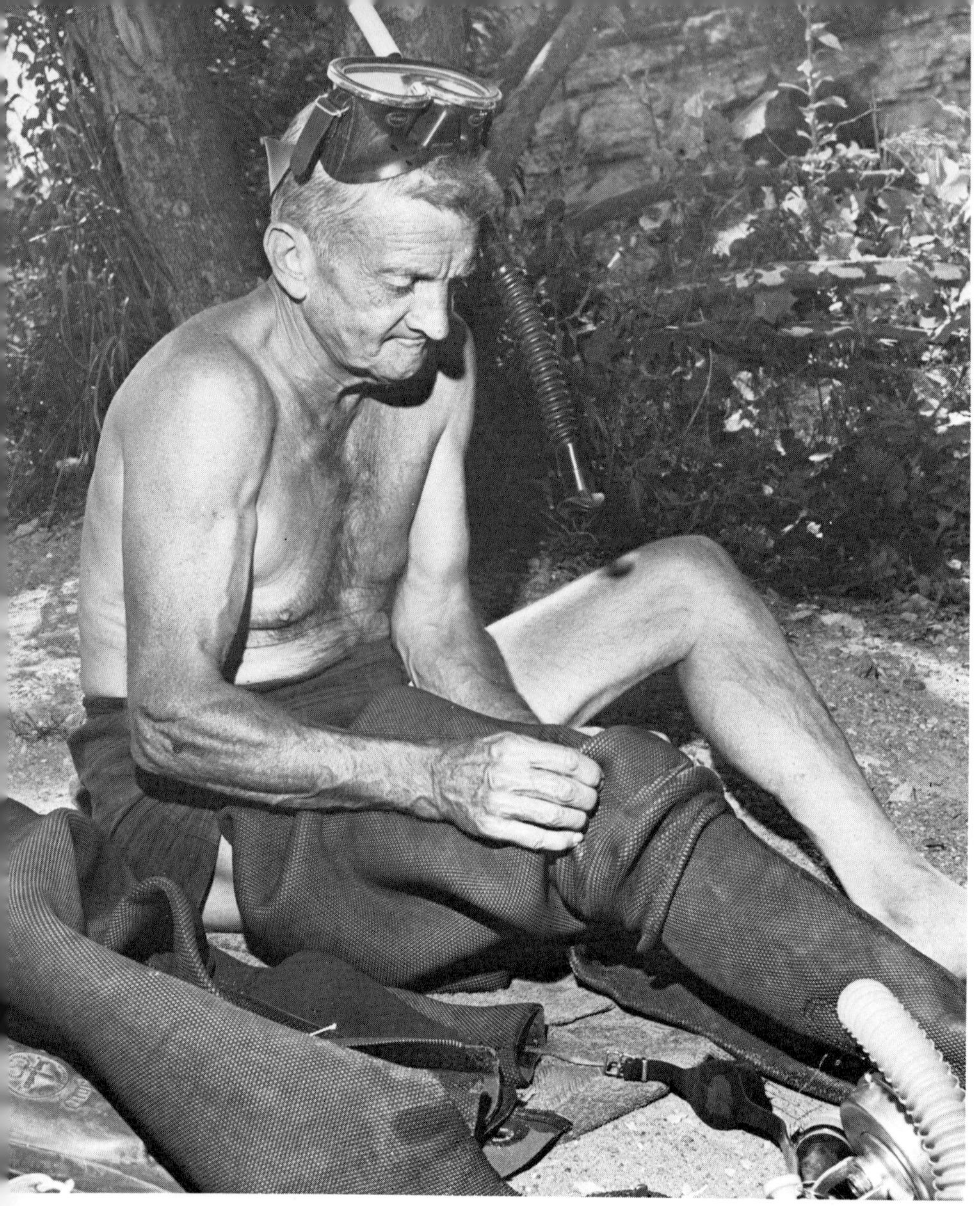

Photo courtesy of *Columbia Missourian*

Figure 10–5 Time for a New Activity.

easy to adapt to the process of aging. The writer for example can often proceed at his own pace and continue to work well into the late years of his life. Likewise, many individuals in professions can continue to be useful in a work way despite the fact that they are very old.

Belbin (1972) accepts the idea that there are two basic modes of dealing with retirement: disengagement and remaining active. For those who disengage, a routine way of life is sought, and the individual learns to restrict his environment greatly so that his behavior depends heavily on old learning. He avoids new learning and consequently suffers some loss in perceptual discrimination. This is a process that may speed up irreversible physiological deterioration. The success of such an approach will depend on the previous personality of the individual and the degree to which his environment supports this kind of adaptation. The second typical pattern that Belbin speaks of involves remaining active and attempting to reorganize one's life-style by adopting new interests and maintaining a capacity for learning. Such an approach is likely to typify the individual whose preretirement style has been of this sort.

The success of an active strategy in dealing with retirement is seen to depend on the availability of an opportunity to reorganize one's life, a willingness to take advantage of such opportunities, and the capacity to respond appropriately when such opportunities arise in the environment. Belbin suggests a number of options for the retiree who wishes to maintain a high level of activity even though he is growing older and has dropped out of the work force. One such option is beginning a new career. To be successful at this, people should have skills from earlier careers which are relatively easily transferred. For example, the previously successful businessman may be able to set up a very small-scale enterprise that will meet his needs for something useful to do without being overly taxing. Some individuals who have maintained an intellectual curiosity through life may in retirement find the time to take up a new subject and to become thoroughly versed in an area about which they have had curiosity but not the time to be anything more than a dilettante. Another possibility is to use previously learned occupational skills in new settings. For example, retirees may be extraordinarily useful in Peace Corps activities where their skills may be needed in underdeveloped societies. Another possibility is to engage in part-time work. One tested example involving this approach is for firms to create "communal workshops" for retirees. In such cases, those who have retired from a firm are used in part-time jobs to do repairs or to be available in case of emergencies. Retirees can fill in on temporary jobs or in some instances have been permitted to market their own products. Another type of activity for the retiree involves participation in new types of social groups such as retirement clubs.

In all of the examples of activities that the retired person may engage in, it is necessary that society adopt attitudes and help to create institutions that can facilitate the retiree's taking on a new set of activities. Furthermore there is great need for society to become more sensitive to the adjustment problems of the retiree and review the entire retirement process from several different points of view. Doubtless such attitudinal changes could achieve much with respect to meeting the social needs of retirees who have, by and large, been ignored up to now.

Carp (1972) makes the very cogent point that when our society thinks about growth and development it tends to focus its interest on childhood and adolescence. Certainly those stages that extend beyond the achievement of maturity are not seen as periods during which development continues to take place. Growth is a process that is seen to occur only in those life periods during which some sort of increase is clearly noted, and the term is not used for those life phases beyond the stages of youth and adolescence because one doesn't expect any increment to take place and, in fact, losses of various abilities seem to predominate.

Carp points out that this may be a very naive view of the whole process of development. Whether an increment or a decrement of some kind is most prominent at any point in life probably depends on what aspects of behavior one is choosing to observe. And often we tend to study what is easy to see or to measure rather than take the trouble to develop the techniques for investigating what is important. Thus the idea that only the earliest phases of life are characterized by growth and development and only the later ones are typified by deterioration and decrement may be greatly oversimplified. What seems to be more to the point is that the process of development always involves losses as well as gains throughout the course of life. Psychological development, for example, requires giving up many old habits as well as the acquisition of new ones. In fact, the child who fails to give up old habits is seen to be "fixated" or immature. Early ways of perceiving the world and reacting to it are replaced by new ones that are more appropriate to the particular stage of the child's life. The youngster who continues to value food above all other things, who persists in needing to have immediate gratification, and who remains entirely self-interested does not grow psychologically. To achieve such growth, he must begin to see value in objects other than food. He must be able to put up with a certain degree of discomfort for a period of time, and he must learn the satisfaction of helping others if he is to become mature.

Going further, Carp indicates that we have a rather clear picture of what development ought to be like from conception through adolescence. Consistently the popular point of view looks to the future, and at every point the individual is required to give up old ways of behaving and accept new ones. However, for those stages of life extending beyond adulthood we have little conception of individual life stages and have done relatively little thinking about them. The older person has no notion of what he ought to behave like and is unclear about the standards that will be used to judge his behavior. The one thing that seems clear is that there is a general expectation that he will decline. This negative expectation probably arises because there are no good age-appropriate standards for the elderly and also because there is a tendency to apply the standards used with younger people when evaluating behaviors of the older adult. Those over 50 tend often to look back on the early years of their adult life as "the good old days." On the other hand, it is possible to regard the period of the early to middle 50's as the potentially most rewarding time of life. It is at this time that a person has finished raising his children and has met most of the responsibilities associated with them. He has probably also become materially comfortable, so that he is in a position to provide himself with many of the pleasures that he may have valued most earlier in his life but never allowed himself to have. If one takes this point of view, life's best time occurs during the 50's and perhaps even the subsequent years when, in many ways, the fewest changes will be experienced. From this point of view, middle age and retirement would not be looked to as a prelude to the end, but as a period to look forward to when potential fulfillment is possible. If such a hopeful and optimistic view is taken about the period of life when retirement normally takes place, it is entirely possible that many important public policy changes could be brought about, as suggested by Butler (1972), both to help society to better meet the retiree's needs and to gain some real advantages for society from what the retiree is capable of contributing.

Butler points out that estimates of the gross national product in the United States by 1985 indicate a per capita rise from a little over $3000 to almost $6000 dollars even taking into account population increases. The significance of this figure is that society will be faced with several choices concerning human activity. Under such circumstances considerably less need for work will be experienced, making possible choices between a 22-hour work week, a 27-week work year, the placement of a significant proportion of the population in education programs, or even retirement at as early an age as 38. In effect, the needs of the economy as well as of the individual will require a redistribution of education, work, and leisure throughout the life cycle. The nature of this redistribution needs to be based on far better information than is presently available.

Up to now retirement has been adopted in industrial and postindustrial societies in order to minimize the disruption occurring through the death of the elderly. In effect, society attempts to avoid being dependent on those who are a high death risk by disengaging from them. This disengagement has until now been timed rather arbitrarily. The possibility of a more flexible approach to retirement has not been seriously entertained because the information we would need to support such a system is not available. It might also be argued that retirement is a system that protects society from outmoded policies, outdated skills and ideas. However, in many respects, retirement is not applied in those instances where the most might be at stake with respect to these issues. Many individuals who make the most critical decisions, even concerning matters of life and death, are not forced to retire in our society. For example, physicians, politicians, Supreme Court justices, and the like, are not required to retire at some arbitrary time in life.

In keeping with Butler's projections concerning the economic state of this country and as well as in keeping with the more optimistic view of the value of the aging and retired individual, it is probably vitally important that our society reorganize itself in such a way that the economic, leisure, educational, and psychological needs of the older person and the retired individual be better met. Butler feels that life's practical realities require that our society improve on income provisions for the retiree so that he can feel a sense of economic security, be housed decently, and have access to high-quality health care. Having such basics satisfied will make possible adaptation in a variety of other realms. With respect to the area of leisure, Butler indicates that public education is necessary to train people to use their free time to enhance their sensibilities toward other people, the arts, and the very process of learning itself. This sense of leisure should probably begin in childhood in order to sensitize the individual to become receptive both to his own inner life as well as to stimulation from outside. In the area of education, Butler feels that colleges and universities must expand opportunities for education throughout the life process. Important goals for such programs would be retraining, providing opportunity to learn new careers and new skills, and preparing people for meaningful leisure pursuits.

In order to avoid the sense of uselessness which often plagues the older person, meaningful roles must be developed for the elderly by matching their skills with the needs of the particular community in which they live. Such matching might be accomplished by local councils that maintain registries of retired people and their skills, and are also in touch with the community's needs so that useful skills of the elderly can be applied in meaningful ways. Such a program need not necessarily be restricted to older people because many who are in the earlier stages of the life cycle can also benefit from such an approach.

Summary

1. In the middle and later years of life the individual struggles with a conflict between ego integrity and despair as described by Erikson.
2. The nature of the problems faced in middle age are a function of one's overall adjustment to life as well as the general life circumstances under which he lives. Virtually all must deal with the awareness that he is growing older and that life's ambitions are not likely to be entirely fulfilled, with the gradual breaking up of the family as children grow up, marry, and move away, with the physical decline

that characterizes aging, and with the growing awareness that death is approaching.

3. At a time when a variety of serious losses are experienced, serious maladjustment to middle age often takes the form of depression along with considerable anger and agitation. Another common maladjustment involves paranoid symptomatology.
4. Those who tend to be most seriously maladjusted in middle age have led a relatively cloistered life, singlemindedly devoted to the people and activities that are being lost in middle age. Optimal adjustment to middle age tends to be achieved by those who find satisfaction and esteem in a variety of activities and interpersonal contacts.
5. The later years of life, usually associated with retirement, are characterized by a gradually progressive physical decline. Retirement is instituted by society as a means of protecting itself and of ensuring maximum output from its members. When retirement is enforced on the basis of some arbitrary age limit, it turns out to be an inefficient practice because of the wide variability among individuals with respect to biological cycles.
6. Retirement creates a variety of problems for individuals including economic problems, a reduction in the options concerning the types of activities he might engage in, and a set of negative expectations on the part of the society in which he lives concerning what his role ought to be. All of these factors are extraordinarily demanding on one's sense of self-respect.
7. Two prominent theories are advanced to explain how optimal adaptation to adjustment takes place: activity theory and disengagement theory. Studies devoted to assessing the validity of these theories indicate that each has some utility in explaining good adjustment to the later years but probably as a function of the personality of the particular individual.
8. The aged and the retired have a variety of social needs that are not well satisfied, given the current set of social attitudes concerning the aged. Our whole outlook on the later years of life tends to be a negative one in which only decline and death are regarded as significant, with the positive features of this phase of life being totally ignored.

Words to Remember

Activity Theory
Depression
Despair
Disengagement Theory
Ego Integrity
Menopause
Paranoia

Part III
Problems in Adjustment: Atypical Behavior

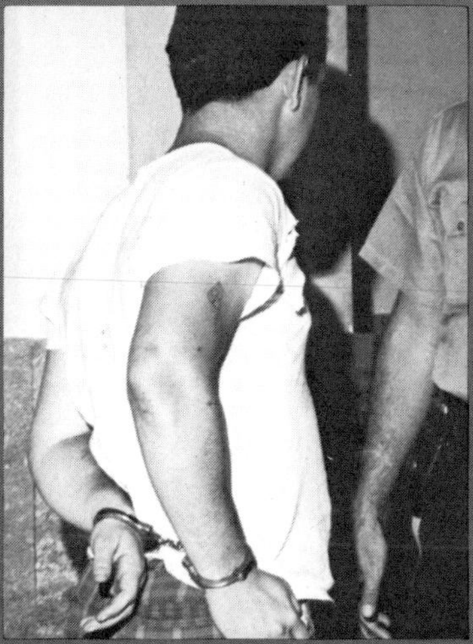

11. Personality Disorders

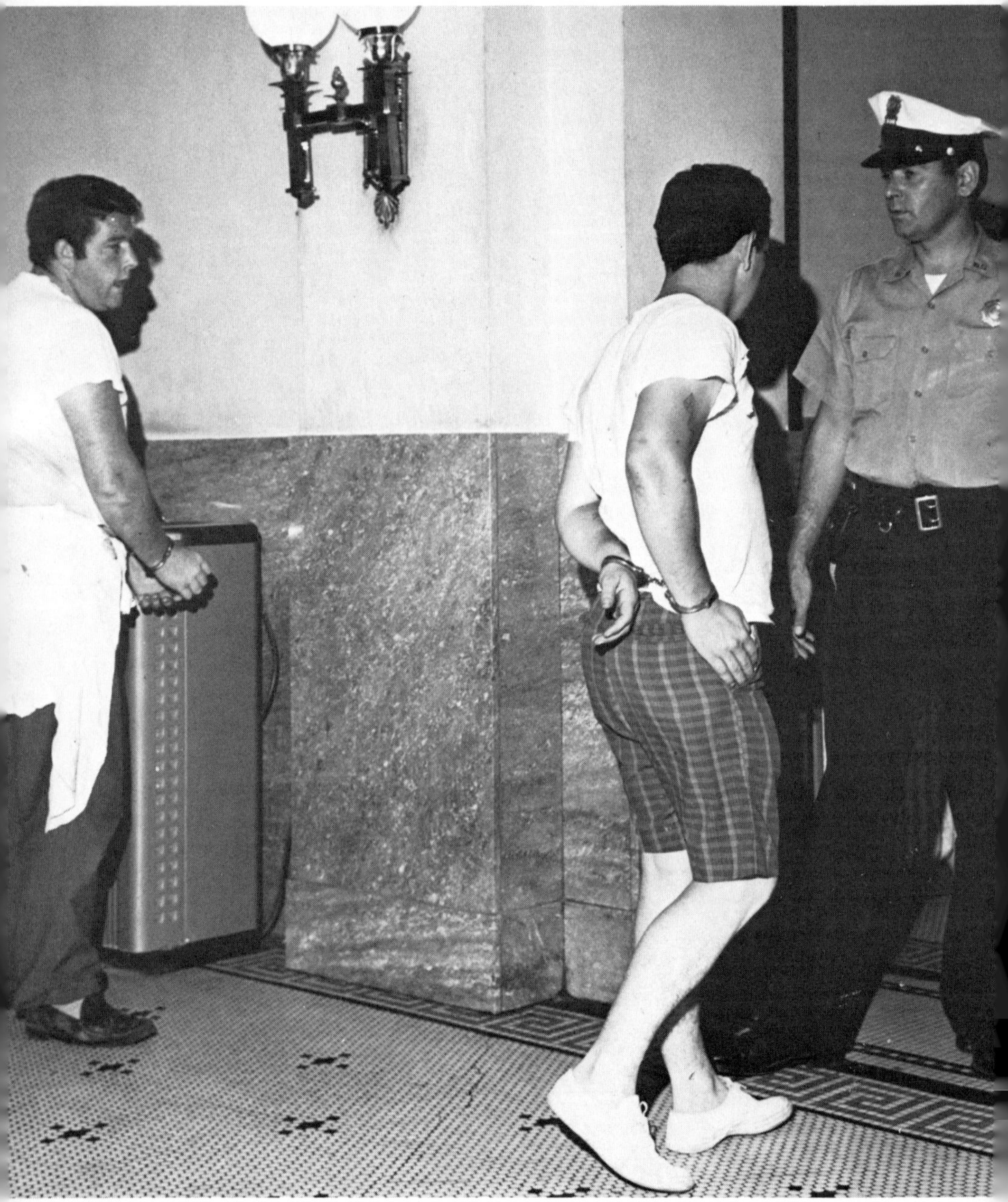

Photo courtesy of *Columbia Missourian*

Objectives

After studying this chapter the reader should be able to:

1. Define *personality disorder.*
2. Discuss addiction in terms of both the physical effects and the psychological effects.
3. Discuss the effects of *set* and *setting* on drug use and abuse.
4. List three categories of drinking behavior and describe the four stages in the development of alcoholism.
5. Describe psychopathic personality in terms of behavioral patterns and discuss treatment and rehabilitation programs for the psychopath.

The diagnosis of personality disorder is very widely used with outpatients at mental health clinics. Most of the behavior that falls within this category is far less dramatic in nature than are the psychoses or the psychoneuroses. Typically such behavior is, of course, less disabling than a psychosis, but it may be equally as disruptive to one's life as a psychoneurosis.

Basically a personality disorder involves long-standing behavioral patterns which the individual believes reflect his "personality," rather than a special problem in adjustment that has recently begun to trouble him. For that reason the person suffering a personality disorder typically does not see himself as being "sick" or terribly distressed. If he does realize his difficulty, he suffers from a dull ache rather than from the sharp pain that typifies the psychoneurotic disorder. For example, the schizoid personality may regard himself as being a naturally shy, withdrawn, somewhat seclusive person; the passive-aggressive personality may see himself as naturally a somewhat dependent individual who likes to have others make decisions for him; and the compulsive personality sees himself as simply being a "fussbudget" who is, by nature, very meticulous and careful about details and needs to order his life in a very precise and specific way. Such individuals do not generally see these characterological traits as being serious problems to themselves. At times, however, these personal qualities become a serious problem for the people living around them and for this reason the individual may seek treatment.

A person with a personality disorder is not greatly dissatisfied with himself and is less well motivated to change his behavior than is the psychoneurotic suffering from extreme anxiety or from the inconvenient behaviors he uses to avoid anxiety. Many who suffer from personality disorders are more similar to the normal personality than either psychotics or psychoneurotics.

We will consider two types of general personality disorders that involve dramatically deviant behavior. Like other personality disorders, however, these behaviors are not seen by the person who engages in them as being terribly onerous or anxiety producing in and of themselves. Referred to here are certain addictions and various kinds of antisocial behaviors. Typically the addict or the antisocial personality is more distressed by the reactions of other members of society to their behavior than they are to the fact that they use alcohol or drugs to excess or that they disregard the rules of the society in which they live. Both classes of behavior will be considered separately.

Addictions

In the literal sense, "addiction" refers to a habitual tendency to desire to do or use something. Oftentimes, we describe someone as addicted to his work, to a hobby, to televised football, or even to peanuts. In such cases we are referring to the observation that the particular person seems unable to limit himself with respect to some behavior; once he begins, it seems as if he cannot stop. Such addictions, while fairly common and at times the basis of personal or interpersonal problems, have received relatively little attention from mental health professionals. Concern with the development and consequences of addictive behavior has focused much more intensively upon the effects of prolonged use of chemical substances to achieve some altered psychological state.

Addictions to chemical substances are much more common than is generally assumed. Every day, large segments of the "normal" population regularly consume caffeine, tobacco, and alcohol. Many people in our culture use a variety of prescription and nonprescription drugs to reduce the discomforts of assorted physical and mental conditions. We are concerned in this chapter with the effects addictions have upon psychological adjustment and hence shall focus upon those substances *whose regular use has been of some concern to mental health professionals.* In discussing addictions, we shall consider the consequences of continued use of a substance in terms of both physiological and psychological consequences.

Addiction, in the physiological sense, refers to an alteration of the biochemical state of the body following prolonged use of a substance. This chemical alteration of bodily processes produces a state of *physical dependence* in which continued use of the substance is necessary to maintain an internal equilibrium. Once dependence is established, any attempt to return suddenly to the original nonuse status will result in the experience of *withdrawal* or *the abstinence syndrome.* While the severity varies with the substance used, withdrawal is an illness that occurs as the body strives to establish a new chemical balance. The typical abstinence syndrome includes fatigue, loss of appetite, nausea, hot and cold flashes, and increases in blood pressure. A person undergoing such as experience is often restless, irritable, unable to sleep, and feels a strong craving for whatever chemical substance he has been using. As his body gradually becomes accustomed to no longer having that substance, these symptoms decrease and a degree of physiological balance is regained. Yet another sign that a particular substance is physically addictive is the development of *tolerance.* As the addict continues to use the substance, the effects of a given dose gradually diminishes. It becomes necessary to use more of the drug in order to obtain the originally experienced alteration in one's physiological state and to avoid the onset of withdrawal. In summary, we define a substance as *physically addictive* if three conditions are met: dependency, tolerance, and withdrawal.

Addictions, however, are not limited to substances that produce physical dependency. Although not leading to tolerance or withdrawal, some substances have been found to produce habituation or *psychological dependencies* in people. Once regular use has been established, the addict feels a very strong craving or desire for the substance and becomes restless, irritable, anxious, and uncomfortable until he meets that need. As will be seen, both physical and psychological dependencies can result in significant problems in adjustment.

DRUGS AND PERSONALITY

Definitions of what constitutes a drug vary as a function of who is making the definition and what aspects of the drug effects are being emphasized. Physicians, for example, are concerned with drugs in terms of their potential for treating or diagnosing illnesses without producing undesirable side effects. More popularly a drug might be defined as a chemical substance that has a profound effect on mood, perception, or consciousness and can potentially be misused to the detriment of society. Considering the wide range of substances that have come into use in recent years, the broadest possible definition of the term *drug* is probably the most useful. Such a definition might be "any substance that by its chemical nature alters structure or function in the living organism" (Nowlis, 1969, p. 5). This allows one to consider the use of various substances that have been accepted by society over a period of many years such as alcohol and tobacco as well as some that have come into very recent use such as banana skins and glue.

Our attention here will be mainly on the drugs that have attracted those of college age, with some discussion of the youth drug subculture. This subject is a controversial one, even among professionals. Interest in the effects of drugs on behavior and experience dates back to the early days of scientific psychology. Primitive men discovered the powers of mind-altering drugs, and as societies matured and trade routes developed, the use of drugs spread from their place of origin to other parts of the world. Cohen (1968) reminds us that opium was used by gifted, prominent Englishmen during the nineteenth century. In the United States around the turn of the century, "laughing gas" or nitrous oxide, chloroform, and ether were used by members of the academic community. William James described his experiences with the inhalation of nitrous oxide and ether. Present-day experimentation with drugs is novel only in that many young people, often from privileged families, are engaged in it. A small percentage become a part of the drug subculture; some, because of an initial instability, become so seriously disturbed that they require professional help. Drug use, however, is not synonymous with drug abuse or addiction.

CLASSIFICATION OF DRUGS

It is not definitely known to what extent the widespread prescription of medications by some physicians for treating emotional difficulties has influenced the use of drugs among people in the United States. It is suspected, however, that significant numbers experience negative psychological consequences as a result of abusing legally obtained medications. Jarvik (1967), in classifying drugs used in the treatment of mentally ill persons, sets up four categories of those most frequently used (see table on pages 313 to 317).

Following Jarvik's classification, *psychogenics* are those drugs that produce changes in mood, thinking, and behavior. The term "psychological states" involves delusions and distorted perceptions. Other terms are used, such as "psychedelic" or "mind altering." Some of these drugs have been used experimentally by psychotherapists, but it is too early to generalize about their therapeutic values. One rather well-known drug in this category is lysergic acid diethylamide (LSD); another is marijuana, which is usually smoked and is more widely used than the others in the category. They are all classified as physically nonaddictive, but may, with continued use, lead to psychological dependence.

A secondary category of drugs is the *stimulants,* which produce an elevated mood, increased confidence and alertness, and reduced or delayed fatigue. In general they are physically addictive. On this list is benzedrine, which is widely used. In addition to caffeine and nicotine, which are mild in effect, the amphetamines are also stimulants. Amphetamines, sometimes called "uppers" as opposed to tranquilizers or "downers," are prescribed by physicians to elevate mood, increase alertness, and reduce feelings of fatigue. Large doses lead to hallucinations, disorientation, and paranoid states (Griffith, 1966). "Speed" is the name given to amphetamines (especially methedrine) by members of the drug subculture when the drug is injected intravenously. It both attracts and frightens members of the subculture as evidenced by the commonly heard catchphrase, "Speed kills." The drug can produce significant negative side effects including potential genetic abnormalities in the offspring of its users, severe personality changes, and possible psychotic reactions (Lemere, 1966).

A third drug category is the *sedatives.* They are, in general, depressants in low doses and hypnotics in large doses. They have been used to treat emotional stress, insomnia, and anxiety. Alcohol, potassium bromide, and phenobarbital, which are in this category, are all widely used. All are ingested, and all but the bromides are physically addictive.

A fourth category is *analgesics* or *narcotics.* Of the various drugs in this category, those that have gained the most notoriety are the derivatives of opium—morphine and heroin. Heroin was, until recent years, used most frequently by the lower social classes. Its use has now moved into all classes and age groups. It is injected and is highly addictive. Following injection of a "fix," the effect is euphoria and contentment, accompanied by a reduction of sex desire and initiative. As tolerance increases and withdrawal becomes a problem, the addict's life becomes centered on acquiring the drug at all costs. This compulsion forces the addict to commit crimes—petty or great—to get the large amounts of money necessary to obtain the drug. For the addict the drug is an escape from the social conditions of his environment and from society's demands for achievement. Currently the majority of users are teenagers and young adults, in part because the death rate for long-term users is extremely high.

Cocaine is another drug falling into this general classification. In our culture it was originally used medically as a local anesthetic and saw some illicit use at the turn of the century. In recent years it has reappeared on the drug scene, where it is called "snow" or, when mixed with heroin, "speedball." In large doses it is a violent stimulant and euphoriant that provokes hallucinations. The body does not develop tolerance for it, but depression occurs as the drug effect wanes.

Below is a table that summarizes and expands information given above.

Major Drugs Most Often Abused *

Morphine (an opium derivative)
Pharmacologic classification Central nervous system depressant
Controls Narcotic (per Harrison Act, 1914)
Medical use To relieve pain

* Adapted from Dept. of Defense, U.S. Government Printing Office. *Drug Abuse; Game Without Winners*, 1968.

Potential for physical dependence Yes
Potential for psychological dependence Yes
Tolerance Yes
Possible effects when abused Drowsiness or stupor, pinpoint pupils
How taken when abused Orally or by injection
Comments Morphine is the standard against which other narcotic analgesics are compared. Legally available on prescription only.

Heroin (a morphine derivative)
Pharmacologic classification Depressant
Controls Narcotic (per Harrison Act, 1914)
Medical use To relieve pain
Potential for physical dependence Yes
Potential for psychological dependence Yes
Tolerance Yes
Possible effects when abused Same as morphine
How taken when abused Sniffed or by injection
Comments Not legally available in United States. Used medically in some countries for relief of pain.

Codeine (an opium derivative)
Pharmacologic classification Depressant
Controls Narcotic (per Harrison Act, 1914)
Medical use To relieve pain and coughing
Potential for physical dependence Yes
Potential for psychological dependence Yes
Tolerance Yes
Possible effects when abused Drowsiness, pinpoint pupils
How taken when abused Orally (usually as cough syrup)
Comments Preparations containing specified minimal amounts of codeine are classified as "exempt" narcotics and can be obtained without prescription in some states.

Paregoric (preparation containing opium)
Pharmacologic classification Depressant
Controls Narcotic (per Harrison Act, 1914)
Medical use For sedation and to counteract diarrhea
Potential for physical dependence Yes
Potential for psychological dependence Yes
Tolerance Yes
Possible effects when abused Same as morphine
How taken when abused Orally or by injection
Comments Paregoric is often boiled to concentrate narcotic content prior to injection. Classified as an exempt narcotic. In some states may be obtained without prescription.

Merperidine (synthetic morphinelike drug)
Pharmacologic classification Depressant

Controls Narcotic (brought under Harrison Act in 1944)
Medical use To relieve pain
Potential for physical dependence Yes
Potential for psychological dependence Yes
Tolerance Yes
Possible effects when abused Similar to morphine, except that at higher doses, excitation, tremors, and convulsions occur
How taken when abused Orally or by injection
Comments Shorter acting than morphine. Frequent dosing required. Withdrawal symptoms appear quickly. Prescription only.

Methadone (synthetic morphinelike drug)
Pharmacologic classification Depressant
Controls Narcotic (a 1953 amendment to the Harrison Act brought drugs like methadone under control)
Medical use To relieve pain
Potential for physical dependence Yes
Potential for psychological dependence Yes
Tolerance Yes
Possible effects when abused Same as morphine
How taken when abused Orally or by injection
Comments Longer acting than morphine. Withdrawal symptoms develop more slowly, are less intense and more prolonged. Prescription only.

Cocaine
Pharmacologic classification Central nervous system stimulant
Controls Narcotic (per Harrison Act, 1914)
Medical use Local anesthetic
Potential for physical dependence No
Potential for psychological dependence Yes
Tolerance No
Possible effects when abused Extreme excitation, tremors, hallucinations
How taken when abused Sniffed or by injection
Comments Although cocaine does not have the narcotic properties of morphine, it has been classified as a narcotic by law because its abuse potential necessitates the same stringent control measures.

Marijuana
Pharmacologic classification Hallucinogen
Controls Narcotic (per Marijuana Tax Act, 1937, plus subsequent restrictive legislation which covered marijuana and narcotics together)
Medical use None
Potential for physical dependence No
Potential for psychological dependence Yes
Tolerance No
Possible effects when abused Drowsiness or excitability, dilated pupils, talkativeness, laughter, hallucinations
How taken when abused Smoked or orally

Comments From a legal control standpoint, marijuana is treated as a narcotic. It is almost never legally available in the United States.

Barbiturates (e.g., amobarbital, pentobarbital, secobarbital)
Pharmacologic classification Depressant
Controls Controlled drug products (per Drug Abuse Control Amendments, 1965)
Medical use For sedation, sleep-producing, epilepsy, high blood pressure
Potential for physical dependence Yes
Potential for psychological dependence Yes
Tolerance Yes
Possible effects when abused Drowsiness, staggering, slurred speech
How taken when abused Orally or by injection
Comments Prescription only. Original prescription expires after 6 months. Only 5 refills permitted within this period. Dependence generally occurs only with the use of high doses for a protracted period of time.

Amphetamine drugs (e.g., amphetamine, dextroamphetamine, methamphetamine—also known as desoxyephedrine)
Pharmacologic classification Stimulant
Controls Controlled drug products (per Drug Abuse Control Amendments, 1965. Methamphetamine added to list of controlled drugs in May, 1966.)
Medical use For mild depression, anti-appetite, narcolepsy
Potential for physical dependence No
Potential for psychological dependence Yes
Tolerance Yes
Possible effects when abused Excitation, dilated pupils, tremors, talkativeness, hallucinations
How taken when abused Orally or by injection
Comments Prescription only. Original prescription expires after 6 months. Only 5 refills permitted within this period.

LSD (also mescaline [peyote], psilocybin, DMT)
Pharmacologic classification Hallucinogen
Controls (Brought under Drug Abuse Control Amendments in September, 1966)
Medical use (Medical research only)
Potential for physical dependence No
Potential for psychological dependence Yes
Tolerance Yes
Possible effects when abused Excitation, hallucinations, rambling speech
How taken when abused Orally or by injection
Comments In 1966, LSD was brought under the control of Drug Abuse Control Amendments of 1965. Control under one of the International Narcotics Conventions is being considered. Not legally available except for medical research.

Glue (also paint thinner, lighter fluid)
Pharmacologic classification Depressant
Controls No federal controls. Glue sales restricted in some states.
Medical use None
Potential for physical dependence Unknown
Potential for psychological dependence Yes
Tolerance Yes
Possible effects when abused Staggering, drowsiness, slurred speech, stupor
How taken when abused Inhaled
Comments Freely available as commercial products, except that some states have laws forbidding the sale of glue to persons under 18.

Aspects of Drug Effects

SET, SETTING, AND PERSONALITY

Experimenters have long been aware that factors other than the drug chemical action influence the objective—to say nothing of the subjective—reactions to drugs. One of these factors in the person's *set* as he uses the drug. *Set* refers to the individual's expectations of what a particular drug will do for him. Personality organization is one of many influences on set; recent experiences also produce certain expectations about what a drug's effect will be. One person smokes a marijuana "joint" and feels only drowsiness or nausea, while another experiences a pleasant distortion in his sense of time and space. At this point in the book, you know that individuals differ greatly in their emotional stability, personality integration, or ego strength—to use several terms that refer to the same characteristic—and these differences account partly for the wide variety of drug effects reported by drug users.

Setting refers to the total physical and social environment in which drugs are taken. The laboratory, with all of its controls and scientific aura, has a very different meaning to the person taking a drug than does a darkened, smoky room filled with friends and loud music. For this reason alone laboratory drug effects differ from those in real-life situations.

The use of marijuana, barbiturates, amphetamines, and LSD (the drugs most frequently used by young people) has caused great alarm among conventional members of society. This alarm, according to those who have considerable knowledge of the effects of these drugs, seems out of proportion, especially if their use and effects are compared, for example, with the known frequency of use and negative consequences of regular use of alcohol and cigarettes. It is estimated that acute alcoholics number in the millions (6,500,000) in this country, and the Surgeon

General's Office, as well as numerous scientific laboratories, have established the dangers of acquiring certain forms of cancer following continued tobacco use. Moody (1969), in *Christianity and Crisis,* points out that the harsh legal penalties for the possession of marijuana, a nonaddictive drug, can bring a noncriminal person into direct and potentially long-term contacts with criminals and thus present more serious social dangers than the drug itself. Health scientists decry the punitive and severely legalistic posture toward all drug use when it is at the expense of rehabilitative efforts.

The reason for the inconsistency in public reaction between the acceptability of alcohol and cigarettes as compared to drugs is understandable in part, given the current state of misinformation about the drugs with which young people experiment. Also, it must be recognized that the frequency and acceptance with which cigarettes and alcohol are used in socially prestigious circles and their contribution to the national economy contribute significantly to their continued legitimacy. In addition, the association of drugs with people who dress unconventionally and who protest conspicuously against our present society damages the reputation of young users in the eyes of the conventional and politically powerful majority. Another less emotional reason is that many strongly addictive substances, such as opium and its derivative heroin, were not thought to be addictive when they first came into use but were eventually found to cause serious social problems.

The "tasters" are those who try marijuana or LSD in their search for new experiences. They differ from the "heads," the more committed drug experimenters who use drugs as part of their general pattern of life. Keniston (1966) points out that the tasters and heads must be separated from the addicts, whose lives are dominated by drugs. Some experimenters apparently become bored with the drug subculture and reenter the mainstream of American life, although hard data on what happens to such individuals are not available. Some, without condemning apparently nonaddictive drugs, band together to educate others about the dangers of using hard drugs.

EXPERIMENTS ON MARIJUANA

Carefully conducted experiments on the effects of marijuana on human beings are very rare. The voluminous literature on the use of this drug consists largely of anecdotes, uncontrolled observations, and secondhand accounts. It includes reports on drug use in other countries where the *set* and *setting* are widely different from an American community.

One carefully controlled experiment used as subjects nine 21- to 26-year-old males who smoked marijuana under pleasant laboratory conditions (Weil, Zinberg, & Nelson, 1968). A placebo containing ingredients that had no drug effect was also given to the subjects. During the session neither the subjects nor the experimenters knew whether the marijuana or the placebo was being smoked, an important control absent from most previous research with marijuana.

Both physical and psychological effects of the drug were recorded. Pupil size, blood sugar levels, and respiratory rates were observed. Following marijuana use, subjects showed a moderate increase in heart rate, with no effect on pupil size, blood sugar level, or respiratory rate; thus, very little physical effect was found in this experiment. After intoxication, the subjects' time sense was significantly slowed. Five minutes seemed more like 10 or 12 minutes. The authors conclude from the results on their small sample of subjects that in terms of medical danger marijuana appears to be a relatively harmless intoxicant.

Several intellectual and psychomotor tests were used on the subjects, who had never previously tried marijuana. The results indicated minimal subjective reactions in these pleasant settings, despite the fact that the doses were high enough to make the whites of the subjects' eyes turn red. The experimenters concluded that the usual doses of marijuana do not impair a user's ability to perform competently tasks of ordinary complexity. Higher-than-usual doses in novice smokers might be expected, from these results, to cause decrements in performance. Other studies have, however, shown significant impairment in subjects' ability to drive an automobile under the influence of that drug. The long-range effects of continual use of the drug have not been measured and are at present unknown.

In another aspect of this research eight heavy marijuana users were tested only on high doses. The effects on the regular users were qualitatively different, as reported below. These differences indicate the influence which previous experience (probably in special settings) has on the drug effect (Figure 11–1). It seems that the marijuana high is a more subtle and subjectively determined experience than alcoholic intoxication. The drug itself has no general stimulating or depressive effect on the nervous system. The only way the experimenters knew the subjects were high was from their descriptions of their feelings.

When the heavy-user subjects were encouraged to talk, before they smoked marijuana they told of past events; after smoking, more of their discussion was about events occurring in their immediate environment. These statements resembled free association more than everyday logical speech and their images were more dreamlike than usual. Clearly, however, the debate on the merits or evils of marijuana should focus on its long-range social and psychiatric effects, for which there are at present no hard data.

Young people often raise the question of whether marijuana is as dangerous in our culture as alcohol. The definitive answer to this ques-

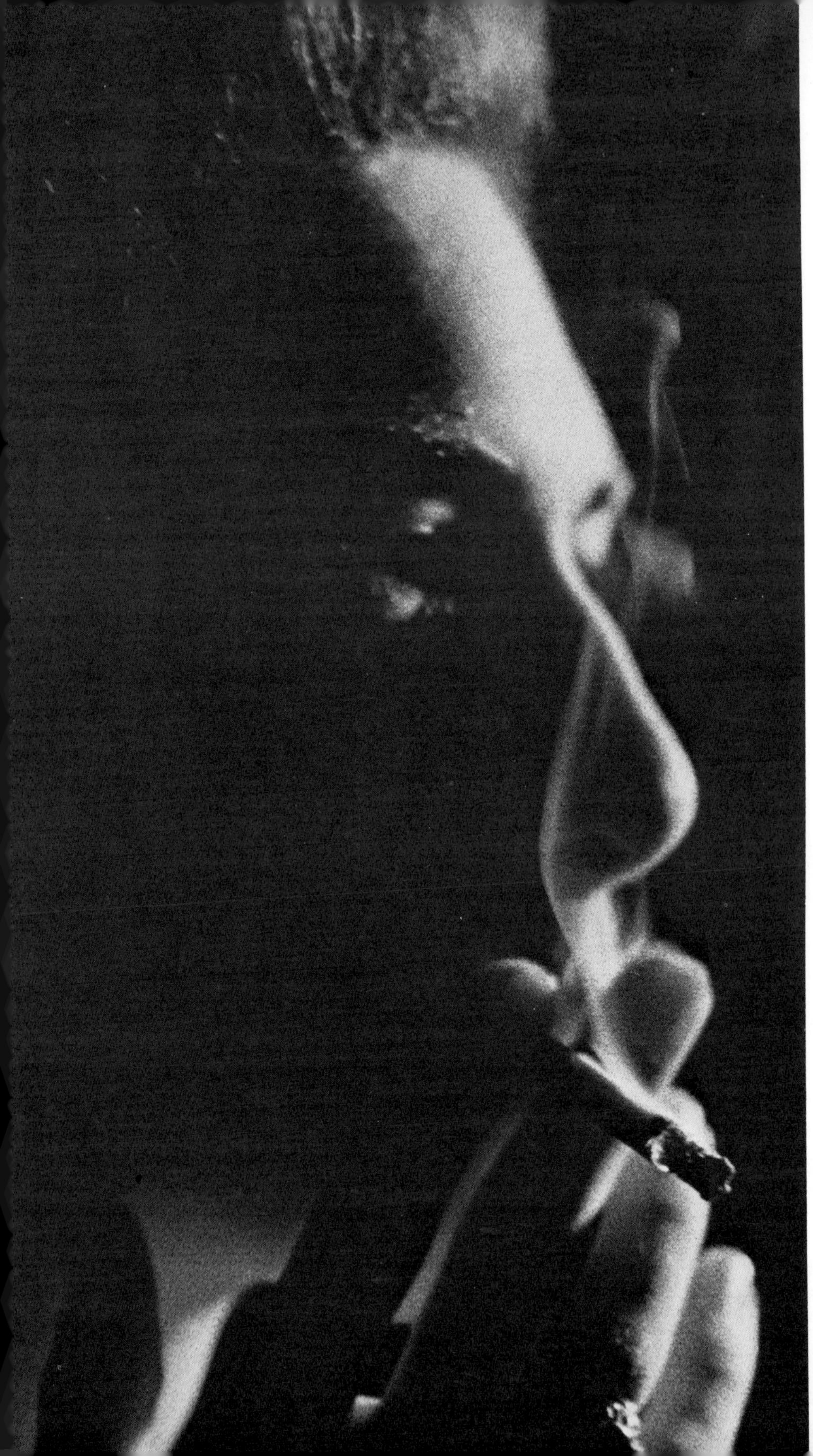

tion will require extensive research. Some such studies are now in progress. One such researcher, Grinspoon (1969), in his recent review of the status of marijuana, judges that it is less dangerous than alcohol and tobacco and, therefore, questions the continued insistence on the use of harsh legal measures against its users.

LSD

LSD (lysergic acid diethylamide), as mentioned earlier, has been called a "psychotogenic" or a "psychotomimetic" drug. These labels were used initially because the state produced by the drug appeared to mimic the typical states of the mentally ill or psychotic person. However, it is now known that the similarities between the psychotic and drug states are only superficial. The physiological effects of an LSD "trip" are relatively mild, as contrasted with the drastic psychological changes brought about by the drug. The increase in blood pressure and heart rate is not great, nor is the increase in blood sugar. Other sporadic symptoms that may occur are nausea, chills, flushes, irregular breathing, sweating of the palms, or trembling of extremities. The pupils of the eyes are widely dilated. The subject usually does not care for food while he is high, because of the vividness of his mental life, but after the drug has worn off he is typically quite hungry. Sleep can be suspended for the length of the episode, that is, for 8 to 10 hours. The psychological effects include distortion of experience (see Figure 11–2), often viewed as hallucinations; objects become bright, colors appear intense, and illusions, which change rapidly in color and form, remain extremely vivid. The subject experiences *depersonalization,* a bizarre separation from the body —a pseudoindependence that gives the illusion of being on the sidelines and seeing one's self in action.

Most of the experiences have been described as extreme, and sometimes the term "profound" is used. Some individuals report *insights* and say they see life in greater depth. Often accompanying this notion of profundity is the *sense of euphoria.* To some people, however, the bizarre quality of the perceptions and the deep emotional experience are more like a bad dream than a great adventure. The experience in such instances may be so terrifying as to produce panic (Huxley, 1954) and, in the emotionally unstable, may precipitate a serious psychotic episode.

LSD has been used clinically, with some encouraging results, by Jensen and Ramsey (1963) in the treatment of alcoholism. Some therapists report an improvement in ego strength and a reduction in depression and in hypochondriasis (Savage, Savage, Fademan, & Harman,

Figure 11–1 A Satisfying Smoke.

Photo by Chris T. Quillen

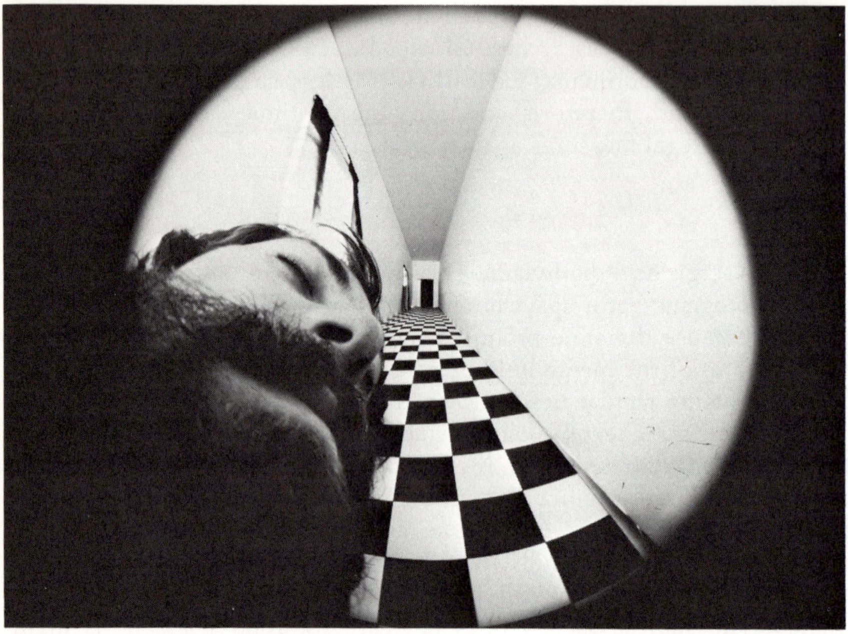

Photo by J. Brian King

Figure 11–2 Perceptual Changes Are Common Among LSD Users.

1964). It should be stated at this point that when LSD is given in carefully measured dosages by professionals, the individual is systematically prepared for the experience. A professional remains with the subject during the entire period, and the drug experience is woven into the whole psychotherapeutic process. The focus of the entire set and setting is toward self-improvement.

Cole, Jones, and Klerman (1961) question whether the new insights from psychotherapy with LSD can be attributed to a drug-induced frame of the mind or a therapist-induced mystical experience similar to religious conversions. Several factors, according to Cole and his colleagues, make this psychotherapy venture quite controversial. The issue of the use of LSD is highly charged with emotion. Controlled research has not been done on many of the questions raised by the use of LSD, and there remains the possibility that prolonged psychotic episodes or aberrant behavior will be precipitated by the use of psychotomimetic agents.

Individuals with certain physical disabilities are routinely screened out of responsible LSD experiments. These disabilities include heart defects, liver malfunction, and suspected epilepsy. Most of the professional writers in this field recommend caution in the use of LSD without the professional assistance of a qualified physician. Some men of the drug culture like Ken (introduced below) report that none of their group has "freaked out" or become psychotic, yet others who are acquainted with some of Ken's fellow users know students who have suffered serious repercussions from the drugs. Numerous reports have been made about *flashbacks* in which the LSD user suddenly and repeatedly reexperiences a "trip" without warning, even though the drug has not been further ingested. The determinants of this phenomenon are not understood completely, yet LSD use does appear to lead to potentially serious psychological problems.

Cole (1961) also points out that clinicians have been unsuccessful in predicting whether patients will respond to the drug in positive or negative ways. Blum (1964) estimates that at least two of a hundred users become so disturbed that they must be hospitalized with a diagnosis of psychosis. These workers caution potential users that reactions to the drug are not currently predictable and thus involve a risk of precipitating personality disturbances in those who experiment with it.

Pros and Cons of Marijuana and LSD Use

Lazarus (1969) reviews the arguments that are usually given against the use of such drugs as marijuana and LSD and presents some objections to each argument. Here are some of those arguments, for and against a greater permissiveness in the use of drugs.

1. One concern that many psychologists share is that drugs are a form of *escape;* then their use becomes for many people a *self-defeating mechanism.* Temporarily, the user forgets his cares and responsibilities. He's not coping rationally with personal problems. The individual, as well as society, is likely to suffer, especially since many otherwise intelligent and able people resort to drugs. The counterargument is that large numbers of people escape in other unproductive but less easily identifiable ways. Advocates of freedom to use marijuana point out that although illegal, is is less harmful in effect than alcohol or tobacco.

2. Although the drugs are not physically *addictive* in nature they lead many users to become psychologically dependent and to adopt a way of life that is difficult to abandon. The counterargument is that many of the people who persist in using illegal drugs deviate more from social norms than the average person *before* beginning to use the drugs.

3. These drugs are at present illegal. To obtain pot as well as hard drugs, the user must associate with people who operate outside the law. Those who argue for the legalizing of marijuana state that the law places users and tasters of marijuana in the criminal sector of society and should be changed for that reason as well as for the mild nature of the drug. Changing laws takes much time, and those that pertain to pot will

not be easily altered because of its adverse image in the opinions of members of the establishment.

4. With a reality-distorting alteration of consciousness some possibility exists that the individual will act in a way to endanger his own life or that of others. Certain drugs block normal ego controls. The counterargument is that people who act dangerously under drugs harbor pathological tendencies in their undrugged condition; their dangerous behavior could erupt at any time even without drugs.

DRUG USE AND STUDENTS

Blum (1966) suggests that drug users are more interested in what's happening in their consciousness than in what is happening in the outer world. Mamlet (1967) states that the goals and activities of members of the drug subculture are incompatible with those of the intellectual community. He adds that, contrary to the mind-expanding claims made for drugs by proponents of their use, drugs are *consciousness limiting* because of the narrowness of the drug community and the contempt for nonusers.

Others argue that drug use must be considered in relation to the total atmosphere of the academic community. Keniston (1966), for example, admonishes educators not to regard anyone who has used drugs as a moral leper, but rather to observe that many users express values compatible with the so-called "normal" American college student. Colleges place greater emphasis on intellectual and cognitive activities than on emotional and affective expression. Some of the deviation of students from the standards of the college establishment lies in their reversal of these emphases. Moreover, as students live in today's mass-media culture, the exposure to repetitive, demanding stimuli is psychologically numbing and may lead to the search for distracting behaviors.

On the negative side, some users get more protection from drugs than they bargained for. They become alienated from contemporary society, in which they see elements of cruelty and ugliness. Drug use may be an avenue for searching for personal and social meaning and humanistic values—an aim for legitimate goals through unwise means. Keniston maintains that there are better and more lasting ways to attain depth of experience and to find meaning in life than through drugs.

DRUG REHABILITATION

Aside from professional specialists and clinics especially designed to deal with drug addicts there are numerous projects for the rehabilitation of former addicts. One is called Synanon, a kind of community group therapy that reaches out into the broader society. The name

Synanon is a neologism coined by a newly arrived addict who attempted to say two words foreign to him: "symposium" and "seminar." He blurted out, "I want to get into another one of those symp—sem—synanons" (Yablonsky, 1965, p. 1x). The group is a community of former addicts who are now trying to lead constructive lives. They live in cities scattered over the United States, where they had been feared and rejected by a cross section of citizens who gradually became acquainted with their aims and have given their support. A group such as Synanon to achieve modification of behavior in the addicts must provide emphatic and continuous reinforcement of desired behavior from the more effective members. Synanon members have not limited their efforts to their own groups but expand them through numerous speaking engagements to inform the public about their program and methods. In addition local groups in college communities and cities counsel and work with people having drug problems.

One Student Who Experimented with Drugs—Ken

Ken's case is chosen because he is one of those drug users who feel they can take or leave the drug culture. Although Ken was known by me for several years, most of this report is based on Ken's own observations. They tally with those of a number of articulate and confident members of an organization of former and present drug users on the periphery of the campus.

Ken is a 20-year-old junior majoring in psychology. He has planned his course selections to prepare him for the field of advertising and public relations. During high school he enjoyed prestige and popularity, but he rejected in part the culture to which he belonged. In college, he appears on the campus in blue jeans, sandals without socks, and other odd assortments of clothing (usually clean), with a string of beads around his neck. He wears his hair and sideburns chin length. He walks with a free stride, developed when he was on athletic teams in high school. On the campus, he may be seen walking with some of his friends, who may or may not be similarly dressed. He is an essentially good-looking young man of average build. Ken is friendly, person-oriented, energetic, open, and frank, and additionally seems to be fairly well integrated with clearly articulated values and a positive self-concept. His family is affluent (at least upper middle class), living in a prestigious suburb of a midwestern city. His father was also from a wealthy background, but the family "fortune" was lost when his father was young, so it became necessary for him to work his way back up the financial ladder. Ken is the youngest of four children, and he describes his relationship with his parents and siblings as very good.

Ken apparently had appropriate encouragement to succeed early in life. He was active in sports and learned to box. He has always done well on various *ability* tests and in challenging courses such as mathematics. He graduated in the upper half of his high school class, went to a private university, but there, as a pledge in a fraternity he disliked, he barely made passing grades. He ended the year on probation. He then transferred to a small junior college where he had a good year—earning a grade point average of 3.8 on the 4.0 scale. He felt very good about this. Still he recognized that he didn't usually work up to his full potential, despite strong motivation to achieve and a rather clear idea of the general vocational area he wished to enter. He hoped to do creative work in the public relations field and expected to succeed in it. He saw himself as being generally motivated toward ends rather than means. "I can gauge myself best by what I produce. When I was making good grades it was very satisfying to me, but I am the kind of person who works only on what interests me."

One of the big factors in Ken's life was a tendency to be overweight at puberty and the ease with which he gained weight afterwards. He hated being fat, but he tolerated the banter it attracted and actually had some ambivalence about it. While he didn't like being thought of as a fat boy, it gave him a bigness and a uniqueness that he enjoyed. Dieting was very unpleasant because he enjoyed eating and sitting around drinking beer. An important event in his life during adolescence was a motorcycle accident in which he broke his leg; for 8 or 9 months he was in a wheelchair or on crutches. His physician said that unless he dieted and reduced considerably, he would have to walk with canes when he reached 35 or 40. This prospect motivated him to diet and he lost enough weight to change his physical appearance totally. He gave up beer drinking, and this, together with his dislike of the fraternity—especially the hazing, which consisted of doing odd jobs at odd hours for the older members—led him into the drug subculture.

In talking about his feelings toward the fraternity, Ken said, "I hated to pay for the privilege of being in a fraternity and have to work all the time, too." He also resented having to "love" his fraternity brothers when, for many of the members, he had no positive feelings—not even respect. His high standards regarding his relationships to other people led him to be frank always in telling others what he liked and disliked.

Making friends had never been difficult, but Ken liked to select them on the basis of social and character traits, and not on the basis of mutual group membership. He had never wanted to be a campus leader, although he did not withdraw completely from the group, particularly if some change was needed. He has always liked to study people, and this now includes observing people's reaction to him as he expresses his individualism in his hair and clothing styles. He states, "I feel that I must be an individual, but it's true—one can go to extremes." In fact, Ken appears to be a bit irresponsible and mildly exhibitionistic. One of the girls who worked in the "head shop" where he also worked said, "He wanders in here at will; he never keeps regular hours." But despite poor work habits, Ken makes interesting salable objects so the store retains him as an employee. At times he parks illegally and puts a used parking ticket on his windshield.

Ken believes that what he has gained from the drug subculture is open, frank communication and a sensitivity to the feelings of others. He has learned through these associations not to fear his own warm feelings toward others or their feelings toward him. "I have no doubt about my masculinity and I don't have to prove it, but being masculine doesn't prevent me from caring about others or dressing differently from others or doing things for my friends and helping them. Keeping myself physically fit by lifting weights is not to prove my masculinity."

As a high school student and a college freshman he was very much like the other students; he dated, participated in groups, and spoke his mind in fraternity meetings and group gatherings. When he transferred to the state university, however, he found friends both among the "straights" and the drug subculture. His first use of drugs was with a friend who was leaving for military service, at which time he smoked marijuana, but felt no effect. Later, he smoked with a good-humored friend who created a pleasant atmosphere for the experience. This time, Kent felt giddy and the whole episode took on such a pleasingly amusing aspect that marijuana replaced the beer he had been drinking. In answer to the question, "What do you get out of it?" he replied that marijuana made him more sensitive to things and people and when he "turned on" with people he was experiencing what they were. He stated he felt no antipathy for the "establishment"; as a matter of fact, he plans to become a part of it.

Being part of the subculture is like living in a small town. You have an intimate relationship with other people who have attitudes similar to your own. When asked if being in the drug community involves any dangers, he said, "Well, one might lose one's identity or blow one's mind, although I haven't seen this happen in this community. It is true that some use drugs as an escape, others just like the feeling and experiences which drugs produce—that's my reason for using them. I don't take drugs to forget problems; in fact, I lay off drugs when I have a problem to solve. Rationality is very important to me. I think I have learned to care more about people and to know that everyone has feelings, and I take them into account. I've learned to be more humane. My ultimate goal is to be a real human being. Since I will be working with people (in advertising) I think this association has made me more sensitive to people as unique individuals."

On one occasion while on drugs, Ken contracted an infection that made him dizzy, and he experienced complete exhaustion. For a time he feared this was an aftereffect of drugs. Although he recovered quickly after his illness was properly diagnosed and treated, he remained very anxious, thought he had "blown his mind," and avoided the use of drugs for a while.

"My emotional adjustment is not static. I guess, since I have taken drugs, I cannot be called completely well adjusted, but I think there's some growth that has taken place. There are various kinds of protest. The subculture doesn't seem to be political, but it is a protest against social restraints. The greatest danger of being in the subculture, from my standpoint, is in being unproductive, and for this reason I'm going to get a haircut, take a job this summer, and drop drugs. When I'm taking drugs it uses up so much of the time that is required to do my school work that I feel crowded. I'm in school for a reason. I feel I'm a fundamentally responsible person; I wouldn't have taken acid (LSD) in the first place if I'd known it was acid. I thought it was something else."

When asked, "Are the people in this subculture different from the students you know in the fraternity?" Ken said, "Well there are individuals in both groups and individuals can't be described in terms of groups. Those who have dropped out of school and are completely on drugs are certainly different."

He was asked, "How can you explain why those in this subculture take on a different hair style and dress?" To which he replied, "It's the atmosphere of freedom—let your hair be what it is naturally, dress like you feel like dressing. Drugs lower your defenses. You're not afraid of being what you really are and feel. Then, drugs let you perceive things more clearly and you see things for themselves." He added that he didn't find any more sex activity within the drug culture than in other cultures. In fact, it seemed to him to be less. "Boys will sleep with girls but have no sexual intercourse. I have seen no homosexuality in the subculture."

KEN—FOLLOW-UP

Two years lapsed after graduation; Ken returned to the campus for a visit. He was 25 years of age at this time. He had been to visit his parents in a nearby city. He expressed his satisfaction with how they were enjoying life in semiretirement.

Ken's hair (below-shoulder length) was the longest it had ever been and he was dressed casually but tastefully. He had a responsible job as assistant manager in a nationally known music recording company, which he had held for 1½ years. He admired his boss and associates and said it would take an income of $23,000 a year to move him. He worked long hours and enjoyed the people (many of whom were performers) he met in his work. He was his usual casual, open self and stated that he had no personal problems.

Alcohol and Alcoholism

As pointed out earlier, alcohol is classified with the sedatives and hypnotics. It appears to be a stimulant because it generally gives the drinker a feeling of well-being; unpleasant realities are minimized and confidence increased. But the presence of alcohol in the blood has been related to impairment of visual motor activity and the lethal effect of the drunken driver, loose on our highways, is finally being publicized (Figure 11–3).

Excessive drinking is a serious national problem. From 5 to 6.5 million Americans, it is estimated, drink excessively (Irwin, 1968). This figure

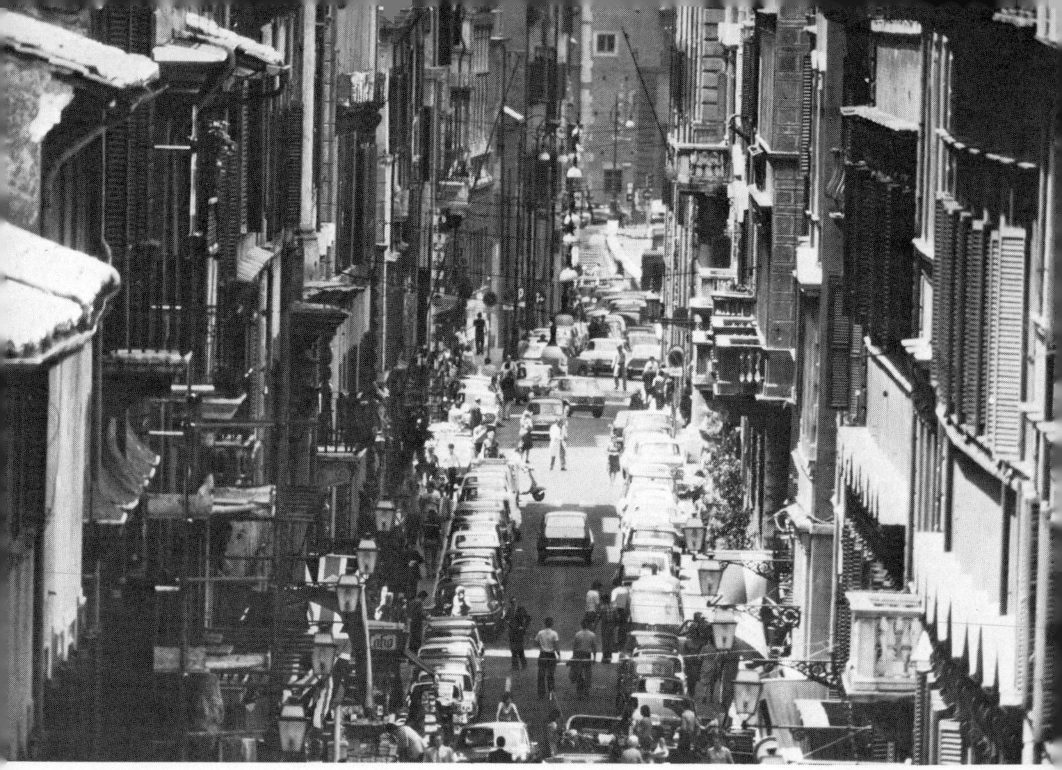

Photo by J. Brian King

Figure 11–3 No Place for a Drunken Driver.

is doubtless much greater at this reading. Some heavy drinkers exercise a modicum of control over their alcohol consumption and manage to carry on their work, interact with their families, and maintain some degree of social adjustment. The chronic alcoholic, however, has lost all control, especially after a period of excessive drinking. Such individuals are not only found on "skid row" but also in important professional, executive, and supervisory positions.

ALCOHOL AND CONFLICT

The manner in which alcohol and barbiturates allow an organism to approach an intense conflict is shown in two experiments with cats. Masserman and Yum (1946) directed a blast of air at each cat as it approached its food. Hunger motivated the cat to go to the food, yet the blast of air discouraged it; the hungry cat suffered conflict as he experienced this acute approach-avoidance situation. Eventually, though hungry, the cat no longer tried to obtain food, even when the air blast no longer occurred. Then, doses of alcohol, which normal cats will not tolerate, were placed in the cats' milk. After drinking the "toddy" the cat could go to the food. The alcohol enabled it to perform an act it could not achieve previously. A similar result was found with the use of sodium amytol, a barbiturate. In this experiment kittens were helped

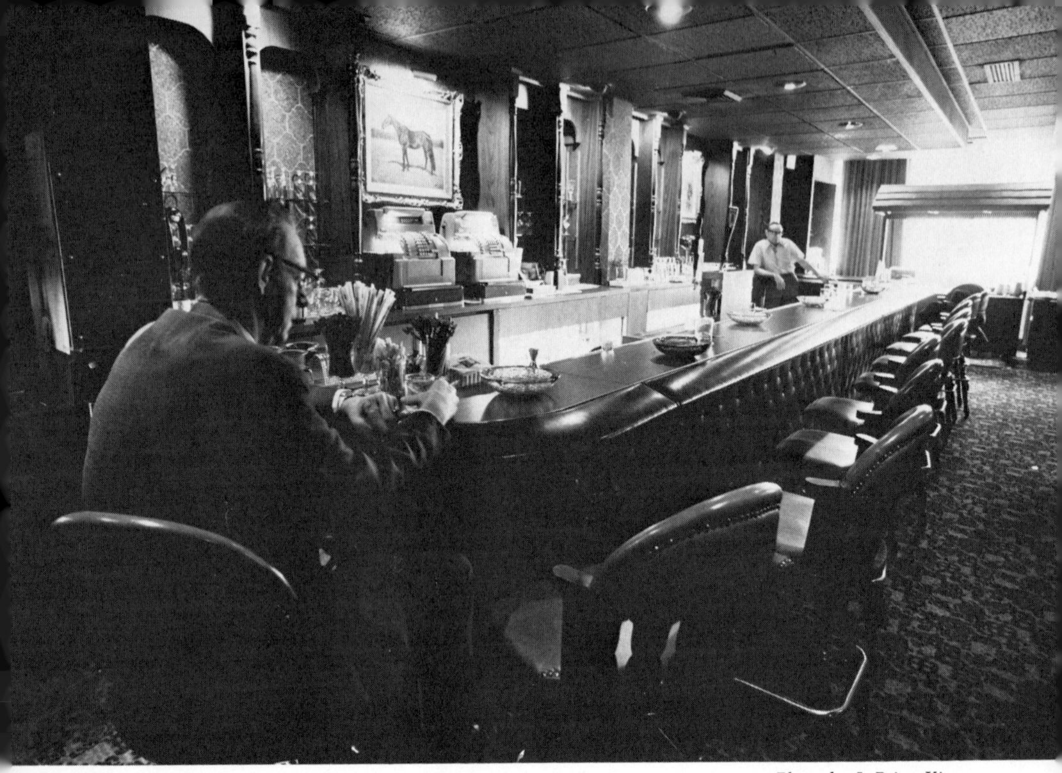

Photo by J. Brian King

Figure 11–4 A Place for Social Drinking.

to overcome another conflict, which was produced by associating a painful electric shock with the food box (Bailey & Miller, 1952).

Three kinds of drinking have been observed: (1) *facilitative,* which is moderate, occurs in social gatherings, and warms interpersonal relations (Figure 11–4); (2) *integrative,* which occurs on festive occasions and in religious ceremonies; and (3) *escapist* drinking, which is used to drown the dread of life's frustrations (Ruch, 1967). Typically the heavy drinker has moved from social and ceremonial drinking to increased consumption of alcohol. This sometimes extends to morning drinking and drinking to the point of blacking out or failing to remember what happened during his drinking. Eventually one drink starts a chain reaction over which the drinker has no control. He may then reach a point at which alcoholism is the dominant purpose in his life.

In his work with alcoholics, Jellinek (1960) identified four distinct stages in the development of alcoholism: (1) The *prealcoholic phase* marked primarily by the use of alcohol in social situations to obtain some relief. At this stage, the drinker experiences more satisfaction from alcohol than one would normally expect. (2) The *prodromal phase,* in which the person begins to drink simply to reduce anxiety. The drinker is able to consume larger quantities of alcohol than had earlier been the case and may experience periods of *alcoholic blackouts,* or periods of amnesia begin to appear. Drinking becomes a more central part of one's life and often the drinker will "sneak" drinks during the day. (3) The *crucial phase* is reached when drinking becomes a more frequent event with marked decreases in behavioral control. The person can no longer control his intake (although he can control the onset of drinking) and may regularly go "on a binge" for days or weeks at a time. (4) The final *chronic phase,* in which the person is clearly addicted to alcohol and consumes alcohol at all times of the day or night. Tolerance decreases somewhat, as significant physical and cognitive symptoms of alcohol abuse become apparent.

In recent years alcoholics under 30 are found also to use tranquilizers, stimulant drugs, or barbiturates. When used by people under the influence of alcohol, other drugs carry increased effect and the user becomes more easily addicted to them (Anon., 1968). It must also be recognized that mixing alcohol with other drugs can cause severe biochemical reactions in the body which may lead to serious illness or even death.

PERSONALITY AND ALCOHOLISM

Alcoholism in a given individual is a complex phenomenon. Only a small percentage of those who use alcohol become alcoholics. The biological, psychological, and sociocultural factors that operate in the use and effects of alcohol are broadly individual. Some say that they lost control over their use of alcohol in their first experience with it (Figure 11–5). A few researchers have suggested that a genetic biological factor may be at work in such cases. There is evidence to show that sociocultural factors operate in alcoholism. Alcoholism is low among Jews, Mormons, and Muslims, and high among the Irish (Catanzaro, 1967). Bandura (1969) interprets these data on cultural differences as evidence that alcoholism is primarily a learned pattern of behavior rather than a result of a particular predisposition. He points to the low alcoholism rates among Jews, who probably experience no less psychological stress than members of other ethnic groups having high alcoholism rates.

On the other hand, studies have been appearing since the 1930s claiming to show differences between alcoholics and nonalcoholics in various personality characteristics. Many early studies have been criticized on methodological grounds. Later studies report that alcoholics are not homogeneous and that categories of alcoholism must be devised before reliable group characteristics can be determined (Sutherland, Schroeder, & Tordella, 1950). Syme (1957), however, argues that it may be premature to claim that there is no alcoholic personality prior to alcoholism. In support of this position, a number of independent Minnesota Multiphasic Personality Inventory (MMPI) studies consistently report high "psychopathic deviate" scores for alcoholics. Psychopathic deviate scores

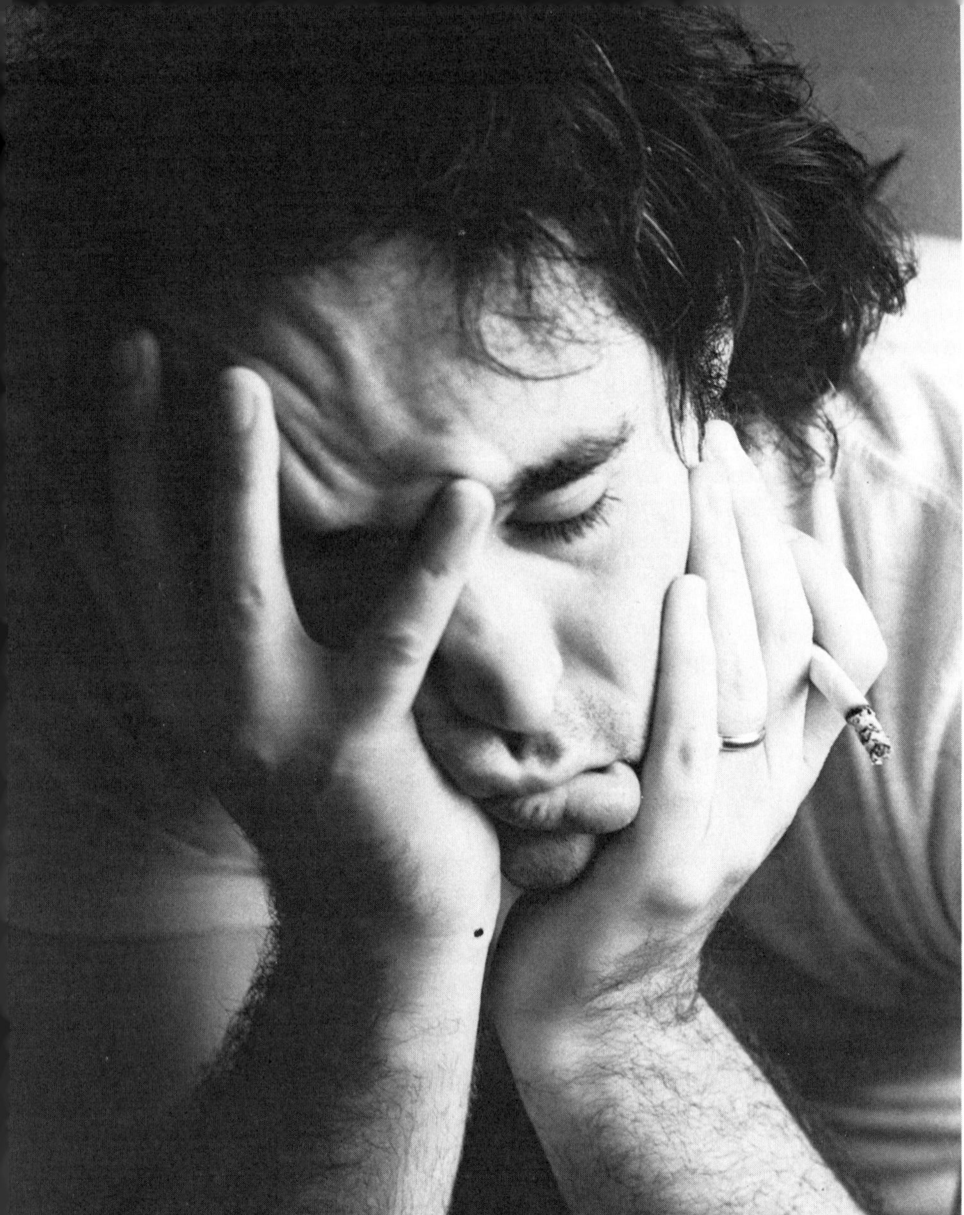

Photo by J. Brian King

Figure 11–5 Hung Over.

are derived from test items reflecting rebelliousness, conflict with parents, and lack of concern about behavior (Jones, 1968). Jones's data show that this acting out and assertive behavior predated, at least to some degree, the inappropriate drinking behavior and it may be considered a predisposing factor rather than the effect of the use of alcohol.

McCord and McCord (1964) report a long-term observation of 29 boys who, while they were a part of a larger group, differed from the rest of the group in that they become alcoholic as adults. Early observations of this kind present a retrospective bias. Compared with boys who did not become alcoholic, these 29 boys (later alcoholics) were "self-contained," outwardly self-confident, not fearful, indifferent to their siblings, disapproving of their mothers, aggressive, sadistic, and subject to sexual anxiety (Figure 11–6). When they became adults they exhibited some different characteristics: they tended to feel victimized by society and were extremely dependent; they avoided group activities and expressed feelings of grandiosity—apparently a compensatory response. As men they tended to reject their sons and either played a passive role in the family or became dictatorial. They disciplined their sons in an erratic, punitive, or lax manner, and engaged in intense family conflict more frequently than the majority of men. Most of them placed pleasure or enjoyment above other values in their lives.

Blane (1968) states that certain adjectives are frequently used to describe alcoholics. The most common are *dependent, hostile, denying, impulsive,* and *inadequate.* Recent studies have shown that *various* pat-

Figure 11–6 The Result of Impulsive Behavior.

Photo by J. Brian King

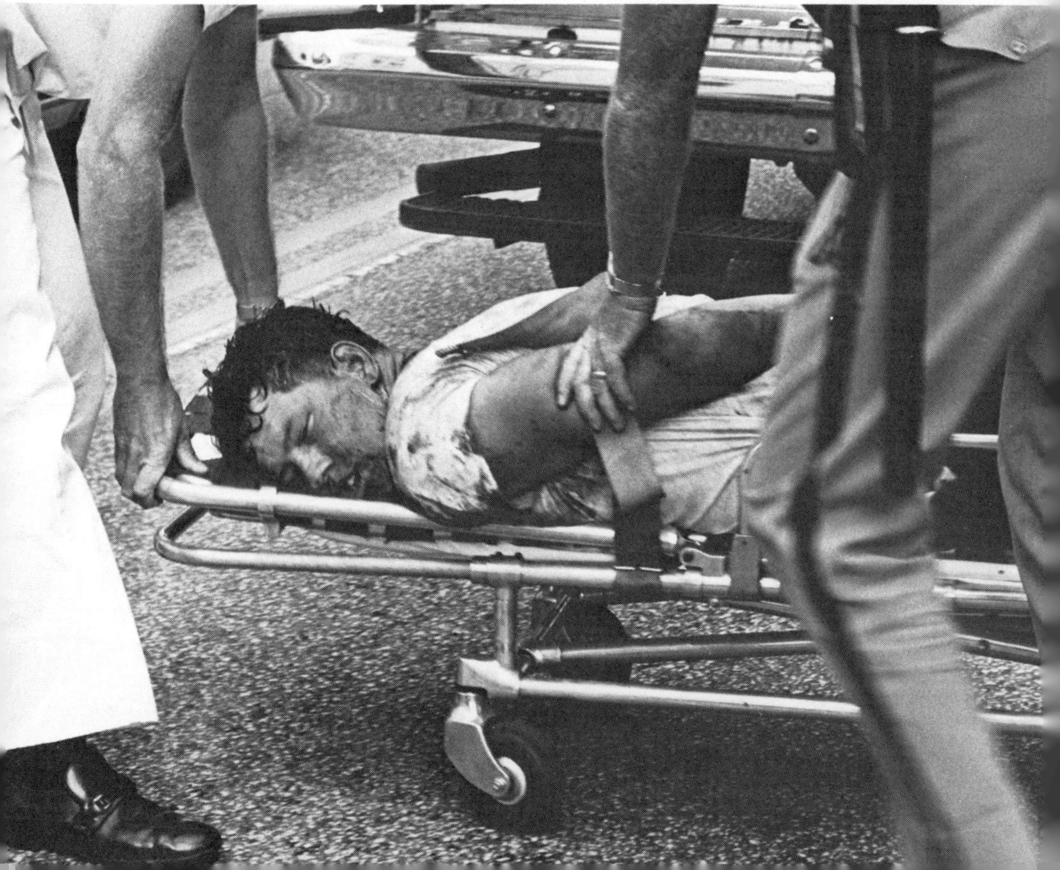

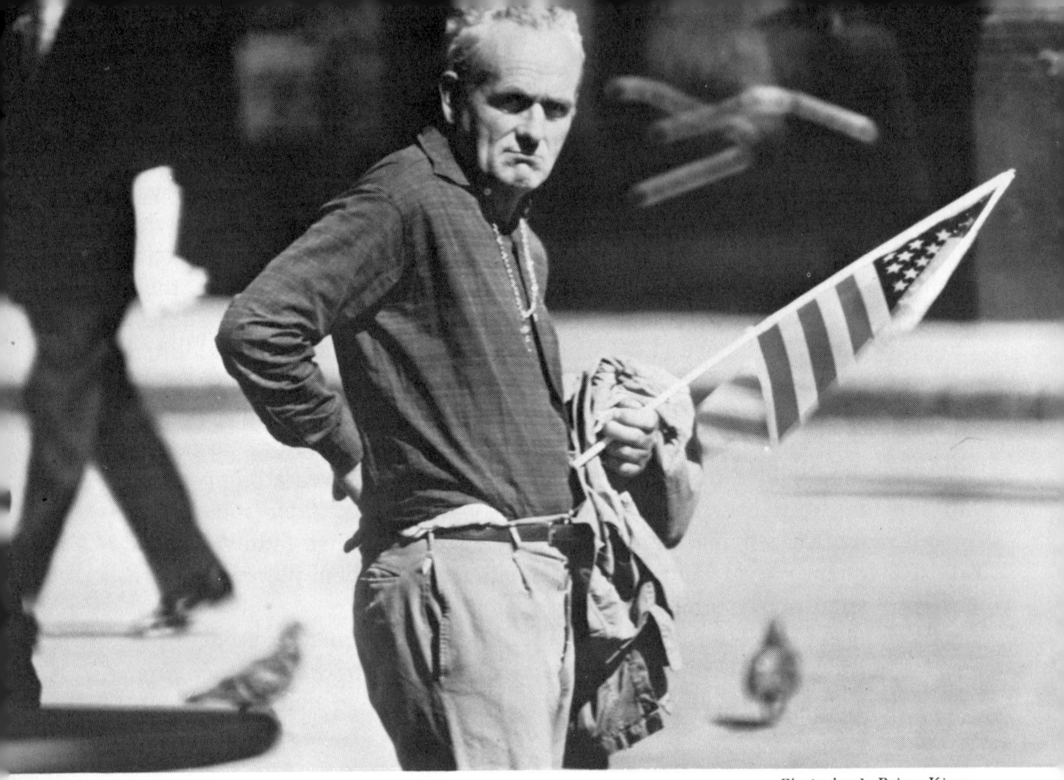

Photo by J. Brian King

Figure 11–7 A Dropout from Conventional Society.

terns are found among the alcoholics studied. Lawlis and Rubin (1971) differentiated alcoholics admitted to the alcoholic ward of a state hospital into three groups: (a) those with an inhibited neurotic syndrome; (b) those with a sociopathic (or psychopathic) syndrome; and (c) those with an aggressive neurotic syndrome. Partington and Johnson (1969), using several sources of data, could discern five patterns—some of them similar to those above. One observation almost all the investigators, reviewed by Wolfgang (1972), report about alcoholics is their poor self-concept. This is revealed in indicators of low self-esteem, lack of self-confidence, and feelings of worthlessness, inadequacy, and self-doubt.

REHABILITATING THE ALCOHOLIC

An alcoholic is not readily converted to complete abstinence. The skid row drinker has dropped out of conventional society and is rejected by it (Figure 11–7). The escape of other alcoholics from different life situations includes the denial of their alcoholism. They often show a persistent disinclination to seek professional assistance. As various professional members of the community come to understand alcoholism as a disability rather than as moral dereliction they can cooperate to establish rehabilitation services of a medical, psychological, and spiritual nature (Catanzaro, 1967).

Behavior modification methods designed to rehabilitate the alcoholic consist in associating aversive or very unpleasant experiences with stimuli that invite the alcoholic to drink. For example, the alcoholic will be offered an alcoholic beverage and invited to look at it, smell it, taste it, then spit it out. At a later session, while he is at the peak of nausea produced by a drug, he is asked to drink some alcohol. Numerous experiments to modify alcoholics' behavior have been conducted; follow-up results vary greatly with respect to the percentages of complete abstinence. Bandura (1969) presents a table showing the percentages of complete abstinence that have been published by various investigators. These run from 23 percent with a two-month follow-up by one experimenter to 96 percent with a fifteen-month follow-up by another experimenter. In general, the abstinence rates are very high immediately following treatment; reversion to drinking is greatest between 6 and 12 months afterward. In many cases reconditioning methods must be supplemented with other programs if sobriety is to be maintained.

Sobriety rates of alcoholics increase with age, with stable employment histories, with middle- and upper-class status, and—most important—with membership in abstinence clubs (Bandura, 1969).

Important also for staying sober is the acquisition of certain behavior competencies that will yield *gratification while sober.* The alcoholic, for example, may not have educational, vocational, and social skills that will give him daily satisfactions when he is sober. Narrol (1967) used reinforcement techniques to promote vocational activities in hospitalized alcoholics. A simulated "token" economy was set up in which the patient could earn points for working. These points could be used for clothing, hospital leaves, recreational opportunities, and so forth. Projects of this type are promising in theory, particularly if they continue for a long period of time and if a realistic transition can be made from hospital wards to the kind of real society to which the alcoholic must eventually move.

Some years ago a lay movement was started by rehabilitated alcoholics, largely because professional treatment failed in so many instances to produce lasting effects. It is called *Alcoholics Anonymous* and has grown greatly in reputation as well as membership and success throughout the years. A book describing the project appeared in 1942 (Anon., 1942). Several features of the program account for its outstanding success with alcoholics. In this association, alcoholics are regarded as persons who can be rehabilitated, particularly as they help one another through frequent meetings and through a philosophy of life that emphasizes both faith and good works. The movement is nonsectarian but frankly religious. The guilt-ridden, demoralized, middle-class alcoholic is given a sense of hope when he is approached by a former alcoholic who has now attained sobriety. He is enlisted in a program of helping other alcoholics become sober. The emphasis in the group is not on denying the existence of the problem but on frankly facing the constant tendency to turn to alcohol for an escape from problems. In this personal organization, he is helped by his ex-alcoholic friends and by his family to find other behavior to satisfy him in times of stress. One of the goals of AA is inner serenity, which involves a feeling of peace with oneself, one's fellow man, and one's God. This is an appeal the alcoholic can accept and work toward. At the meetings of AA, he hears testimonials, which support his hope to change his habits, and suggestions for satisfying behaviors he can substitute for his defense mechanism—alcohol.

Psychopathic Personality

Some delinquents and antisocial individuals have been classified as *psychopathic personalities.* They are generally described as irresponsible, poor in establishing meaningful human relations, and unwilling to accept blame. Furthermore they resist professional assistance (Cleckley, 1959). The concept of psychopathy has raised controversy in the behavioral sciences and has sometimes been called a wastebasket into which cases are tossed when they cannot easily be diagnosed otherwise. The persons so classified usually aggravate those trying to help them, are widely heterogeneous in personal and social identities, and commit a broad variety of offenses. They are characterized as aloof, solitary, weak in personality integration, "without a conscience," free from anxiety, attention-seeking, irresponsible, demanding, and initially impressive to those who deal with them. The initial good impression leads others to characterize them as charming until the antisocial behavior becomes manifest. Many of the corrective methods attempted early were not effective in bringing about any basic changes, and therefore some therapists concluded that people with this syndrome are incorrigible.

Some authors see value in the use of the concept *psychopath,* if proper criteria can be devised. However, individuals who have been cautiously classified *psychopathic personality* in terms of the above description, account for only a small percentage of those sent to corrective and penal institutions. Psychopaths annoy and disappoint those around them, but few go to prison.

Tests of psychopathic individuals are reviewed by Pennington (1966). Pennington has further divided criminal offenders into the *pure psychopath* (P) and the *antisocial character neurotic* (ACN). Basing his classifications on social histories, observed behavior, and test scores, Pennington furnishes some evidence that the two groups can be clinically and psychometrically (by means of tests) differentiated on several counts. The psychopath (P) shows *deprivation of affection* [1] in the early years as contrasted with the antisocial character neurotic (ACN), who has experienced more overindulgence and not as much deprivation. P *has*

[1] The italicized terms describe P as contrasted with ACN.

been a problem to others from the earliest years; ACN exhibits antisocial conduct usually in the teens. P is a *troublemaker in prison;* ACN often has a good prison record. P tends to be a *social isolate* and commits minor crimes; ACN is somewhat more sociable but commits more serious crimes. They differ in *sex drive*—weak in P and average to strong in ACN. P appears *calm and unconcerned;* ACN is tense, anxious, and remorseful upon occasion. P indicates *no verbalized insight,* whereas ACN verabilzes superficial insight. P has *tenuous emotional ties* with people and situations; ACN occasionally has strong ties, but often with the wrong persons and situations. P shows *psychological deficit* on tests of symbol manipulation, but this is not found in ACN. They differ in their scores on a mechanical aptitude test—below average for P but some high scores for ACN. P is *rarely athletic,* whereas ACN is usually athletic. In P, behavior appears unmotivated and sometimes bizarre; ACN's motivation is suggested by his superficial views of his activities. They differ in *remote memory:* It is excellent for P, but not for ACN, who has some memory blanks. The ACN thus shows some neurotic traits; P seems *devoid of worry and emotional ties* with people, and the usual interests in his peers are weak.

GENETIC FACTORS AND ANTISOCIAL BEHAVIOR

In most discussions of the antisocial personality, considerable emphasis has been placed on environmental factors. Recent findings of certain genetic characteristics among criminals in several different countries have suggested that some antisocial personalities may have deviant chromosome patterns.

Among prison populations it has been found that about 3.5 percent, as compared with fewer than 1 percent in the normal population, have an extra Y chromosome. Instead of their cells having 22 pairs of chromosomes per cell and typical XY chromosomal pairs, certain individuals have cells with an XYY pattern. These individuals are more often above average in height, below average in IQ, and aggressive and antisocial in behavior. It is too early to come to any conclusions about the genetic aspects of criminals; from previous knowledge it seems clear that experience is an influential interacting factor in criminality. A good brief review of some of the findings in this area is presented by Sanford and Wrightsman (1970).

The hypothesis that the way an individual views and interacts with the world around him is an expression of his self-concept has been studied by Fitts and Hammer (1969). They found that the delinquent has a poor self-concept as the alcoholic (see p. 334) and others displaying antisocial behavior. He lacks self-respect, is confused and uncertain in his self-picture, and is inconsistent in his self-regard. His personality is poorly integrated and he does not possess the strength to cope with frustration and stress.

Change in self-concept is difficult to accomplish, and incarceration alone does not improve it. A total well-designed program of rehabilitation, particularly one involving maximum participation by the delinquent in and responsibility for the operation of the program does lead to improvement. Delinquents need firm but fair controls, but above all they need to be treated as persons of worth and value.

TREATMENT OF THE PSYCHOPATH

Professionals who deal with antisocial and disturbed individuals are reluctant to treat psychopaths, mainly because of the client's lack of cooperation and his inadequate emotional involvement in his misbehavior. The psychopath's irresponsibility has seemed to evoke a certain amount of professional irresponsibility. A variety of approaches have been used in the hope of changing their behavior, including isolation and punishment, electroshock, lobotomy, and psychotherapy of various types. Currently professionals are achieving most success with appropriate psychotherapy and milieu therapy. Prevention of psychopathy, though difficult, is highly important because much evidence indicates that many delinquent children have been reared by delinquent parents.

Usually milieu therapy takes place in an institution that has been organized as a *therapeutic community.* Self-governing environments, coupled with group psychotherapy, and paternalistic discipline settings have been used to reinforce a total effort that employs any techniques that will build frustration tolerance and improve perception of reality. It is now believed that for some psychopathic individuals improvement in behavior is a possibility (Pennington, 1966).

Recently *behavior modification techniques* have been applied to psychopaths. Cohen, Filipczak, Bis, Cohen, Goldiamond, and Larkin (1968) have used institution reinforcement practices in programs to overcome the delinquent's educational and vocational deficits. In our society, which requires some education and skills, these deficits prevent the delinquent from obtaining socially reinforcing jobs. The youths in the Cohen program earned points for academic achievement that could be exchanged for improved living conditions, meals, wide variety of food, entertainment, and leisure activities. Cohen and his associates have been encouraged by their results.

Summary

1. Personality disorders are characterized by long-standing, troublesome behavior patterns which the individual has accepted as "natural" aspects of his personality. Symptoms include excessive dependency, immaturity, compulsiveness, suspiciousness, as well as addictions and antisocial behavior.

2. Addictions are seen as irresistible yearnings to behave in a certain way or to use certain substances. Drug addiction is characterized by *dependence, tolerance,* and the suffering of an *abstinence syndrome* when withdrawal is attempted.
3. Drugs are classified as *psychogenics, stimulants, sedatives,* and *analgesics.*
4. Specific drug effects may depend on the set of the drug user and the setting in which drugs are used.
5. Public reactions to the use of marijuana and LSD was discussed. Experimental evidence on the effects of marijuana and LSD was cited and the need for further research before definitive conclusions can be made was emphasized.
6. Alcohol is seen to be a sedative, and addiction to this substance to reduce conflicts is a widespread national problem. Although no single personality structure seems to predispose to alcoholism, sociocultural factors do seem to play a significant role.
7. Rehabilitation of the alcoholic is a difficult task because of motivational inadequacies. Behavior modification techniques have shown some success as has Alcoholics Anonymous.
8. Psychopathic personalities are delinquent, antisocial personalities who are irresponsible, and unable to establish meaningful interpersonal relations. Not all those who commit criminal acts are properly labeled psychopaths, and studies have been reported to differentiate between pure psychopaths and antisocial characters.
9. Some recent, though inconclusive, findings suggest that genetic factors may be an important cause of psychopathy.
10. His lack of apparent motivation for change makes the psychopath an unattractive candidate for psychotherapy. Milieu therapy and behavior modification techniques have been applied with some encouraging results.

Words to Remember

Amphetamines
Analgesic Drug
Chronic Phase
Crucial Phase
Dependency
Depressant Drug
Drug Abuse
Drug Addiction
Head
Hypnotic Drug
Milieu Therapy
Narcotic Drug
Personality Disorder
Psychogenic Drug
Psychopath
Psychopathy
Sedative Drug
Set
Stimulant Drug
Synanon
Taster
Tolerance
Withdrawal Syndrome

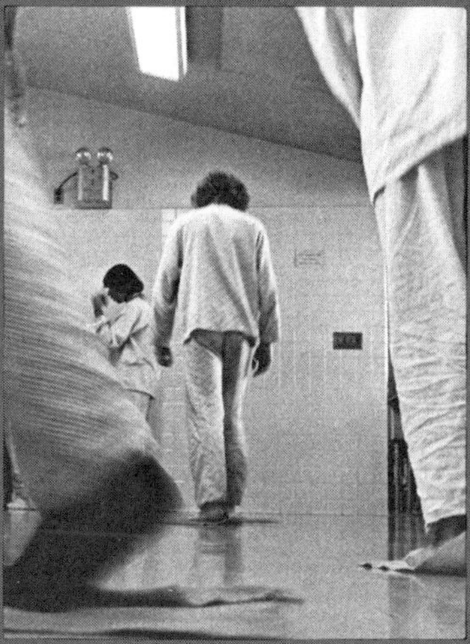

12. Psychosis, Neurosis, and Psychosomatic Disorders

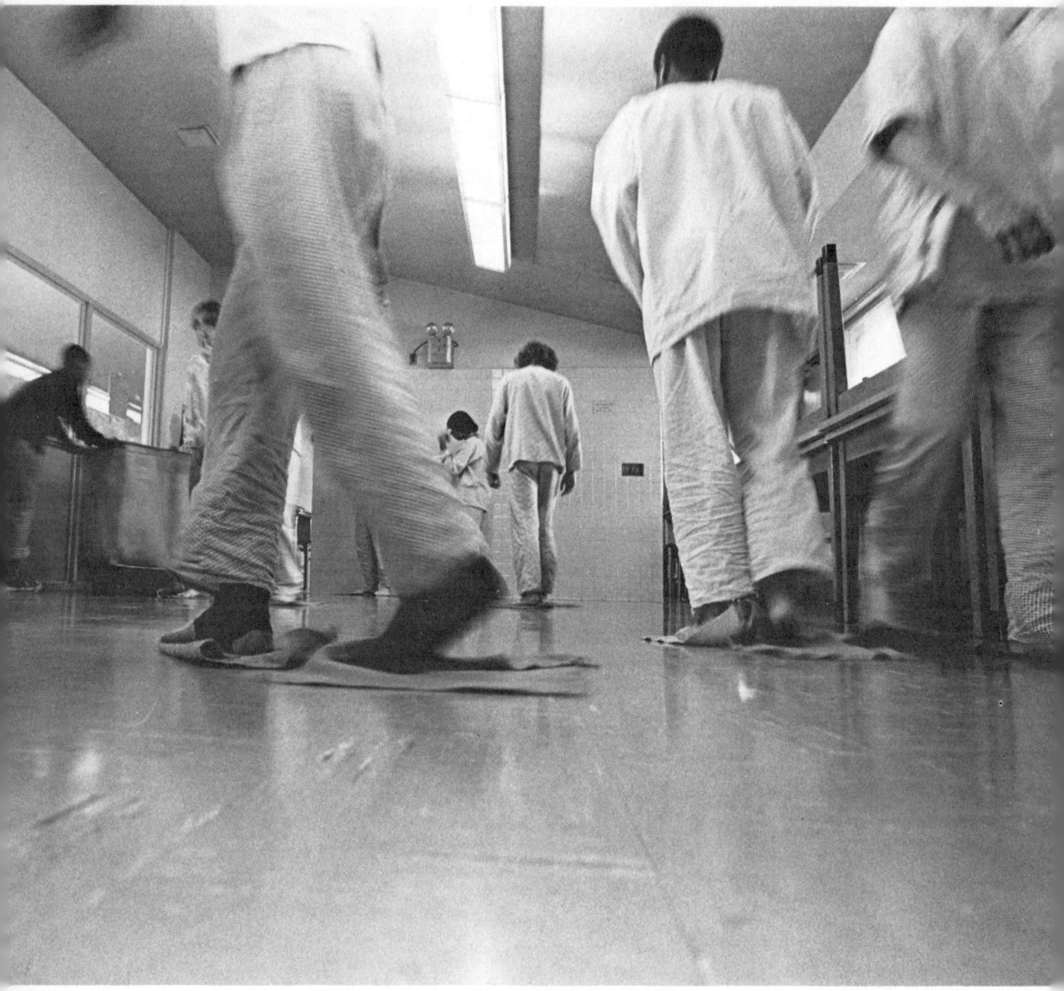

Photo by J. Brian King

Objectives

After studying this chapter the reader should be able to:

1. Define *psychosis.*
2. Describe the behavioral aspects of the four major types of schizophrenia.
3. Describe affective disorders.
4. Define *psychoneurosis.*
5. Describe the major theoretical positions that attempt to explain the causes of neurotic behavior.

The two most obvious and dramatic types of maladjustment are the *psychoses* and *psychoneuroses.* By definition, psychoses are the most extreme of the behavior disorders, usually so disabling that the afflicted individual is unable to care for himself and often must be institutionalized. As will be seen, the observable symptoms of psychosis are often extraordinarily unusual, realistically inappropriate, and thus very difficult for the observer to understand. These symptoms may be so strange as to be called "bizarre." Psychoneurotic disorders, by contrast, are not as disabling, since they typically involve less of a break with reality than is true of the psychoses. Still, they are extraordinarily uncomfortable for the afflicted person and sometimes result in behaviors which are felt to be a nuisance at best and extremely upsetting at worst. While not very common, it is possible that one can be so disabled by a psychoneurosis as to require hospitalization.

Psychosis

The general term *psychosis* encompasses a number of separate disorders all involving extreme disability in adjustment. The most prominent of the psychotic disorders is *schizophrenia* and the *affective psychoses.* Collectively, these two groups of disorders form the *functional* psychoses and are distinguished from the *organic* psychoses. This distinction reflects the assumption of many mental health specialists that the former are determined primarily by psychological causes, whereas the latter have their etiology in some physiological malfunction of the brain.

SCHIZOPHRENIA

Schizophrenia is perhaps the best known and certainly the most widely researched of the functional psychoses. At the same time, it is probably the least well understood. Schizophrenia is characterized by a limited number of "fundamental" symptoms which are assumed to be present in all who suffer from the disorder and also by other "accessory" symptoms which may or may not be present depending upon the nature of the schizophrenic disorder. Included among the fundamental symptoms are cognitive (i.e., thinking) and affective dysfunctions. The thought disorder observed among schizophrenics involves a tendency to think in such a highly personal way that the logic typifying normal thought is no longer present. As a result, ideas may be condensed in ways which are understandable only to the schizophrenic. Dissociation may be present as ideas strung together very loosely with no apparent ties among them. Chains of thought are disrupted by inappropriate intrusions, hence the schizophrenic frequently loses control of his ability to consider a problem or situation rationally. One could list a variety of other examples of thought disorder all of which would have in common the fact that in his thinking the schizophrenic is no longer concerned with the logical rules that must be followed in order to make ideas understandable to other people.

The affective disorder seen in schizophrenia primarily involves a display of feelings that are grossly inappropriate to the particular situation in which they occur. Examples might include uproarious laughter on sad occasions, uncontrollable weeping on happy occasions, or, most commonly, simply a lack of any kind of emotional reaction despite intense provocation. This absence of an affective reaction in the schizophrenic is often referred to as "bland" affect, or schizophrenic apathy. In such a state, the individual appears to have given up all involvement with the people and things around him and to have simply withdrawn whatever feelings he might have ever had toward them. People who interact with many schizophrenics often begin to feel that they are less than thinking, feeling people and are instead cold and mechanical beings.

Classically four categories of schizophrenia have been identified: the simple type, the paranoid type, the catatonic type, and the hebephrenic type. The simple schizophrenic is an individual who lives an isolated life functioning at a level well below what he seemed to be initially capable of in terms of his intelligence. Often, he will live alone and subsist on a marginal level. When employed, he may work at a menial job that keeps him away from other people and provides little more than the bare necessities of life. The hermit who shuns people and rummages around in wastecans to fulfill his needs is an example of what may be a simple schizophrenic. Often the laborers and helpers working around traveling carnivals include simple schizophrenics. These are people who because of their disorder are no longer capable of functioning at a higher level than they are achieving but can still care for themselves and often can exist outside of institutions without the help of others. Studies of the history of such individuals reveal that they appeared quite normal up until the time of adolescence when other youngsters begin to think about their future and what they want out of life. In adolescence the developing simple schizophrenic seems to be completely devoid of ideas about his future and, what is even more serious, he seems completely unconcerned about the fact. His concern rests with getting by from day to day and he, therefore, does only as much as is necessary for that purpose.

The paranoid schizophrenic is characterized primarily by *delusions* (i.e., a misinterpretation of events and the behavior of others) of persecution and/or grandiosity. The former refers to the overwhelming belief that the people around him are "out to get" him. The latter refers to the delusion that he is an extraordinarily important person and thus he may sometimes feel that he is being picked on because of his superiority to those around him. Typically persons suffering from paranoid disorders are fairly intelligent people who, at times, can convince others about their imagined problems. The paranoid's persecutors may be people among his own family, his neighbors, or his colleagues at work. He may also fear large organizations who are at some considerable distance from his immediate world such as the FBI, the Communist Party, or the Masons. In addition, it is not uncommon for the paranoid schizophrenic to suffer *hallucinations*. Hallucinations involve the experiencing of sensations when there are not outside stimuli to cause them. They may occur in any of the sense modalities. Thus, one may hear voices or sounds when there is no one around, or one may see things when there are no external visual stimuli. Hallucinations may also involve the senses of smell and touch, although these are rare.

Catatonic schizophrenia is characterized by peculiar motor symptoms and a tendency to be mute. In this form of schizophrenia the patient often sits in a very rigid detached manner, refusing to speak to or even acknowledge the presence of those around him. When he does speak, he uses words quite sparingly; in extreme cases, not a word will be said by him for days. Also in extreme cases, the patient behaves as though he is without a will of his own. He will remain for hours in whatever position he happens to be. Thus the catatonic patient can be placed in peculiar positions which will be retained over long periods of time. This tendency to simply go along with whatever physical position is imposed on one has been called *waxy flexibility*. Occasionally the catatonic will display an excited state during which he can be extremely dangerous because, in his excitement, he can be indiscriminately violent toward people or things around him.

The hebephrenic form of schizophrenia is characterized by what seems to be extraordinary regression and childishness. The hebephrenic seems to live in a world that is completely his own. Frequently he will laugh inappropriately as though in response to some internal stimulus of which an observer is totally unaware. Not uncommonly the hebephrenic will hallucinate continually for long periods of time and be entirely oblivious to the world around him. Furthermore, in his regressed state the hebephrenic will often fail to look after his personal needs and may wet and soil his clothing and eat his food like an infant.

THE LONGITUDINAL DIMENSION IN SCHIZOPHRENIA

In addition to categorizing schizophrenia in terms of overt symptomatology, it is possible to distinguish subtypes by considering the history of the disorder. Two distinct categories have been identified when schizophrenia is examined on this basis, the *process* and *reactive* types. The process schizophrenic is one whose history of emotional problems goes back quite a long way in his lifetime. He is an individual who has long tended to withdraw from people in the face of relatively minor life stresses and, as a result, he has never been able to achieve very much. As a youngster the process schizophrenic probably had considerable difficulty getting through school, if he was able to manage it at all. At adolescence, he is likely to have had few friends and to have been unable to develop an interest in the opposite sex. As he grew older it is unlikely that he was able to work at a job very successfully and would not be likely to have had a normal family life. An individual with such a background ordinarily has a very difficult time recovering from a schizophrenic disorder.

The reactive schizophrenic, on the other hand, generally shows a history of appropriate development and fairly adequate emotional adjustment and suffers his disorder as the result of some sudden and very serious stress. In some cases the source of stress may be the events associated with entering or actively serving in military service; for others, the loss of a source of affection (e.g., death or divorce) or some other personal life crisis may precipitate a psychotic episode. Whatever the circumstances, the disorder comes on as the result of a life problem which would be difficult for most people to deal with effectively. Typically the prospect for recovery among reactive schizophrenics is good. It has also been found that the reactive schizophrenic is more responsive physiologically than the process schizophrenic; his blood pressure, for example, responds to a chemical stimulant more readily (King, 1958). Furthermore, he is also more responsive emotionally to anxiety producing stimuli (Reisman, 1960). Both findings suggest the potentially greater effectiveness of attempts to provide treatment through the use of appropriate antipsychotic medication and/or psychotherapy.

EFFORTS TO DETERMINE THE CAUSES OF SCHIZOPHRENIA

Studies to uncover the underlying causes of schizophrenia have been directed toward either internal factors, that is organic or constitutional predispositions within the individual, or external factors, such as the kind of environment within which the schizophrenic grows up. One type of internal force that has been studied as a potential cause of schizophrenia is the biochemistry of those who become schizophrenic. In such studies researchers try to determine whether biochemical substances which cause schizophrenic-like symptoms in normals are found in excess in schizophrenics. For example, drugs such as mescaline and LSD create symptoms in normals which seem like those experienced by the schizophrenic. Therefore, it seems reasonable to assume that perhaps the schizophrenic manufactures his own mescaline or LSD internally in amounts which create disturbing psychological symptoms. From time to time biochemical studies do seem to find an excess of some substance in schizophrenics as compared to control groups.

The problem with these studies is, however, that these biochemical imbalances can result from a variety of factors such as diet, and certain mild chronic diseases. Since the studies of schizophrenics are done on institutionalized patients, and the control subjects for these studies are normal individuals living outside of institutions, it is difficult to determine whether the reported imbalances are caused by institutional living conditions or by the schizophrenic disorder. The fact that findings in one study have rarely been repeated in other similar studies carried on in different locations suggests that the significant biochemical differences that have been found in schizophrenics as compared to normals probably result from factors associated with institutionalization rather than from schizophrenia. Thus the whole line of biochemical research has contributed relatively little to our understanding of schizophrenia.

Another internal factor that has been considered as a possible cause of schizophrenia has been genetic, that is, the assumption that the schizophrenic inherits a constitutional predisposition to the disorder. Many early studies in this area claimed to demonstrate that schizophrenia tends to run in families and that, for example, if one member of an identical twin pair (identical twins have the same genetic makeup) is schizophrenic, there is virtually a 100 percent certainty that the other member of the pair will also be schizophrenic. These studies also indicated that the likelihood of schizophrenia in both members of a nonidentical twin pair drops considerably, and in fact, tends to be no greater than the probability that any two siblings in the same family are schizophrenic. Later, more systematic studies of hereditary factors in schizophrenia reported that there was considerably less likelihood of schizophrenia in both members of an identical pair than the 100 percent suggested earlier, but these later studies still found a relatively significant relationship supporting the genetic hypothesis.

Nonetheless such evidence has been regarded as inconclusive by those who argue that schizophrenia is determined by environmental factors. They claim that identical twins share not only the same genetic makeup but also a very, very similar environment. If environment, and not genetics, is the most important factor causing schizophrenia then both identical twins would be expected to display schizophrenic symptoms if either one of them had such a disorder. Recent studies reported by Rosenthal (1959), however, indicate that identical twins have a higher probability of both having schizophrenic disorders than nontwins even though each identical twin was raised in a different environment. These findings provide an even stronger basis for the genetic theories.

Those who seek to understand the cause of schizophrenia on the basis of factors external to the individual have examined interactions within families which have produced schizophrenics. A variety of approaches have been taken in family studies of schizophrenics. One group of investigators (Bateson, Jackson, Haley, & Weakland, 1956) has been interested in the way members of a schizophrenic's family communicate with each other. Specifically, they have described a pattern known as a "double-bind" that takes place in interactions within a schizophrenic's family, but particularly between the mother and the child who becomes schizophrenic. Double-bind messages are characterized by the fact that two contradictory meanings are communicated at the same time. For example, one might tell another person that he loves him but in such a tone of voice as to raise doubt as to whether he really means it. As a result the listener doesn't quite understand what message he is receiving, what thought or feeling is being sent, and thus is at a loss to know how to respond to it. This group of researchers feels that one long-range effect of growing up in a setting where people are communicating double-bind messages is to become a double-bind communicator oneself in order to avoid ever taking a firm position on any issue.

Other researchers (Lidz, Fleck, & Cornelison, 1965) have studied families of schizophrenics and report finding a high degree of instability among them. High percentages of schizophrenics are said to come from homes where one parent has been lost early in the schizophrenic's life, either through death or divorce. When both parents were present, the home often is characterized by serious discord between the parents, who may themselves be psychotic or seriously disturbed in some other way. These studies suggest that the strange behavior of the schizophrenic is understandable as the result of early exposure to very strange behavior in the important adults around him.

The same investigators have reported that in the families of some schizophrenics they observed a situation which they defined as *marital schism.* In marital schism each parent is immersed in his own problems to such an extent that he cannot adopt a role which reciprocates that of the other parent. Each parent wants his own way and tries to force the other one to give in to him; thus they fail to support each other in any way. As a result threats of separation and divorce are frequent. In moving from crisis to crisis, these parents are driven further and further apart emotionally. Basic family problems are therefore rarely solved. Another pattern reported by these investigators is *marital skew.* In such cases, one parent is very dominant and the other is very submissive. Often the dominant partner is somewhat disturbed. Since the "weak" parent is quite submissive, the child is unaware that the parent who sets the tone for how family life is to be lived is in any way abnormal. In modeling the dominant parent, the child gradually adopts the maladaptive behavior patterns.

Another set of investigators (Wynne, Ryckoff, Day, & Hirsch, 1958) have studied family processes in schizophrenia and have identified what they feel are certain unique characteristics of such families. Their focus is on a process called *pseudomutuality.* This process is characterized by a very strong investment in maintaining the idea that a close meaningful relationship exists between all family members. Family members feel strongly about at least giving the appearance that they fit together even if the individuality of one or more of them must be destroyed in order to maintain this illusion. Under such circumstances when any one family member attempts to assert his own personal identity the entire group becomes tense because the myth that all are trying to maintain is threatened. A major problem of pseudomutuality that predisposes individuals to schizophrenia is that the identity of each family member becomes blurred, and this makes relationships outside the family very difficult. Normally a person sees himself as a part of both a family group and a larger social group. Much home training should prepare a person to function as part of this larger social unit. The family of the preschizophrenic, however, seems to see itself as a self-sufficient unit, and most of its energy is devoted to maintaining its own integrity. As a result the youngster growing up in this family learns very little that is useful in dealing with the larger society. And since he cannot successfully avoid the outside world, many of his serious psychological problems are thought to result from this.

Although the family studies of schizophrenics have provided some interesting hypotheses concerning the potential causes of the disorder, they have been far from conclusive. One problem is that in virtually all cases schizophrenic families have not been compared to normal families, so that it is very difficult to know whether or not a pattern found among families producing schizophrenics occurs equally often in families that produce reasonably normal children. Without such information one cannot comfortably say that the family itself causes the disorder. Another problem with family studies of schizophrenia is that it is not clear whether the pattern observed in a family having a schizophrenic member has been present throughout the schizophrenic's life or whether it developed after the schizophrenic became manifestly disturbed. It is entirely conceivable that the presence of a very disturbed member has an effect on family styles which itself causes the observed relationships that seem unique or unusual. In such a case the suspect family relationships would not have caused the disorder but in fact would have been caused by it.

SCHIZOPHRENIA AS A FUNCTION OF BOTH CONSTITUTIONAL AND ENVIRONMENTAL FACTORS

In recent years the theory has been advanced (Meehl, 1962; Rosenthal, Wender, Kety, Schulsinger, Welner, & Østergaard, 1968) that to become schizophrenic one must both be born with a constitutional predisposition for the disorder and also grow up in a particularly stressful environment. It is assumed by these theorists that individuals who are free of the crucial predisposing factors will never become schizophrenic no matter how difficult an environment they experience in their development. Similarly, those born with a constitutional vulnerability for schizophrenia but fortunate enough to grow up in a setting that is not very demanding will also avoid becoming schizophrenic.

In an effort to understand the various factors that may contribute to the development of schizophrenia, studies have been done of children who were born to schizophrenic mothers but were adopted into families where there was no schizophrenia and of children born to normal mothers who were adopted into families where the adoptive mother became schizophrenic. These groups of adoptees have been examined as adults to determine their psychological state. It was assumed that if environment were particularly significant for the development of the disorder, those adoptees reared in families where there was schizophrenia would show more psychological disturbance than would those individuals born to schizophrenic mothers but raised in families where there was no schizophrenia. The reverse would be true if biology were particularly significant. Rosenthal et al. (1968) found that more psychological disturbance, in particular schizophrenia or schizophrenic-like disorders, was present in those individuals having a biological mother who was schizophrenic than was the case among adoptees reared in homes where the adoptive mother was schizophrenic. Somewhat similar findings were reported by Heston and Denney (1968), who also studied adoptees.

Results of the adoptees studies suggest rather conclusively that some constitutional factors operate in the development of schizophrenia, although they do not yet clearly identify what these factors are. They also fail to demonstrate what contribution environmental factors make to the development of schizophrenia. A recent study reported by Sameroff and Zax (1973) indicates that schizophrenic mothers are more likely than normals to have birth difficulties, which may contribute to some type of constitutional predisposition to serious mental disorder in their infants. These authors also report, however, that the same is true for children born to depressed mothers. Furthermore the chronicity of the mother's illness seems to be more of a factor in the occurrence of birth complications than is the specific diagnosis. Further studies of the nature of the damage caused by birth complications might help to shed greater light on our understanding of the etiology of schizophrenia.

AFFECTIVE PSYCHOSIS

The term "affect" used as a noun means emotion, and the disorders that are classified as affective psychoses are extreme disturbances of mood involving either deep depression or uncontrollable elation and activity. *Depression* is the symptom most commonly seen in affective psychoses. The very depressed individual generally feels deeply downcast, thinks only of pessimistic, unhappy things, is full of self-blame for all sorts of presumed past indiscretions or bad behavior, and often moves and thinks quite slowly. The severe depressive fails to keep up with daily responsibilities or frequently to even look after his own personal needs (Figure 12–1). Not uncommonly, sleep is disturbed, so that although the depressive can fall asleep, he awakens very easily and is unable to get back to sleep. Appetite diminishes and there may be a serious weight loss. In some cases the depressive thought content is present, but it is accompanied by restlessness and nervous agitation. This type of depressive, unlike the typical case, is very anxious and jumpy. He paces quite a bit, wrings his hands, pounds his head against the wall, moans in despair, and is very dramatic in his agitation.

Depression may come about for two reasons; in many cases it is a reaction to a terribly distressing event, perhaps a death in the family or a serious injury from an accident or some such. In these instances it is quite normal to become upset, and the depressive at first is not recognized as being seriously disturbed. In the person with a depressive psychosis, however, the upset persists long after the normal individual would have recovered. In other cases the depression seems to arise without any apparently significant stimulus, and the person who suffers this form of depression commonly experiences a cyclic pattern of mood changes. He may go through periods of depression which eventually clear, seemingly spontaneously, and after a period of apparent normality

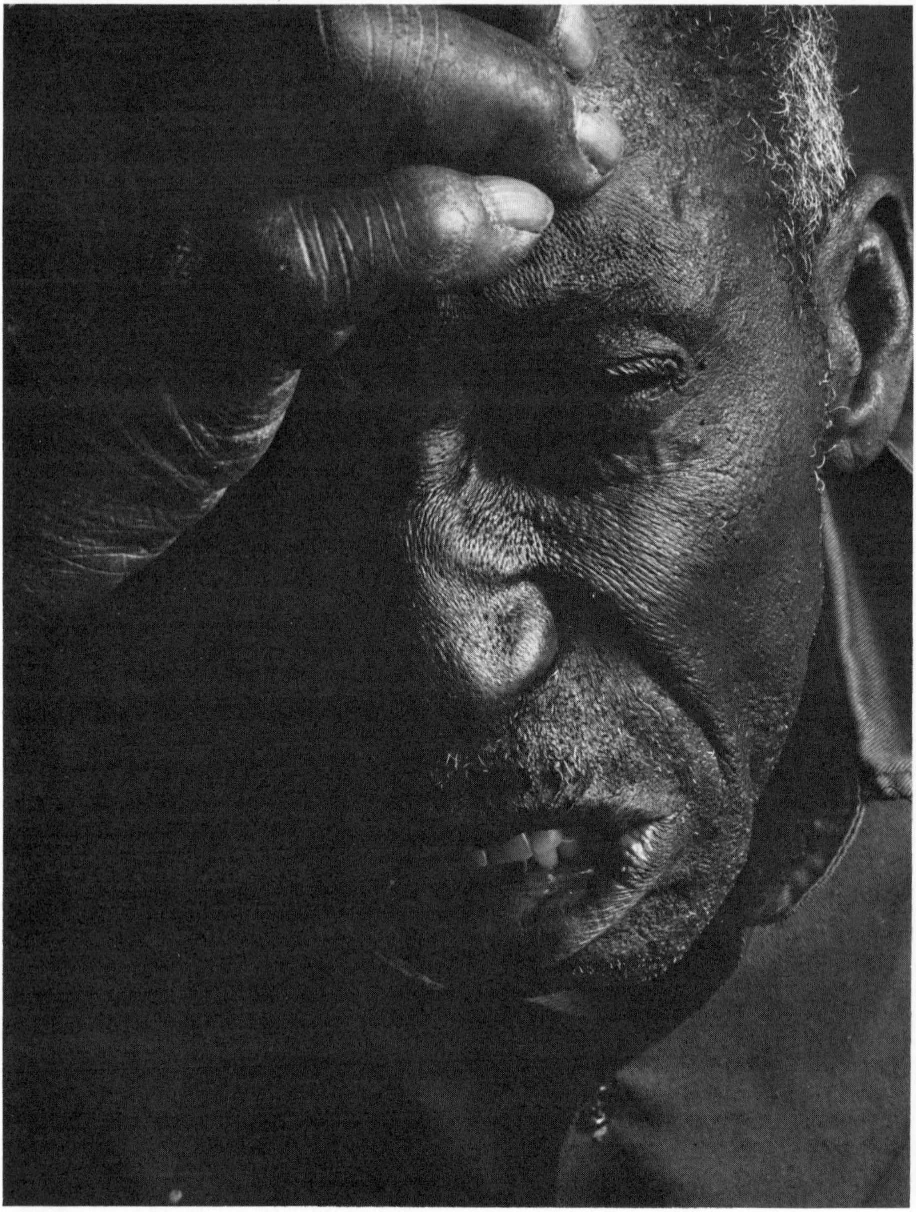

Photo by J. Brian King

Figure 12–1 The Agony of Depression.

become depressed again. Such cyclic cases represent what is meant by *manic depressive psychosis.*

The *manic* phase of a manic depressive disorder involves hyperactivity, a very "high" mood state in which the person seems extraordinarily happy, talkative and expansive. Such individuals display so much energy that others find it hard to keep up with them. They are often amusing, but they seem unable to stick to any particular topic and give you the feeling that they must be active merely for activity's own sake. It is almost as if to stop acting would lead to something dreadful. In the most extreme cases such individuals can drive themselves into a state of complete physical exhaustion, even to the point of death unless someone intervenes and sedates them. Extreme manic states like some depressions tend to occur cyclically.

Some manic depressives go from cycles of depression to normality back to depression. Others go from cycles of mania back to normality back to mania. A third pattern is to swing all the way from serious depression to serious mania.

SUICIDE

A very serious threat in all cases of affective psychosis is the possibility of suicide. Those subject to agitated depressions, often people in the stages of menopause or the male climacteric, are especially serious suicidal risks. Depression and suicide however are risks for individuals of any age group at which particularly difficult stresses and adjustment problems must be managed. As might be expected, the risk for suicide increases as the individual grows older and is highest among those in their old age. The suicide rate among college students is higher than it is for their contemporaries who are not in college. Considering all deaths among college students, suicide accounts for about one-third, a figure exceeded only by accidents as a cause for death in this group (Havighurst, 1969).

Not all deaths from apparent self-destruction have death as a goal. Most suicidal people are undecided about living, and suicidal threats and attempts are often desperate calls for help. This ambivalence about living is most apparent in *suicidal attempts* that do not result in death. More men than women commit suicide, but more women make attempts that fail. Hostility and aggression have long been recognized as basic characteristics of suicide—in fact, suicide is seen as an example of aggression that has been inhibited and then turned inward. Other emotions are causal in suicide—self-blame, the feeling of being lost (disintegration of values), fear, despair, and helplessness.

Suicide is a highly complex behavior with multiple causations that differ with individuals. Statistical data are in large supply, and they provide some surface understanding of suicide. Suicide rates are correlated (found more frequently associated) with the following factors: male sex, increasing age, widowhood, single and divorced state, childlessness, high population density, residence in big cities, a high standard of living, economic crisis, alcohol consumption, history of a broken home in childhood, mental disorder, and physical illness. Conversely low suicide rates are related to female sex, youth, low population density (though not extremely low), rural occupation, religious devoutness, the married state, a large number of children, membership in the lower social-economic classes, and war (Stengel, 1964).

These factors, and even the emotions leading to suicide, do not adequately reveal the person's struggle with memories of rejection, lack of deep and continual need satisfaction, conflicts, guilts, depressions, self-hatred, lack of real love or unifying emotions, and hopelessness about the future.

Menninger (1938) has said that the suicidal gesture is thus a cry not only of distress, not only a cry for help, not only a prayer, but it is a pleading: "I want to live; help me to find a way to live." This cry is heard not only from the mentally ill who attempt to take their lives, but from the deeply unhappy, the severely upset (emotionally), and those who have temporarily lost hope. This finding about suicide argues for the importance of detection, prevention, and multiprofessional treatment of persons in a suicidal state of mind.

Theories About the Cause of Affective Psychosis. As in the case with schizophrenia, two types of theories are advanced about the etiology of affective psychoses. One type stresses internal factors, and the other stresses external factors. As is true in schizophrenia, one type of internal factor that has been examined as the potential cause of affective psychosis is the biochemistry of the manic depressive. Although some biochemical abnormalities have been found which might account for manic depressive disorders, it must be concluded (Beck, 1967) that these results are inconsistent and that the few positive findings that can be confirmed cannot be identified as causing the psychosis but rather may be secondary to problems like poor diet, reduced activity, and increased glandular secretions.

Heredity has also been implicated as a potential cause of manic depressive disorder. While Kallman (1953) has reported a high degree of concurrence of manic depressive psychosis in members of identical twin pairs, Beck (1967) has challenged this study on methodological grounds. Beck has also reviewed the work of others who have studied potential hereditary causes of manic depressive psychosis and finds that concordance rates in these studies are lower than those reported by Kallman. Thus it is impossible to be conclusive about the significance of hereditary factors in affective psychosis.

Studies of families of patients suffering affective psychosis have not actually been done. The closest thing to such a study was done by a group of psychoanalysts (Cohen, Baker, Cohen, Fromm-Reichman, &

Weigert, 1954). Each took several patients suffering manic depressive psychosis into psychotherapy and compared notes with respect to what they had learned from these patients about their early family experiences. On the basis of the therapeutic study of twelve patients, this group of analysts concluded that the manic depressive tended to come from a family that felt isolated in their particular social setting, either because they were minority group members or because economically they could not keep up with those around them. Sometimes serious mental illness in the family caused them to feel alienated from others. In all cases this social isolation was very keenly felt, and much effort went into conforming to accepted social standards in an effort to win the respect of the neighbors. Additionally, there was much emphasis within the family on raising its economic level or winning honors that would bring recognition. Children in these families were brought up to conform rigidly, to behave well, and were looked upon as the means by which the family might pull itself up by its bootstraps. The child's own needs were overlooked in favor of what he might be able to accomplish to elevate the family. Often the need for prestige and for improving family status was inculcated in the child by the mother, who was ambitious and who tended to see the father as a failure.

According to Cohen et al. (1954) in the first year of the manic depressive's life his mother accepts it as her solemn duty to take good care of her child and she looks after him very devotedly providing many comforts and satisfactions. As the child grows and begins to be capable of independence and perhaps even rebelliousness, the mother, a very conventional person, becomes uncomfortable. Toward the end of the first year she shifts her way of dealing with the baby. Just as she accepted it as her duty initially to care for the child, she now sees it as the child's duty to begin to do things for himself and for others as soon as he is capable. She, in effect, demands the kind of conformity from the child that has characterized her own functioning throughout her life. For the premanic depressive this is seen to be a particularly puzzling time of life because he has built a set of positive expectations and feelings about his attentive mother and suddenly is confronted with a whole new set of very negative feelings about this changed mother. Integrating the two sets of feelings and understanding what is going on are a task that is regarded as never being accomplished successfully.

As a child the premanic depressive is often a particularly talented member of the family group, usually the most capable member of the family. Therefore, he is given the special responsibility of raising the family's status. However, he must succeed in this task without cutting himself off from the rest of the family by arousing envy in his siblings. The only way he can manage this is by underselling himself and doing his best to hide his superior ability, particularly within the family.

The adult adjustment of the premanic depressive is characterized by the outward appearance of considerable skill at interacting with other people. Typically he knows a great many people and seems to get along well with them. He has a good sense of humor and seems to be well liked. Actually close observation reveals that his social performance is rather stereotyped, like an act that he has learned to do, and the same script is used indiscriminately with everyone he encounters. Generally people find the act entertaining but the premanic depressive's relationships lack depth, and he displays a minimal ability to understand the needs of others and to reciprocate feelings. People are seen to be objects to be manipulated. A few may be appealed to for the satisfaction of deep dependency needs, but even in these cases little understanding of others and their needs is displayed.

The affective psychosis is touched off in the premanic depressive as the result of some serious loss of emotional support. Often such a loss involves the death or departure of another person, but it may even involve an apparent success such as a promotion at work which cuts him off from a source of emotional support that he felt he needed. Basically the premanic depressive is seen as a person who manages to get along by appealing to others to care for him. As long as such appeals are not excessive and they are satisfied, he remains fairly stable. When he is disappointed, however, his demands become childish and excessive and are, threfore, highly likely to be rejected. This creates a cycle that ends up in deep depression and in many with a need to become extraordinarily active as a way of staving off the depression.

As is the case with the family studies of schizophrenia, one can criticize the study by Cohen et al. (1954) on several grounds. First, the families of the manic depressive patients are not compared to the families of other types of patients or of comparable normals. Therefore, it is impossible to say that what was found to be true for the early experience of the manic depressive might not be equally true for other groups of subjects. Another serious problem is that only 12 patients were studied and it was a particularly select group. All were individuals well motivated to engage in and able to afford intensive psychotherapy. These factors alone indicate that they were striving individuals who had achieved material success. The conclusions drawn by the study group concerning the importance of certain background factors may, therefore, be less evident in the early histories of manic depressives whose social and professional accomplishments are more modest than those in the group studied.

Several follow-up studies of the Cohen et al. (1954) project have been done (Gibson, 1958; Becker, 1960; Becker, Spielberger, & Parker, 1963; Spielberger, Parker, & Becker, 1963). These studies have attempted to introduce what were thought to be necessary controls for adequately understanding the findings of Cohen et al. (1954). A summary of the results of these studies indicates that, in comparison to schizophrenics, manic depressive patients do seem to come from families which emphasize the need to elevate family prestige in which the patient is seen to play a key role. Manic depressives also see themselves as being exposed to greater envy and competitiveness than do schizophrenics and do attempt to undersell themselves. It was also found that manic depressives show more concern about being approved by others than do schizophrenics.

In comparison to normal individuals who had never suffered emotional disorder, manic depressives were also found to have valued achievement more highly, to have displayed more authoritarian attitudes, and more concern with conformity to family attitudes. However, no differences were found between manic depressives and other patient groups such as schizophrenics and neurotic depressives with respect to the degree to which achievement was valued and family values were prized. Thus this raises the question of whether some of the qualities of the manic depressive which are described by Cohen et al. (1954) typify only manic depressives or whether they typify a variety of patient groups.

Psychoneurotic Disorders

The term *neurotic* is part of today's popular vocabulary, although many who use it freely have only a general idea of its meaning. The technical term of which it is a contraction is *psychoneurotic,* one of the traditional classifications of common maladjustment. The psychoneurotic individual suffers severe anxieties and conflicts, and the defense mechanisms he uses to deal with them are self-defeating and themselves become problems. Larry (p. 5), who suffered intense anxiety when he attempted to teach, Katherine (p. 8), whose overpowering fears and preoccupation with perfection were defeating her, and Irwin (p. 46), whose many obsessions incapacitated him, are examples of neurotics. None of the concerns of these people ever materialized. While we are all subject to anxiety and distressing conflicts, and entertain bizarre ideas that obsess us or compulsions that grow out of guilt, in the neurotic these symptoms are so severe that he finds them unendurable.

TYPES OF PSYCHONEUROSES

Several different types of neuroses are identified, although any particular neurotic probably has a mixture of neurotic symptoms. The particular form taken by a neurosis depends upon the ways a person tries to control his anxiety. Some of the most common forms of neurosis involve raw feelings of anxiety, obsessive-compulsiveness, phobias, hysteria and dissociated states, depression and hypochondria.

Anxiety Neurosis. The anxiety neurotic is a generally tense person who is not really aware of what is upsetting him. Some people are tense and apprehensive because they are consciously beset by real pressures. The anxiety neurotic cannot identify such real pressures. In addition he tends to be unsure of himself, so that he has a hard time making decisions. At times, usually only for brief periods, the anxiety neurotic experiences feelings of panic. He may be so upset that his blood races and his heart pounds leading him to fear that he might have a heart attack.

Obsessive-Compulsiveness. The obsessive-compulsive neurotic is one who needs to keep occupied through thinking or behavior in order to remain free of anxiety. The person who uses his thoughts to control anxiety (the obsessive) will generally be preoccupied with useless ideas. He may try to solve mathematical problems in his head. He may dwell on sports statistics. He may make lists in his mind over and over. He may make poker hands out of automobile license plate numbers. Very little of this internal activity is toward some useful, practical end. The primary purpose such thoughts seem to serve is to keep other, disturbing ideas out of his mind.

Those who must engage in useless acts (compulsion) may display a variety of repetitive behaviors. Some of these behaviors seem to be related to a need for safety such as checking over and over before leaving the house to be sure that the lights are out, the gas is turned off on the stove, and the water is not running in the sink. Similarly some people must check repeatedly to be sure that the doors to the house or car are locked. Another class of compulsive acts involves concern for cleanliness, neatness, and appearance. These include frequent handwashing (as in Lady Macbeth) or bathing. Similarly a concern for neatness and order may lead to changing clothes frequently, hair combing over and over, and constant tie straightening, and the like. Many compulsive acts are even less practical and actually involve superstitions. Examples would be having to touch every third or fifth picket on a fence, or having to avoid stepping on the cracks in a sidewalk.

Most obsessive-compulsive neurotics have symptoms of both obsessions and compulsions. It should also be pointed out that many of the thoughts and behaviors described occur in people who are not neurotic. The difference between the neurotic and the normal is that in the former the symptoms take up so much time, and so much anxiety is present in spite of their use that the person cannot manage to keep up with what is expected of him in his daily life (at work or school, in his family and social relationships).

Phobias. Phobic neuroses involve fear of some object or situation that can only be controlled through physical avoidance. Sometimes phobias are pretty specific and result in only mild annoyance or inconvenience. An example would be a fear of large dogs that would prompt a person to cross over to the other side of the street to avoid passing one or that would make it impossible to enter a house where there was a large dog. Another such example would be a fear of riding in elevators. This would prevent one from going to the upper floors of tall buildings, only a minor disability in a small town having few such tall buildings.

On the other hand, one may be phobic about being among large numbers of people or being in open spaces. Such phobias would be very disabling because they would prevent a person from being comfortable whenever he or she left the home or apartment.

Hysteria and Dissociated States. Hysterical neurosis is characterized primarily by the presence of physical complaints, often dramatic ones, that don't make sense organically. These symptoms are usually associated with the senses of touch, sight, hearing, or smell. So, the hysteric may seem to be blind, but unlike the truly blind person he will avoid walking into objects in unfamiliar surroundings. He may lose feeling in some part of the body, so that he cannot feel heat, cold, pressure or pain. He may even complain of paralysis in an arm or leg, although the muscles involved fail to show atrophy as they would in a person who was truly paralyzed.

The organically nonsensical quality of hysterical symptoms is underlined by the fact that they occur in parts of the body that could not be afflicted without involving other parts given the patterns followed by the nerves. For example, a hysteric might complain of a loss of feeling in the hand but nowhere else. To lose feeling in the hand because of organic defect, however, would also require a loss of feeling in part of the arm as well.

It should be emphasized that despite the fact that the hysteric's symptoms are not organically based, neither are they a "put-on." The person really feels convinced that he has them. It is characteristic of hysterics, though, that they don't display the distress one would expect from a person suffering such dramatic and disabling maladies. This may be because the symptoms relieve neurotic anxiety and because they win for him sympathy and relief from unpleasant responsibilities (secondary gain). These are apparently more important than the physical losses suffered.

Dissociation involves a disturbance of consciousness such that the person loses his memory for who he is and what his life situation is. This may last for a short time (a few hours) or a long time (several days or a week). The occasional dramatic case of multiple personality is an example of dissociation in which a person with one kind of personality has brief lapses in which he behaves like a very different kind of person. In some cases a rigid, conforming, upstanding citizen has spells where he behaves like a "swinger," calling himself by a new name that is appropriate to his new identity. When dissociation is longer lasting, also a very rare occurrence, the person loses touch with who he was and the life he had led, and wanders away to a community where he is unknown. There a new identity as well as a new life may be taken up. In some such cases the person even marries and raises a new family.

Depressive Neurosis. Neurotic depression is usually touched off by a distressing external event. It tends to persist, however, well past the time one would expect. In neurotic depression the emotional disorder is not nearly so severe and disabling as it is in the affective psychoses. Generally the person feels sad, cries from time to time, may have some difficulty falling asleep or staying asleep, and finds it hard to enjoy things. On the other hand, the neurotic depressive can usually manage his work, family, and social responsibilities.

Hypochondriacal Neurosis. The hypochondriac is preoccupied with his body and lives in constant fear of becoming ill. He frets over the possibility of contracting diseases or of suffering a disorder in a vital body organ such as the heart, lungs, liver, or kidneys. He doesn't actually have the delusion that he is diseased. But, despite reassurance, he is afraid that he might become so.

THEORIES ABOUT THE CAUSE OF PSYCHONEUROSES

Freud's psychoanalytic theory was one of the oldest and for many years dominant theory about the cause of psychoneurosis. In recent years a number of different views have been taken by theorists identifying themselves as humanists and learning theorists. All theorists attempt to explain essentially the same behavior, although they may differ in what aspects of the observed behavior they emphasize.

The Psychoanalytic Theory. Freud explains the anxiety common to all neuroses on the basis of internal conflict. He feels that in the neurotic there are powerful, but largely unconscious, impulses to behave in a certain way and equally powerful feelings about such behavior that inhibit impulse expression. This internal struggle drains psychic energy, so that any additional psychological problems threaten to upset the person quite seriously. The anxiety of neurosis is felt to signal this dangerous situation. The other behavioral symptoms such as phobias, obsessive-compulsiveness, and the like are defensive maneuvers to ward off the uncomfortable anxiety.

From the psychoanalytic view the roots of psychoneuroses lie fairly deep in the personality structure. Treatment is aimed at helping the neurotic become aware of his troublesome conflict, assisting him in discharging, directly where possible, the demanding impulses, and aiding him in finding indirect, but socially acceptable ways to win still further impulse gratification.

Humanistic Theories. A large number of theorists count themselves as humanists, though they vary somewhat in their emphases and treatment approaches. However, all seem to feel that neuroses, as well as other disorders, arise because society insists that we inhibit many powerful feelings in the course of development. These include the anger resulting from frustration, the loneliness and disappointment resulting from feeling unattractive, and the grief associated with feeling unloved. As these feelings accumulate, defenses must be erected to prevent their expression. These defenses result in distortions of reality and the symptoms that typify neuroses.

For most humanists treatment of neurosis requires the release of the troublesome fund of repressed feelings. It is assumed that once these feelings find open expression, in effect once the dam is broken, there will no longer be a need for defending, and the person will be able to live a more fulfilling life. Different humanists use different techniques for encouraging affective release, as will be described in Chapter 13.

Learning Theory Approaches. Like the humanists, learning or behavior theorists vary with respect to their views of the causes of neuroses and in their treatment approaches. Unlike the psychoanalysts, though, all reject the idea that the roots of such disorders lie in the early years of psychological development. Instead, they stress that symptoms are learned responses to specific upsetting situations which need to be unlearned. And unlike the humanists, the learning theorists are less interested in internal feelings than they are in external behavior.

One learning approach to psychoneurosis is exemplified by Wolpe (1958). He sees neurosis developing as the result of the contiguous association of feelings of anxiety with stimuli that had formerly been neutral. This association comes to result in the feeling of anxiety whenever the previously neutral stimulus arises. Some people are more susceptible to neurosis than others simply because they are so put together constitutionally that they feel anxiety more often or more intensely. Others are especially vulnerable because of their early learning experiences.

Wolpe (1958) like other learning theorists, has a slightly different formulation for the development of the various types of neurotic symptoms. The anxiety neurotic, for example, is seen to have a conditioned anxiety response to subtle but pervasive stimuli, perhaps even internal ones. By contrast, in hysteria he believes that a motor or physical symptom is conditioned in especially stressful times rather than an anxiety response. He believes that this is most likely to happen in particularly extraverted people who are more given to action than to thought. The obsessive-compulsive is seen to learn both anxiety responses as well as obsessive or compulsive symptoms at the same time. To the extent that obsessions and compulsions reduce anxiety, they are learned rapidly. Wolpe's approach to treating neuroses is described in the next chapter.

Another important learning approach to psychoneurosis is based on the work of B. F. Skinner (Ullmann & Krasner, 1969). Skinner's view is that all learning results from reinforcement. If a person does something that leads to a reinforcing consequence, he is likely to repeat it. When the behavior is no longer reinforced, it is eliminated. Thus neurotic behavior is sustained by the reinforcing reactions it produces in the people associated with the neurotic. This point of view is called the *sociopsychological approach* by Ullmann and Krasner (1969), who explain specific neurotic subtypes on slightly differing bases.

For example, the person who is phobic may start out by simply avoiding situations in which he is anxious, either because he is inadequate in them or because they are very frightening. Once this avoidance begins, however, it tends to elicit sympathy and attention from others. This reinforces the phobic behavior and helps to maintain it further. The anxiety neurosis is seen to be a complex phobic reaction. Obsessive-compulsive behavior is reinforcing because it helps the person avoid other behaviors that might be noxious.

From the sociopsychological viewpoint hysteria is a disorder in which the person plays a role that he feels he is expected to perform. Also, it is a role that pays off in that by being "sick" the person receives reinforcement in the form of concern from those around him. Ullmann and Krasner (1969) feel that some people are better than others at playing expected roles, hence they are more susceptible to hysterical disorders. The application of Skinner's approach to changing the behavior of seriously disturbed patients is described in the next chapter.

Psychosomatic Disorders

We are all aware of a close tie between our emotions and certain physiological functions. When we become frightened our heart may pound and our pulse quickens. Disgust may cause the stomach to churn. Extreme sadness results in a flow of tears. Thus there is a unity in the way thoughts, emotions and our physiology function. This can be a great asset. For example, when we feel threatened by danger, there is an automatic increase in blood flow to the nerves and muscles that must cope with the problem, stored energy reserves are released, and the heart beats faster to speed the circulation of the blood. In effect the body is like a nation preparing for war. And the signal that sets the process in motion is the feeling of danger. What happens, however, when the signal is chronically present, the body responds with the proper preparations, but there is no follow-through?

In such a case the body is in a constant state of preparing for a threat that isn't acted on. The heart continues to work harder than it should under normal conditions. The blood keeps circulating faster than normal. And eventually this chronically abnormal physiological state actually causes changes in bodily tissues. Such changes are what are called *psychosomatic disorders.*

TYPES OF PSYCHOSOMATIC DISORDERS

The concept of psychosomatic disorder developed as physicians became aware that there were many illnesses that they could treat symptomatically but whose causes they could not affect with medicine alone. This led to the suspicion that emotional factors play a key role in such cases. In time a large variety of physical disorders came under scrutiny as having possible psychosomatic origins. These included many skin disorders; asthma; hypertension and migraine headaches; ulcers and various stomach disorders; mucous colitis; and constipation. The specific role of emotions in these disorders is still far from clear. Many have been studied extensively by clinicians and researchers, but their findings are still not conclusive. Still, some suspicions and tentative conclusions about a few of the most prevalent of the psychosomatic disorders can be summarized.

Essential Hypertension. This disorder, better known to laymen as high blood pressure, can cause physical changes in the heart muscle and blood vessels. As already described, elevated blood pressure is a common reaction to stress. People vary in susceptibility to this disorder, but the tense, jittery person seems most vulnerable. Studies also show that aggressive feelings elevate blood pressure. What isn't clear is whether hypertension sufferers show blood pressure changes in response to other feelings besides frustrated aggression.

Migraine Headaches. There are many different kinds of headaches, and headache may be caused by any of a number of disorders. The typical migraine sufferer has periodic attacks. These usually begin with some early symptom such as a blind spot, speech difficulty or an abnormal sensation. The headache itself is nearly always concentrated on one side of the head and is accompanied by nausea, vomiting, and sensitivity to light.

Alexander and Szasz (1952) characterize the typical migraine sufferer as being bright, ambitious, hostile and envious, and a compulsive perfectionist. He often seems very conforming despite his ambition, as though he were required to go along with strict behavior patterns that preclude the direct expression of anger. Alexander felt that the headaches occur when this person is very angry and cannot allow himself to express the feeling for fear of alienating his family. Alexander theorized that the migraine sufferer inhibits his feelings before the body can fully prepare to express anger. If the inhibition occurred after some bodily preparations for attack, the resulting symptom would be hypertension rather than migraine. This interesting theory is not yet supported by research evidence.

Peptic Ulcers. Peptic ulcers are inflamed areas on the stomach lining. They are caused by the chronic presence of excess digestive acids in the stomach. Normally acids are sent into the stomach when food is present. Once these acids do the job of digesting the food their secretion ceases. When the acids stay in the stomach too long, they begin to irritate the lining. People who are susceptible to ulcers tend typically to secrete too much acid, often even when the stomach is empty.

One well-known psychological theory by Alexander (1950) to explain acid oversecretion holds that the ulcer sufferer has primitive yearnings for love and affection. Because he feels such feelings are not "grown-up" he must inhibit them. Still, the need for love persists, however, and must find outlets that do not involve overt behavior. In some, it is theorized, the feeling takes its most primitive form, the wish to be fed. Thus the stomach reacts continually as though it were about to receive food.

Research studies on the causes of ulcers (Maher, 1966) seem to indicate that ulcers occur in both humans and animals who are chronically high acid secretors and who undergo prolonged stress. This does not contradict Alexander's theory. However, it does suggest that stresses other than loss or lack of love can produce ulcers in constitutionally predisposed people.

Bronchial Asthma. Asthma is a disorder in the breathing apparatus. Its symptoms include difficult breathing, wheezing, gasping for air, and the feeling of suffocation. It is caused by spasms that reduce the diameter of the bronchia, tubes that send air on its way to the lungs.

A popular view is that a combination of both constitutional factors in the form of allergies and emotional factors cause asthma. The psychoanalytic view of the emotional problem holds that the asthmatic attack, which seems like a stifled cry, is actually a suppressed cry for the mother. This hypothesis seems to be supported by the clinical observation that asthmatics have a hard time crying and that often an attack ends when the asthmatic can break down and cry. Therefore, the feelings that are thought to be important to the asthmatic are strong dependency needs on others that can neither be accepted nor expressed.

Personality studies of asthmatics (Zax & Cowen, 1972) characterize them as very restrained, angry people who find it hard to be overt about their hostility. In general these studies indicate that the more seriously disturbed the personality, the more severe the somatic symptoms. These studies neither support nor contradict the psychoanalytic stress on unacceptable dependency feelings.

Other studies indicate that psychological factors play an important part in asthma but not necessarily deep-lying dependency feelings. For example, cases have been described in which attacks were triggered by contact with flowers—both real and papier-mâché flowers; by the specific hour of the day; or by the sound of a particular song. Such phenomena suggest that psychological conditioning may be as important as physical allergies in prompting asthmatic reactions.

CAUSES OF PSYCHOSOMATIC DISORDERS

Many theories have been offered to explain why certain people suffer psychosomatic disorders at all and why they have the symptoms they do. One of the oldest of these, the *conversion theory*, argues that the psychosomatic symptom symbolizes a neurotic conflict. This theory has not won many adherents.

Another theory, the *personality-profile theory*, holds that certain personality types are prone to certain organic illnesses. From this view specific types of people are subject to a symptomlike peptic ulcer, whereas a different type would be more vulnerable to migraine headaches. Most research fails to support this theory.

Alexander (1950) proposed that it was not personality type but specific emotional states related to specific internal conflicts that determines the type of symptom that appears (the *specific conflict theory*). Thus the chronically angry person will have high blood pressure regardless of what makes him angry or what personality type he is. Persistent yearnings for affection, on the other hand, will lead to other symptoms.

Perhaps the most widely accepted theory of why psychosomatic symptoms arise where they do is the *somatic-weakness hypothesis*. This holds that most people have a vulnerable organ system (an "Achilles' heel").

Because of such a specific weakness, some people are more prone to psychosomatic symptoms than others and, under stress, are more likely to suffer certain symptoms than others. Although the specific nature of the constitutional weaknesses that might be involved is not well defined, many theorists subscribe to a combination of this theory and some other that implicates emotional factors in some way.

RECENT VIEWS OF PSYCHOSOMATIC MEDICINE

Many of the ideas we have already discussed have attempted to explain the development of specific illnesses. More recent theorists and researchers have emphasized a relationship between emotional and psychological factors and general physiological functioning (Zax & Cowen, 1972). For example, one group of researchers has stressed that the experience of suffering a serious loss (of love, a dear one, or a precious possession) leads to a psychological "giving-up" that makes one vulnerable to all types of physical disorders. President Nixon's intensified phlebitis problem following his resignation would be a good example seeming to support this theory.

Another approach, tested primarily in animal studies, proposes that early life experience can predispose one to later physical vulnerability. Thus animals housed individually when young suffered from more weight problems after exposure to stressful conditions than animals that had lived in small groups. Other factors such as handling in early life and mother-litter interactions apparently also are related to later susceptibility to physical disorder.

Quite recently many studies have been done with humans that may help us to understand the causes of psychosomatic disorders and that offer exciting treatment possibilities. This work involves *biofeedback*. Biofeedback refers simply to a number of techniques for actually giving a person information about the ongoing functioning of one of his physiological systems. It has been found (Engel & Shapiro, 1971) that when a person can "see" internal physiological responses that he is otherwise insensitive to, he can change them. He can control his heart rate and blood pressure to some extent, for example, and can reduce respiratory resistance.

One researcher has reasoned that many people with psychosomatic symptoms have learned to react to stress with undetected expenditures of energy that are great enough to have an effect on nervous system functions. As an example, holding the body rigidly may make a person feel vigilant, but it also disturbs his smooth muscle function and upsets his digestion. This can result in ulcers or colitis. Teaching a person through biofeedback to control key internal functions can, therefore, lead to a cure of symptoms.

Interestingly, it had been thought that most internal functions that are now demonstrated to respond to learning through feedback were not under the person's control. Biofeedback studies with humans intended to get at *how* the person exercises internal control reveal that the control that is achieved is not done so on a conscious basis. Many subjects can change their heart rate but can't say how they do it. One subject, when asked to tell how he managed such an internal change simply shrugged and answered, "How do I move my arm?"

Summary

1. Psychoses, the most disabling of the behavior disorders, involve a break with reality. Psychoneuroses, while causing severe discomfort, are not characterized by a loss of touch with the real world.
2. Two major subgroups of psychosis are schizophrenia and the affective psychoses. Fundamental to schizophrenia are thought disorder and an affective disorder involving the expression of grossly inappropriate emotional reactions.
3. Four major types of schizophrenia were described: simple, paranoid, catatonic, and hebephrenic. Along a longitudinal dimension the process and reactive types were described.
4. A variety of underlying potential causes of schizophrenia were discussed. These included biochemical, genetic, and environmental factors. A summary of the evidence provided by a variety of such studies suggests that both constitutional and environmental forces combine to produce schizophrenia.
5. Affective psychoses are characterized by extreme mood states, either deep depression or the height of elation. Such disorders are often cyclical in nature. In some cases the depression leads to suicidal attempts.
6. Studies of the potential causes of affective psychoses have investigated biochemical, genetic, and familial factors. Findings in the biochemical and genetic studies are inconclusive. Some familial patterns seem to be related to the occurrence of affective psychoses but may also predispose individuals to other disorders as well.
7. Psychoneurosis is characterized by anxiety and conflict that are either overt or covered over by defenses that are themselves quite disabling or inconvenient.
8. The various psychoneurotic subtypes include anxiety neurosis, obsessive-compulsive neurosis, phobic neurosis, hysteria and dissociated states, depressive neurosis, and hypochondriacal neurosis.
9. Many theories have been advanced to explain the cause of psychoneuroses. The oldest, the psychoanalytic theory, holds that the

disorder results from internal conflict. The humanists attribute neuroses to feelings stored up because of life's frustrations and inhibitions imposed by society. Learning theorists attribute neuroses to the reinforcement of neurotic behavior patterns.

10. Psychosomatic disorders result from emotionally induced, chronic, abnormal physiological states that cause actual tissue change.
11. Hypertension, migraine, peptic ulcers, and asthma are all examples of disorders strongly suspected of having significant emotional causes.
12. Theories about the causes of psychosomatic disorders attempt to explain why they occur and why they arise in the organs that they do.
13. The oldest, and least respected, theory holds that the psychosomatic symptom symbolizes a neurotic conflict. The personality-profile theory argues that specific personality types are subject to specific psychosomatic symptoms. The specific conflict theory sees the specific symptom as being caused by specific conflicts and the physiological effects of the emotions these conflicts arouse. The somatic-weakness hypothesis proposes that symptoms arise in stressful times in those organ systems that are particularly weak or vulnerable.
14. Recent thinking about psychosomatic medicine suggests that as the result of psychological losses a person "gives up" emotionally and becomes vulnerable to a variety of physical disorders. Another recent approach attributes a key role to early experience in creating vulnerability to psychosomatic disorder. Recent studies involving biofeedback demonstrate that a person can learn to control internal physiological processes related to physical illness.

Words To Remember

Affective Psychosis
Conversion Reaction
Delusion
Dissociative Reaction
Double-Bind
Hallucination
Marital Schism
Marital Skew
Process Schizophrenia
Pseudomutuality
Psychoneurosis
Psychosis
Reactive Schizophrenia
Schizophrenia
Somatic-Weakness Theory
Specific-Conflict Theory
Waxy Flexibility

Part IV
Roads to Enhancing Adjustment

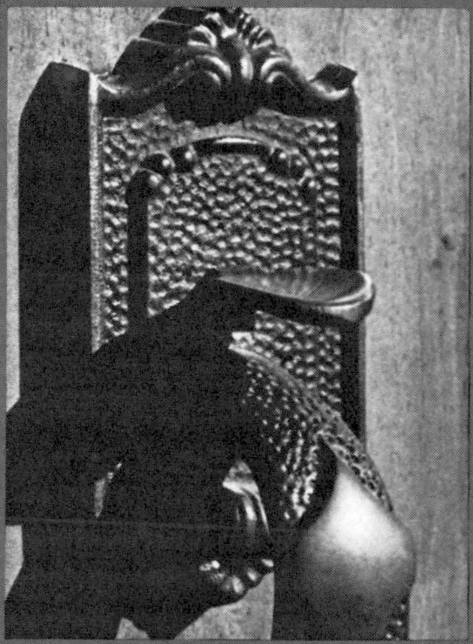

13. Counseling and Psychotherapy

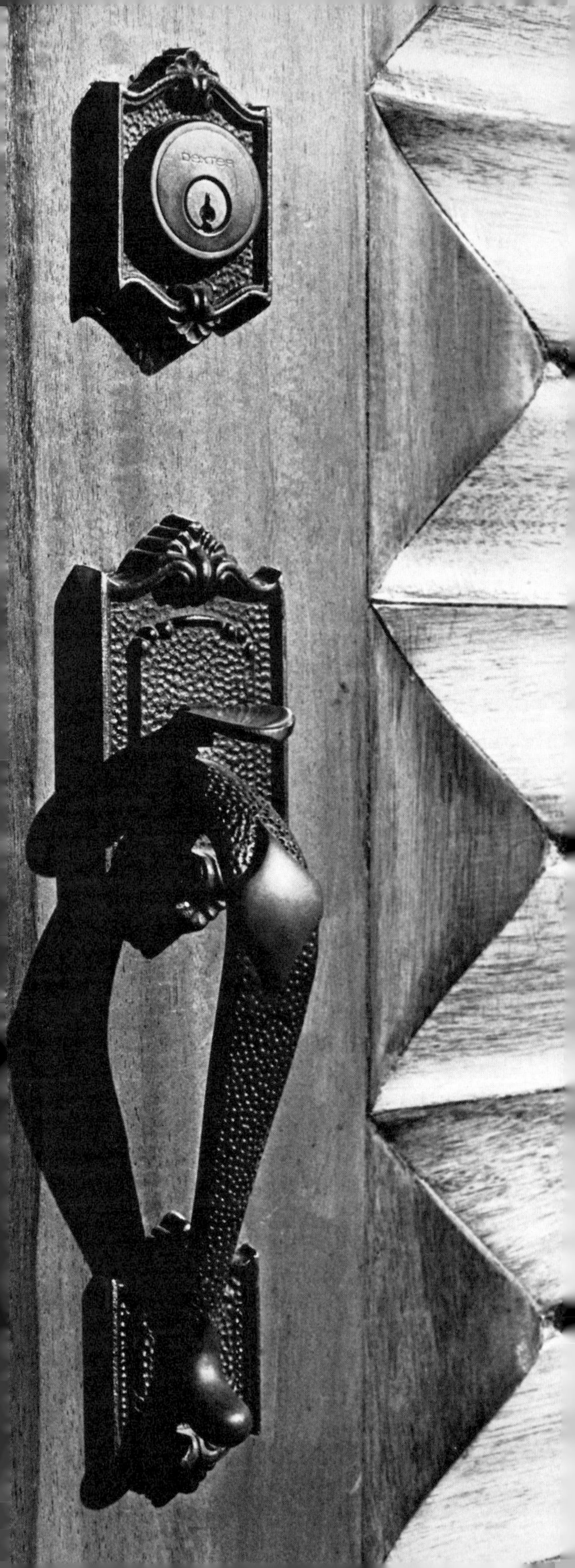
DEXTER

Objectives

After studying this chapter the reader should be able to:

1. List the characteristics that most forms of psychotherapy and counseling have in common.
2. Describe six current therapies in terms of their major techniques and objectives.

By now, the reader surely realizes that at some time in our lives we may all face problems generated by failure to reach our goals (*frustration*) and the *conflict between our needs.* As noted earlier, frustration and conflicts (or even the prospect of these conditions) produce *anxiety,* a distressing state that is a major source of inadequate and self-defeating behaviors. Such behaviors are called *defense mechanisms* because they defend the individual against anxiety and related threats to him as a person. Defenses may themselves become additional problems, however, because they often cause the individual to avoid facing his difficulty and attempting to cope with it rationally.

Now we shall review some of what is known presently about the available means to help us adjust to distressing or disabling problems. What can individuals who are in distress and are unable to meet the requirements of their situation do to lower their level of anxiety, to find the causes of their difficulties, and to change the conditions that led to them? Before we discuss the possibility of seeking professional help, we shall describe the so-called helping or human service professions.

The Helping Professions

To whom can you turn when in need of help to get through an emotional crisis? Who can help you to overcome a state of depression or a constant feeling of inadequacy? The study and treatment of human emotions has so broadened over the years that several professional groups now exist whose research focuses on the reasons for emotional disorder and on identifying the most effective ways to alleviate them. In some places, these groups form "mental health" teams that approach the treatment of a disorder using their respective different skills in an integrated fashion.

Portions of this chapter were contributed by William T. McReynolds.

Photo by J. Brian King

SIMILARITIES BETWEEN THE PROFESSIONS

Let's begin with similarities. Members of each of the helping professions—psychiatrists, clinical and counseling psychologists, psychiatric social workers, and psychiatric nurses—work with those who are to some extent emotionally disturbed. These professions attempt to help individuals adjust to their environment and to reduce the distress they are experiencing. Each of these professions is similar with respect to the type of *relationship* established with clients or patients, the *processes* that operate as the client improves, and many of the *techniques* used (Patterson, 1966).

PERSONNEL

A *psychiatrist* holds an M.D. degree; after completing his medical education, he has taken graduate work and resident training in psychiatry. A related medical field is neurology. In the field of neurology the physician specializes in abnormalities that result from defective functioning of the central (e.g., the brain) and peripheral nervous systems. If the physician practices both neurology and psychiatry, he is known as a *neuropsychiatrist.* As physicians, both neurologists and psychiatrists are legally qualified to prescribe drugs, electroconvulsive shock, and other physical procedures. The psychiatrist may practice psychoanalysis or some other methods of psychotherapy. Although most organized psychoanalytic training institutes in this country require practitioners to hold a degree in medicine, Sigmund Freud, the originator of psychoanalysis and himself a doctor of medicine, did not feel that medical education was essential and acknowledged that some of the most valuable contributions to psychoanalysis came from persons with nonmedical training. An eminent example of Freud's statement is one of the best-known living psychoanalysts, Erik Erikson.

The *clinical psychologist* has completed the curriculum of an accredited department of psychology in a university and usually holds a Ph.D. degree plus a year of supervised clinical practice (internship). Clinical psychology began as a profession by making major contributions to diagnosis through the use of standard psychological tests. Today members of the profession are trained in various therapeutic procedures, including behavior modification, an avowedly psychological technique. The training of a *counseling psychologist* is similar. He holds an accredited doctorate (usually Ph.D.) in a counseling program in a university. His training involves supervised practice with clients who usually come to him with problems of vocational, educational, or emotional origins. As Ph.D.s the clinical and counseling psychologists possess research training, which makes them unique among mental health professionals.

In general, *counselors* or *counseling psychologists* work with normal individuals whose problems center on their development or adjustment. The problems brought to the psychotherapist generally involve more severe symptoms. Despite these differences, it is difficult to draw a hard line between the two groups of workers. They may work in different settings (school vs. other institutions or hospital), or with different methods (interest and ability tests vs. depth interviews and projective tests), but many of their functions overlap.

The *psychiatric social worker* usually holds the M.A. or M.S.W. degree, and his training also includes an internship in a psychiatric seting. He is especially qualified to work in the family situation and to understand the socioeconomic, cultural, and interpersonal realities in the home that give rise to emotional strains. He is also usually qualified to engage in psychotherapy.

Psychiatrists as medical doctors have worked closely with nurses who share their hospital and clinical orientation. Some years ago in response to serious need, nursing developed the specialty of the *psychiatric nurse.* This nurse has specialized education and experience to prepare her to care for the emotionally disturbed patient, and she can perform technical procedures in a mental hospital or clinic, such as administering drugs and carrying out other medically oriented treatments. In recent years the psychiatric nurse has also been trained to engage in group therapy, family counseling, and even individual psychotherapy under professional supervision.

Common Conditions in Psychotherapy and Counseling

Because of individual differences in personality and because of the relatively early stage in the history of the treatment of emotional disorders, there are many different approaches to psychotherapy. Still, certain common conditions are thought to characterize these different approaches. Sundberg and Tyler (1962) have developed a list of these conditions some of which we shall review at this time.

One important condition to be established in the treatment of the disturbed person is the *lowering of his anxiety level* so that he can explore the painful area of his experience; with lowered anxiety he can face his problems more readily and approach their solution. An understanding therapist who seems confident and strong and who obviously accepts a person despite his feelings of guilt or inadequacy can help the client to enhance his problem-solving ability.

Establishing *a strong personal relationship* that can be used for constructive change is also a basic element of therapy. This personal relationship may be desirable for different therapists or counselors who use different methods of treatment (Fiedler, 1950a, b). Studies point to the importance of a *warm and accepting relationship* (Truax and Carkhuff, 1965; Gardner 1964). This condition alone may not bring about personality change, but it is important as a condition in treatment.

A third condition is some kind of *verbal or nonverbal communication* (e.g., the use of toys, fingerpaints, or play with children) that allows the client to establish connections between his own inner and outer world. For therapeutic approaches that emphasize the need for insight, this communication is obviously a necessary precondition. But it is also essential in approaches stressing behavior change.

Last, *some* degree of commitment or *motivation for change* on the part of the client or patient is important. The motivation to seek a therapist, to make an appointment, and to participate actively in treatment derives from the distress the client experiences because of his anxiety, guilt, or resulting symptoms. Once in treatment, difficult and, at times, painful work is done, and cooperation between therapist and patient is necessary for progress to occur.

Goals of Psychotherapy or Counseling

Counseling or therapy may lead to any or all of the following: (1) *rational or cognitive events,* such as solving personal problems or making decisions; (2) *affective* events, such as the development of *self-esteem,* the lowering of fear, and a closer congruence between self-concept and the ideal self; or (3) the achievement of a clearer sense of meaning in life.

Different clients bring different problems to the therapist and are disturbed by different symptoms. Sundberg and Tyler (1962) list these various formulations of the goals of therapy.

1. *Motivation to do the right thing.* These "right things" are behaviors that are accepted by the patient and that he respects. This motive may be regarded by the sophisticated as a simplistic goal, but it is a goal that is valued alike by some counselors and some clients.
2. *Reduction of emotional tension* by facilitating the expression of feelings. Called *catharsis,* this process consists of talking out, or acting out emotionally, feelings that have been disturbing.
3. *Release of the potential for growth.* This goal emphasizes the possibilities for development. Either existing blocks to personal development are removed or the client is encouraged to discover avenues of growth and creativity that are presently open to him.
4. *Habit change.* Through the learning process, undesirable or ineffective habits have been formed. The therapeutic process includes modification and replacement of undesirable habits with effective ones.

5. *Modification of cognitive structures* or mistaken ideas. Misconceptions held by the patient about the nature of things and about himself that interfere with his adjustment are examined and hopefully corrected.
6. *Self-knowledge.* This goal includes the interpretation of aptitude and interest tests as well as the discovery of previously unrecognized attitudes, needs, or traits.
7. *Better interpersonal relationships.* This goal is the opposite of isolation and estrangement from others. It consists of establishing better communication and relationships with others who are significant in one's life.

A given counselor may have several of these goals in mind in dealing with a client. Also, there may be "unconscious" or underlying influences (aversions, withdrawal from situations, or overreactions) that may have caused the client's problems, and their modification will give rise to the need for several of these goals. The major goal of psychotherapy is to help the client to behave rationally and effectively.

Approaches to Psychotherapy

INSIGHT THERAPY

In the insight therapies, talk is the major vehicle of treatment, the patient, and often his past, being a major subject of discussion. The therapeutic session is different from the usual social interaction in that the talk is focused on the patient, his needs, his defenses, and there is much probing to understand deep-lying motives for behavior. The client or patient at first is unaware of what is really causing his distress or complaints. Unknown or unconscious forces in his life (conflicts, anxieties, defenses) are preventing his directing his life in terms of his conscious goals; he tends to lack awareness; he may be immature and self-centered. In insight therapy the client comes to talk freely, and as he talks to understand and bring under control the destructive inner forces so that he gains greater rational control over his life.

PSYCHOANALYSIS AND PSYCHOANALYTIC PSYCHOTHERAPY

The treatment procedure worked out by Freud is based on the belief that a person's emotional problems have their roots in the early stages of psychological development. Insistent, unsatisfied impulses are seen to clash with internal prohibitions to create a conflict state. Although unconscious, these internal forces and struggles exercise a powerful effect on behavior. Successful treatment requires the exposure and defusing of unconscious impulses and the establishment of effective coping techniques.

Psychoanalysis is a long and intensive treatment process. The patient is seen for four or even five days each week and a complete analysis is rarely finished in less than two years. Analyses lasting four or five years are not uncommon. The basic rule in psychoanalysis is that the patient must say whatever comes into his mind, holding back nothing, no matter how embarrassing or trivial it may seem. This is what is meant by *free association*. The analyst's role is to offer himself as a blank screen onto which the patient can project feelings that he had toward people who were significant to him in the past. This is what is known as *transference*.

The course of a psychoanalysis can be described as involving three distinct phases. The first involves the removal of defenses erected by the ego to prevent the expression of unacceptable impulses. The ego, in its effort to maximize adjustment, sets up defenses in the form of repression and various types of distortions (see Chapter 4) to control impulses whose direct expressions are seen to have potentially adverse consequences. Even when the person feels unhappy or has troublesome symptoms related to these defenses, he does not easily give them up. So, much analytic time is devoted to clearing away defenses against impulse expression.

In the second analytic phase, impulses find free expression and are "worked through." This means, for example, that unacceptable, unconscious anger toward a loved one is expressed over and over in its many forms until it loses its emotional force, and its source is understood.

The final analytic phase involves a rebuilding of defenses. The new defenses, hopefully, will have fewer troublesome unconscious impulses to deal with because an intellectual awareness and insight will have resulted from the first two treatment phases. Ideally the new defenses will allow some form of impulse expression, perhaps indirect or partially direct, so that emotional forces will not have to be dammed up entirely.

While the three phases described characterize psychoanalysis in general, it should not be assumed that in any particular case they follow in a neat time sequence. In reality there is a mixing of all three phases during much of the treatment. Breaking down of defenses is generally typical of the early treatment stages and rebuilding of coping mechanisms is most often seen in the late stages. Still, the possibilities for various mixtures are almost infinite.

Much insight psychotherapy follows the principles and processes that characterize psychoanalysis but focuses on specific personality problems. Such an approach does not attempt the ambitious personality reconstruction seen in psychoanalysis. This type of insight therapy, often called *psychoanalytic psychotherapy*, consequently takes less time than psychoanalysis and is conducted less intensively. The case of Vincent is a good example of psychoanalytic psychotherapy. Its outcome seems to have typified what occurs in successful instances of such an approach.

The Case of Vincent

Vincent is an attractive twenty-one year old. He is one of several sons in a middle-class family and seems to relate well to others. He came to the counselor on his own and expressed serious concerns about his "problem." He explained that he was troubled about his strong aggressive tendency, particularly when it was directed against his girl friend. He was inordinately jealous of her. When she paid attention to others in his presence, he became so incensed that he felt a strong impulse to shake her physically and otherwise assault her. Yet he also realized and feared the effect that his behavior was having on their relationship. He also felt guilty about his jealousy. This was the second girl with whom he had had these impulses. Vincent noted that the girls were rather similar; both had difficulties getting along with their fathers, and were very affectionate. The occurrence of a second stormy relationship between him and a girl was very depressing to him and motivated him to seek help.

Vincent did not seem to have any difficulty in building a relationship with the counselor. He knew that he needed help and therefore he revealed himself quite openly and readily.

In his early life, a great deal of sibling rivalry and jealousy had taken place between Vincent and his brothers. As Vincent described it, the home atmosphere was stormy. Vincent recalled that his mother had placed the motto on the wall in his room "Keep your temper; nobody else wants it." In spite of such warning, temper tantrums were the means he used to release tension and to gain power over his brothers and the other members of the family. He remembers feeling inferior, highly sensitive, and self-conscious as a teen ager. He was reluctant to go out for fear that others would detect some sign that he masturbated.

After several therapy sessions, Vincent recalled significantly that as a boy he was afraid of the bullies in the school yard. While he was not one of the people they pushed around, he feared they might do so. The fear of the harm others could do to him has been with him all his life. His attitude was that "just as they could take my ball away from me as a child, they could now take my girl." Even presently he rarely walks comfortably into a crowd without examining it first to see who's in it. He is so leery of others' attitudes toward him that he studies alone. Once while in college, he attended midnight mass in his home town with his girl friend and saw some of the bullies from his boyhood. One said, "Oh, look whose here, little Vince and his girl." His reaction to this was inward rage and the feeling they could take her from him. This fear of losing his girl to someone else is, he thinks, basic to his jealousy. He still has the low self-esteem he had as a boy despite considerable academic achievement.

In school he was successful, earned good grades, and was apparently a good writer. The assignments he completed in his writing courses expressed much aggression—probable evidence of his daily frustration at not reaching his high expectation. During his psychotherapy he alluded to suicidal thoughts and revealed he had once actually taken pills of some sort as a suicidal attempt. He also, in an attempt to see his girl friend and talk with her, kicked her door in. He had to pay for it "in two ways: $50 and the shame of being regarded as 'a little off.' "

The therapist regarded his relationship with Vince as generally good, but the client often attempted to manipulate the therapist and to use the therapy situation to resolve his surface difficulties—especially to find ways to win back his girl friend, who had broken off with him. The therapist used the sessions to encourage Vincent to express his feelings, particularly those other than anger. In the process, Vincent came to discuss his sadness, and the therapist urged him to express it, to cry if he wanted to, and to accept this crying as permissible.

The interviews were used to build an honest, meaningful relationship that could be generalized to other relationships outside the interview. The therapist tried to help Vincent to learn to extend his trust to others in order to build better and deeper relations with others. Some of the changes that were hoped for by the therapist and that did occur during therapy were Vincent's firmer control over aggressive behavior, a reduction of his attempts to manipulate others in interpersonal relationships, and a weakening of a tendency to disrupt good interpersonal relations.

Vincent has expressed well many of his own reactions to insight therapy which reflect many of the changes typically resulting from such an approach: "Psychotherapy has been a long and sometimes frustrating process for me, but because of it I am able to see myself in a new perspective. There are some things that the psychologist cannot change, I suppose, for I still love that girl very much. But I now see that there were things in our relationship that would have torn up any compatibility we could have found. I don't think it could ever have worked.

"This new perspective of myself; it makes me know my true feelings. I now see that I get angry when there's nothing to get angry about. Maybe I feel insecure or feel hurt, but instead of admitting it to myself (maybe even letting myself cry!), I cover it up by showing anger. What I am learning to do is identify my true feelings and see through my false reactions—that anger bit—before they get me into trouble. I then let my real feelings show in an appropriate fashion. I think I have always realized that I was substituting false reactions for real ones, but I never could admit it to myself. If anything, psychotherapy has made me face the facts and really look at myself.

"Other things help, too. I see myself in other people now and so get a better view of my behavior. I get outside of myself, so to speak. One thing that happened to me really made a difference in my outlook, and I wish everyone could have the same experience. I saw myself on a videotaped television interview and was shocked to see myself as others do. It wasn't all bad. My biggest impression was that I came on as much more intelligent and articulate than I ever thought I did. I'll never forget it.

"Another way I have seen myself is in literature. Often I can identify with a character or with a description of a character. For example, this passage from an English essay, 'The Fate of Pleasure,' by Lionel Trilling (1963):

> It has always been true of some men that to pleasure they have preferred what the world called unpleasure. They imposed upon themselves difficult and painful tasks, they committed themselves to strange, "unnatural" modes of life, they sought out distressing emotions, in order to know psychic energies which are not to be summoned up in felicity. These psychic energies, even when they are experienced in self-destruction, are a means of self-definition and self-affirmation . . . it is the choice of the hero, the saint, and martyr and in some cultures, the artist.

I think this states the nature of the relationship I had with my girl. When we first met, she dated many guys while I dated only her. So I set myself up as the hero (getting her was like slaying the dragon), the saint (I dated no one else), the martyr (I felt she was purposely hurting me by dating others), and even the artist (I put a lot of my feeling into short stories and poems). And who wants these 'unpleasures?' Maybe somebody who needs psychotherapy.

"What I must do now is recognize these forces or drives that are in me before they can cause me trouble. This may mean, among other things, that I will have to avoid certain people and situations. In a different situation, with a different type of girl, these forces may not be aroused. I can't change me, but I can learn to live with myself. The process of psychotherapy has been difficult, and I still have much to learn. But I am twice the man I was for this experience. One might say I've had a 'baptism of fire,' or that I'm a 'sadder but wiser man' for all that I have been through."

RATIONAL-EMOTIVE THERAPY

Another therapeutic approach that stresses insight along with changing one's way of thinking about oneself is the *rational-emotive therapy* of Albert Ellis (Ellis & Harper, 1961). Ellis holds that many unpleasant emotional states stem from irrational self-instruction rather than objective reality. The individual in such a case is making wrong assumptions about himself and the world. One becomes anxious, depressed, guilty, or hostile not necessarily because of what is happening to him but how he interprets this external event or what he tells himself it means. Many people have irrational ideas that result in their interpretation of events in such a way as to make them emotional and unhappy.

Ellis maintains we can achieve better personal adjustment if we use the "A-B-C technique" when we are suffering from anxiety, depression, fear, or unrealistic guilt. A is the objective situation, what is really happening—a person's action or an event. C is the subjective feeling we have—anxiety, guilt, depression. B is the interpretation of the objective situation, possibly irrational or erroneous. Ellis suggests his clients ask themselves "Is anxiety, guilt, or unhappiness really due to A (the objective situation) or to what I am telling myself, how I am interpreting A, rather than what A really is?" Ellis then suggests the client examine his irrational interpretation (B) and change it. He is to ask himself what are the wrong assumptions about himself and the world. He is to see these assumptions as irrational and is to work constantly with the therapist on changing them.

Example

C. A person is depressed.
A. He is not making the grades necessary to get into the medical school.
B. Is he telling himself medicine is the only field in which he'll be happy, or medicine is the most appropriate field for him in view of his abilities and habits. Is this erroneous in this case? Can't it be corrected?

Example

C. The individual is worried over the kind of sex thoughts he has.
A. He sees himself as a weak, undesirable person whom others would reject if they really knew him.
B. Are not the sex thoughts the rational consequences of his humanity and the kind of background he's had? Should he evaluate his total selfhood in terms of sex thoughts? Are there not some typical and acceptable outlets for his sex urges? Is he really atypical? Do most people really care what his inner life is, or would they reject him if they knew what he knew? Isn't he being irrational on this subject? Can he perceive the irrationality of his thinking and change it with psychological assistance to more realistic assumptions?

Some frequently found irrational ideas that need to be corrected according to Ellis are:

— One needs to be loved and approved by almost everyone for everything one does.
— One needs to be thoroughly adequate and achieving in all possible aspects.
— Most people are bad, wicked, and villainous and should be severely blamed and punished.
— When things are not going the way one would like them it is terrible, horrible, and catastrophic.
— Unhappiness is externally caused and people have little or no ability to control their sorrows.
— The past is all-important in determining what happens in our lives.

CLIENT-CENTERED COUNSELING AND PSYCHOTHERAPY

Client-centered therapy is *nondirective* in that the counselor does not take major responsibility for directing the session. He does not diagnose the client, interpret his behavior, reassure him, or make suggestions as to what he should do. It is *client-centered* in that the client is responsible for exploring his feelings and personality, arriving at insight, and making decisions. The therapist listens empathically to the patient's feelings, presents attitudes, behavior, and decisions, and attempts to create an atmosphere within which free self-exploration can take place. The therapist is quite active in showing the client "unconditional" positive regard, and reflects the client's feelings as a means of helping him to clarify them. No judgment is made of the client's behavior. In the earlier interviews the client reveals much about himself that is negative. As therapy proceeds, positive statements begin to emerge, and the client gains a more accepting sense of himself.

Important to client-centered therapy is the general attitude of the therapist, his view of the nature of man and what is important in man's readjustment. The client-centered therapist respects his client as a worthy person capable of development or growth. The client's unhappiness, immaturity, self-defeating behavior, or aggression are regarded as due to the fact that he is conflicted over the need to behave in such a way as to satisfy others and thereby win positive regard, or to satisfy his own need to actualize. Overcoming this conflict requires a therapist who can convey positive regard for the client's efforts to self-actualize. In essence, then, this approach is future oriented and does not dwell on events of the past as do the insight therapies (Rogers, 1959, 1964, 1967).

Client-centered counseling has been used with satisfactory results with college students and relatively normal persons who are struggling with marital, vocational, or identity conflicts. It has been helpful in treating mild neuroses; and, obviously, is most effective with the client who is verbal and has initiative. It is less so if the patient is highly dependent, or has severe behavior problems.

BEHAVIOR MODIFICATION

The behavior modifier approaches the problem of eliminating undesirable behavior within the learning framework. From this point of view, undesirable responses (symptoms such as anxiety) are learned according to the usual principles of learning, as discussed earlier in Chapter 5. Thus through extinction, counterconditioning, and so forth, behavior can be modified in socially desirable directions. The neurotic's anxiety can be conditioned "out" by arranging for the pairing of fear- or anxiety-arousing stimuli with pleasant or relaxing experiences (see the description of systematic desensitization below) or by repeated exposure to fearful stimuli until fear responses subside (that is, extinction). The behavior therapist may make use of a number of learning principles, including operant and respondent conditioning, extinction, modeling, and punishment, to change behavior. The important characteristic to remember about the behavior therapy approach to clinical problems is that there is a definite tendency to rely on experimentally established behavior change procedures, usually learning principles, in the modification of behavior. In addition there tends to be a focus on overt, observable behaviors, both because changes in these behaviors are most readily apparent and because the learning principles governing the acquisition and change of overt behaviors are best known.

Examples of Behavior Therapy

Let us consider several illustrative cases. Lovaas and Simmons (1969) have described one of the most striking examples of the use of conditioning procedures to alter an undesirable, even life-threatening behavior. The patients were three severely retarded children who, like many severely retarded or emotionally disturbed children, engaged in much self-destructive, self-mutilative behavior. The children would self-inflict blows to their heads by either hitting themselves with their fists or knees or banging their heads against beds, chairs, walls, and other stationary objects. Much tissue damage had been done by the head banging, and each child was described as being well scarred. Physical restraints and pads were necessary to block the self-destructive behavior and preclude further serious threat to life. Lovaas and Simmons sought to eliminate the head banging first by extinction. Two of the children were allowed to hurt themselves repeatedly without contact or intervention from hospital personnel. Although this method eventually proved effective in reducing the self-destruction, it took many thousands of such blows to complete the extinction process successfully. It was obvious that such a long and potentially harmful approach could not be used with children whose self-destructive acts were more harmful.

In a search for a more rapid and effective behavior modification procedure, Lovaas and Simmons (1969) tried punishment. Each of the three children was given painful electric shocks immediately following a self-destructive act. The subsequent behavior was both immediate and long lasting. After only a few punishment trials the children ceased their head banging and immediately began to show general behavioral improvements. After several punishment trials in varying situations and in the presence of different hospital personnel the reduction in self-destructive acts became stable across situations (that is, generalized) and over time. Further, general behavioral improvements in play behavior and cooperation with staff suggested that the children had been freed of a self-defeating as well as destructive behavior pattern.

"TOKEN ECONOMY" HOSPITAL WARD

A second example of behavior therapy procedures and one that has spurred widespread application of similar procedures is provided by Ayllon and Azrin (1965). Utilizing operant reinforcement procedures to promote the rehabilitation and social retraining of chronic hospitalized mental patients, Ayllon and Azrin established the first "token economy" hospital ward treatment plan.

The patients were 44 chronic mental patients who, as a group, averaged more than 15 years of continuous hospitalization. Before treatment, patient behavior was limited mostly to body maintenance; most or all patients just lay around the ward all day, sleeping, smoking, eating at prearranged times, and little else. Most were receiving no formal therapy, the hospital professional staff having long before given up hope of their rehabilitation. Treatment geared to move patients out of their lethargic withdrawal into meaningful social interaction involved the reinforcement of on-ward and off-ward work activities with desirable hospital privileges, luxuries, and preferred commodities. To enable hospital staff to reinforce cooperative patients, promptly and effectively, tokens were used as secondary reinforcers that could be traded for luxuries, privileges, or commodities. Thus, at prespecified times of the day patients received poker-chip-like tokens during or immediately following performance of certain minimal on- or off-ward duties (mopping the floor, working in the laundry, personal grooming, and hygiene). At other predetermined times they were allowed to use the tokens they had earned to "buy" such luxuries as choice of personal bedrooms and furniture, the freedom to leave the ward and walk around the hospital grounds, access to a television set or movie being shown, and personal items such as consumables (candy, cigarettes) and clothing. Patients' performance of the reinforced work behavior greatly increased soon after introduction of the token reinforcement program and was shown to vary markedly with subsequent experimental changes in reinforcement practices.

Many token economy mental hospital programs have replicated and extended Ayllon and Azrin's (1965) findings. Atthowe and Krasner (1968) and McReynolds and Coleman (1971), for instance, have shown how token reinforcement procedures can be used to retrain severely regressed mental patients to dress, groom, and feed themselves as well as become involved in therapeutic, recreational, and work activities. In addition work is presently under way to develop token reinforcement programs that will lead to patients' eventual discharge from the hospital and readjustment to the larger "token" (monetary) reinforcement system of the outside world.

SYSTEMATIC DESENSITIZATION

A third widely studied and applied behavior therapy technique, purportedly based on the respondent conditioning paradigm, is Wolpe's systematic desensitization. The desensitization procedure was developed as a treatment for phobic fears. Relaxation, according to Wolpe, is a fear-inhibiting response that can be counterconditioned to fear-arousing stimuli (bugs, heights, giving speeches, etc.) such that the feared object or situation no longer causes distress.

Desensitization, then, involves three procedures: (1) training in deep muscle relaxation resembling many hypnosis induction procedures; (2) devising a systematic program of gradual exposure to fear objects or situations either in the form of imagined or real-life encounters; and (3) simultaneous relaxation and graded exposure. The beneficial effects of systematic desensitization have been repeatedly demonstrated in research with fearful college students, including those with fears of snakes and other small animals and anxiety about giving speeches and taking tests. Lang, Lazovik, and Reynolds (1965), for instance, used desensitization to help students overcome their extreme fear of snakes. After treatment, many subjects were able to touch or hold a harmless snake, whereas subjects in a control group continued their fearful avoidance.

Similarly, Paul (1966) showed that students who were anxious about giving speeches before even small audiences overcame this problem to a great extent following several weeks of desensitization. Anxious students given a more Freudian, insight-oriented therapy or control experiences showed comparatively little reduction in their speech anxiety. Whether desensitization will work as well with more severely disturbed, neurotic individuals is not known; initial work along these lines (McReynolds, 1969) is somewhat discouraging.

According to Wolpe's formulations, desensitization is a *counterconditioning technique,* with relaxation being (counter) conditioned to phobic stimuli, thereby displacing all fear responses. However, this explanation of desensitization involves several assumptions, including one that muscle relaxation opposes fear, which other thinkers in the area have rejected. At present, the proper theoretical account of systematic desensitization is greatly disputed. The issues involved are complex and prohibit more than cursory mention in our overview of the technique.

IMITATION LEARNING

Research on imitation learning has also provided an empirical base for new therapy techniques. The most extensive applications of modeling procedures as a behavior modification technique has been in the area of fear reduction, again working with "phobic" college students and children. Bandura, Grusec, and Menlove (1967) reduced dog phobia in children by having the fearful children observe a child model petting and playing with a dog. In another study, Bandura, Blanchard, and Ritter (1969) showed that snake-fearful students who saw a model handle a harmless snake greatly overcame their own fears, as reflected in their willingness to hold a snake. Further, comparisons of modeling and desensitization treatments for exaggerated fears have shown them to be of equal effectiveness or have favored the modeling "therapy" slightly.

SELF-CONTROL THROUGH BEHAVIOR THERAPY

Self-control behavior therapy procedures provide a final, most engaging example of the application of known learning procedure to human behavior modification. Self-control behavior therapy grew out of the idea that individuals can exert influence over their own behavior by the self-application of reinforcement, punishment, and other procedures affecting learning and performance. In self-reinforcement, for example, a person allows himself certain luxuries or privileges only when certain prespecified behavioral standards or goals are reached. One may make the pact, "I'll work hard this week so I can (allow myself to) go out this weekend." By systematizing such "self-contracts" so that goals and rewards are explicit and precise, we can exercise a great deal of control in areas in which our behavior is unreliable or unpredictable. McReynolds and Church (1972) showed that college students who were taught to make self-contracts concerning adequate study behavior improved their grades significantly in a single semester. Self-contracts entailed both a daily specification of study goals and preplanned reinforcers, such as coffee breaks and dates, which were contingent on goal attainment. Glynn (1970) improved students' learning of history and geography classroom material by allowing them to reinforce their study with candy or toys after completing an assignment. Other forms of self-control, such as self-punishment, management of stimulus conditions, and even self-modeling, are also possible methods, although the development of such procedures awaits further research effort.

EMOTIVE APPROACHES TO PSYCHOTHERAPY

Recent years have seen a rise of interest in humanistic and existential approaches to psychotherapy. These have emerged in reaction to the feeling that our society is so computerized and bureaucratized that the individual and his feelings tend to be overlooked. As a result many people suffer from a nagging loneliness, a sense of alienation from their fellows, a feeling that their lives lack meaning and purpose. Fundamental to the humanistic-existential approaches is the notion that man is free to direct the course of his own therapy and knows best what will be most satisfying for him. Client-centered therapy, which was discussed earlier, obviously falls within this framework. The emotive or cathartic approaches to psychotherapy are also good examples of humanistic outlooks.

The observation that powerful emotional expression can relieve many distressing psychological symptoms is a very old one indeed. Intense emotional expression is part of the ritual of many primitive religions, and it occurs spontaneously and often beneficially in connection with many of the traumatic situations that arise in man's life such as bereavement. In recent years many have advanced the idea that this process of "letting it all hang out" and "spilling one's guts" has potent curative powers, and relatively formal systems of psychotherapy have been organized around this principle. It should be noted that even this idea is not a new one, having been advanced by Breuer and Freud in the late nineteenth century in what was the forerunner of psychoanalysis.

The theory behind many of the emotive therapies holds that throughout his lifetime, man is forced to inhibit many intense feelings which somehow accumulate within his psyche over the years. Ultimately they become difficult to control, and the defenses that must be erected to prevent their expression account for whatever symptoms he feels. Inhibitions are forced upon man by society. At a fairly early point in life most people are encouraged to believe that strong emotional expression is unacceptable. Even children are taught not to cry because it's infantile and not to express strong anger because it's not nice. Thus most individuals grow up under an almost insupportable weight of emotional inhibitions. Janov (1970) goes so far as to assert that all men suffer neuroses unless they have gone through a process that has purged them of the stored-up emotion that has prompted them to be defensive all their lives. The task of therapy from this point of view is relatively straightforward. The patient must be encouraged to let down his defenses sufficiently to release the great store of feeling that he has been saving up, following which defenses will be unnecessary, he will begin to view his situation and the people around him with greater objectivity, and will function much more effectively. Various types of emotive approaches have special emphases which seem only to represent variations on this basic theme.

Wilhelm Reich's Therapeutic Approach

Clearly the forerunner of the modern emotive schools of psychotherapy was Wilhelm Reich, who started out as an orthodox psychoanalyst and made many important contributions to psychoanalytic theory. At first, Reich was particularly impressed in his work by the resistance that patients put up against revealing old memories which are usually associated with strong negative feelings. Eventually he became interested in the form that such resistance took and began to concentrate as much on how a patient said things as he did on what they were saying. This led further to an interest in the way the body was used and the voice was controlled in order to restrain the expression of feeling. Ultimately he arrived at the theory that patients had a great deal of energy bound up in their defenses and that this was because they had to suppress their emotions and were frustrated sexually. Thus a cure was to come about only through a freeing of energy tied up with defenses, and this could be achieved only if suppressed feelings were expressed and sexual release were obtained.

A routine part of Reichian therapy involves physical examinations to assess the degree and nature of muscular rigidity. Treatment sessions ordinarily are carried out with the patient wearing only underwear or a bathing suit, both as a means of overcoming defensiveness and also to provide the therapist with the opportunity to observe the patient's muscles. The Reichian analyst thinks of the body as being divided into seven vertical segments, each of which is controlled by a particular set of muscle groups. Therapy is directed toward breaking down muscular "armor" segment by segment. The segments identified by the Reichians are the ocular, the oral, the cervical, the thoracic, the diaphragmatic, the abdominal, and the pelvic. The technique used to break down the armor in each sector is to encourage the patient to express affect through the muscle groups that are unique to each segment. For example, to overcome the resistance put up by the ocular muscles, the patient is asked to open his eyes widely as though frightened and to force as much emotional expression through the use of the muscles controlling the eyes as he can. The muscles of the oral segment are loosened up by having the patient change his voice pattern or move his mouth and jaw energetically. At times the patient is encouraged to simulate crying for this purpose. This progressive dearmoring of various muscle segments from the top of the body down is thought ultimately to result in the release of the affect that has been responsible for the defensiveness and armoring, and frees the patient to live more naturally, appreciating his own impulses. The ultimate criterion for success in Reich's system is "orgastic potency." Thus, the criterion of health from this point of view is the ability to have a potent orgasm.

Primal Therapy

Primal therapy is a fairly recent system developed by Janov (1970). His theory is quite a simple one. All psychopathology is seen to result from the painful emotions which have been held back, and the cure is simply the reexperiencing of these feelings. In this approach, interest focuses on the very earliest inhibited emotional expressions. Inevitably, from this view, since the growing child is quite helpless and must depend on his parents for a variety of life's necessities, very basic needs are frustrated in the earliest years of life resulting in "primal pain." This includes the feeling of not being loved as much as one would like or not receiving as much stimulation as is needed. Such feelings are invariably held back out of awareness and invariably exercise a negative effect on behavior through life by creating tension. Thus avoidance of anxiety related to this tension becomes an important motivating force in the individual's life. The way to correct this situation is to permit the expression of primal pain.

To promote such expression, the primal therapist sees patients intensively over a three-week period during which he attempts to assist them in recovering the painful inhibitions of the earliest years of life. The process that he engages in during these three weeks when he sees the patient for several hours every day is not specified. However, the goal is clear. This is to induce a "primal" that occurs when the patient actually visualizes the situation from early childhood that was so painful and is able to express the agonizing pain, usually through a primitive scream or speech in childlike language. Ultimately the expression of this primal scream is thought to be the curative mechanism. In primal therapy the three-week period of individual treatment is followed by an extended period of group therapy consisting of a very large number of patients (perhaps 40 to 50 at a time) who essentially participate in weekly meetings during which they continue to experience primals.

Gestalt Therapy

Gestalt therapy was developed by Frederick (Fritz) S. Perls (1969) and was based on the principles of Gestalt psychology. Gestalt psychology emphasizes the wholistic quality of our perceptual experiences such that man has a tendency when perceiving an imperfect or incomplete stimulus to complete it within his own mind. Thus the circle with a small break in it is seen as a perfect circle rather than a ring that is not closed. Perls felt that just as man needs to complete stimuli perceptually, he also has the need to fully experience situations that he encounters. Thus, in any situation where needs or feelings have gone unexpressed, such feelings remain active until they find expression. This process for Perls is like completing a Gestalt or achieving a sense of closure. When the process of achieving closure is blocked, anxiety is the result. This feeling is relieved when catharsis takes place and discharges the blocked feelings. Gestalt therapy involves a set of techniques for encouraging a return to a state in which one discharges affect spontaneously.

A major aspect of Gestalt therapy is the use of procedures designed to undo resistance to expression of feeling. The essence of this approach is to make the patient aware of his own immediate personal experience. By immediate experience, Perls is concerned with what is actually happening moment by moment within the therapy situation. Thus the patient in Gestalt therapy is strongly encouraged to reveal what he is feeling at a precise instant in the same way that the psychoanalytic patient is encouraged to free-associate. For example, in one therapy group, a very inhibited man was tapping his finger on a table while listening to a woman in the group talk endlessly on. When asked if he had any comment on her statements, the man denied that he did but continued to tap his finger. The therapist then asked him to tap more intensely, more loudly, and more vigorously and to continue until he could begin to sense what he was actually feeling at the moment. The patient's anger mounted rather quickly under these circumstances and before long he was pounding on the table and expressing violent disagreement with the woman. This intense concentration on the feelings of the moment inevitably results in considerable emotional expression. The ultimate goal of Gestalt therapy is not simply to rid oneself of certain feelings, but also to do away with the repressive defenses that have held them back and to become aware of how actions have been shaped by these feelings.

THERAPEUTIC GROUP ACTIVITY

Before looking at groups as therapeutic agents, let us recall through an interview with a normal student the influence groups have on all of us.

Katie is an intelligent, well-adjusted, 21-year-old college senior from a large midwestern city, majoring in psychology. She was later elected to Phi Beta Kappa, an honorary society. After graduation she married an able medical student and she took a Master's degree in psychiatric social work. She is presently employed in this vocation. She was told that the purpose of the interview was to enable her to talk freely (with some interrogation) about the positive and negative effects of groups on her personal development. She was asked to begin with those groups that seemed to have a *positive effect* on her. She responded:

> In junior and senior high school I was active in my church youth group. Here in college I am involved in the Committee of Concerned Students, a group entitled by the school newspaper as a group of "clean-cut activists." It consists of both men and women. The group began in 1968 during the primaries as the Committee of Concerned Democrats supporting Gene McCarthy and Robert Kennedy; now it

is focussing on campus and local issues. The other group I have found exciting here on campus is a lecture-discussion group which meets in a church-sponsored coffee house near campus.

In answer to the question, "What specifically do you think these groups did for you?" Katie said:

Part of their function was *social,* especially the church youth group. I made friends and we did fun things. But these groups also offered exciting new experiences and gave me an opportunity to develop myself as a person. I had certain *responsibilities* within these groups, and the groups exposed me to *new ideas.* Through my church group I went to summer conferences and a national youth convention. In these two groups in which I am now participating we are constantly confronted with both ideas and the necessity of taking action on what we believe.

"Let's turn to the groups that had a *less positive influence.* Which ones were they?"

In high school I was a member of a sorority. I didn't like some of the older girls; we seemed to have nothing in common. They were more narrow, boy-minded, and less interested in school. Another factor was that the sorority excluded one of my friends and I knew this really hurt her. In college I was a member of the Student Activities Council. I just sort of felt that participation in both of these was a waste of time.

"Were there any groups from which you felt rejected?"

When I was a college sophomore several of my friends and I decided to go through rush week, a period in which prospective members are looked over, selected, and persuaded to join or are rejected by the fraternities or sororities. It definitely wasn't my "thing." I was uncomfortable in the rush situation. We went through a series of short interviews with strangers all day long at the different houses. I could never think of the right things to say, and I invariably stuck my foot in my mouth. I didn't pledge, and it was a very ego-deflating experience. Only one of my friends did pledge, however; the rest of us survived the humiliation and the whole thing has become a big joke. Now I really feel that I am glad I didn't pledge, but then, that might be subconscious sour grapes. The experience had some value because it did *make me take stock of my personality* and perhaps realize a little more fully *what I was really like to others.*

"Have you been influenced by any less formal groups?"

This may sound silly, but my seventh grade class was really important in my life. When we went to junior high from various grade schools we were put into a track system on the basis of achievement and potential. I was put into an accelerated class, and I remained with this group of kids for the rest of school. We were all from about the same income bracket and had similar values. I guess you could say we were from liberal urban families. Naturally, we became close friends. As a group we were academically oriented and were active in school affairs. We also had somewhat wider interests than just our school activities. For example, one summer several of us did some inner-city recreation work in the black ghetto. It was a pretty awakening experience for us at that time. Almost all of these classmates went on to college, and some of them are still my closest friends. I really think that that atmosphere had a lot to do with my continuing interest in education and the development of my social awareness.

EFFECTS OF GROUPS ON PERSONAL DEVELOPMENT

The interview with Katie gives us an example of how groups, by their special nature, quietly influence the development of the individual both positively and negatively. For a long time various professionals working with youth have made use of groups, with the prospect of increasing the self-esteem of the members, developing new interests and skills, and exploiting the group so that individuals will be supportive of one another. We recognize certain well-established psychological principles operating in groups for human development (Brayfield, 1968). There is considerable *social reinforcement* by peers. Some of Katie's behavior was received well by her friends, other behavior was ignored. Certain members of the group, including attractive young leaders, serve as *models for behavior* whom the students unconsciously imitate. The accelerated school group in which Katie was placed was certainly *reinforcing and challenging*. She and her peers were presented with achievement expectations that they could meet. This *bolstered their self-esteem* and, as Katie indicated, many in the group not only achieved in academic endeavors but became more involved in student activities. They learned to assume more responsibility and actually developed social leadership. In doing all of this they were *satisfying some important needs and motivation.*

Some nonpsychologists have been using groups of various kinds for personal improvement for some time. The commercial courses that pivot on public speaking have been in existence for many years, operating throughout the country. Graduates of such a course see it as having an important positive effect on their development in general. The members of these groups usually go through the process of making brief talks in front of their peers. They begin with biographical statements. As a result of brief weekly talks before their group they extinguish some of their anxiety about speaking in public. Also, being homogeneous in some of their background and aspirations, they support one anothers' efforts. One adult student said he has never made a speech since taking the course, but he thought the course influenced his development in a positive way. He added, "It enabled me to second motions; I couldn't do this before!"

Alcoholics Anonymous is a lay group of former alcoholics. These people have a common purpose, and they meet periodically, usually with enthusiasm. Their emphasis is on frank acceptance of the fact that they have failed to control their drinking and that they need help outside themselves in the form of both religious commitment and commitment to each other. One of their activities is recruiting active alcoholics as members and spending time with them in crises until they become "dry." By and large, the members evaluate the group as successful in their development toward abstinence and responsibility. Many feel that they grow in self-acceptance and in improved relationships with their family. As a result of this movement, other groups have formed to help people with shared problems such as ex-patients, homosexuals, compulsive gamblers, and drug addicts.

Groups, then, effect our development and they have been used successfully for individual improvement in social attitudes and habits. Let us now see how they have been exploited by professionals for the improvement of mental health.

KINDS OF GROUPS

The group may function in a number of different ways as a therapeutic agent. Frank and Powdermaker (1959) classified them as (1) *didactic* groups in which the material is presented by a leader and discussion is encouraged; (2) therapeutic *social clubs,* such as those in a mental hospital, which aim to build patients' skills in social interaction; (3) *inspirational* groups, which use group identification and personal involvement (an example of this is Alcoholics Anonymous); (4) *psychodrama,* where problems in the group are acted out by the patient with other significant persons in his life (the latter roles played by persons in the hospital); (5) *free interaction* groups, the commonest type of therapeutic group. In the sessions the members are encouraged to express their feelings and ideas freely and to interact with each other.

GROUP THERAPY

Soon after the turn of the century an internist in Massachusetts, Joseph Pratt, gathered tubercular patients in groups so that they could discuss the reasons for hygienic measures (Hadden, 1955). This was one of the early publicized uses of the group for therapy. In the thirties this idea spread, and groups of schizophrenics were formed. Moreno introduced the term "group therapy," thereby making the use of the group as a therapeutic instrument extensive and popular (Dreikurs, 1959). Group therapy has since been used for psychotics, neurotics, patients hospitalized for various illnesses, families of patients with emotional disturbances, and others.

Certain college courses such as "Personal Adjustment" have used a modified form of group therapy. The class is divided into small peer groups, which discuss cases or veer off to relevant student personal problems, with the general objectives of group therapy mentioned below. For success, these classes should be conducted by persons trained in psychodynamics to understand the processes involved and to follow up with individual therapy if needed by any participant.

One ingenious use of the group was to gather emotionally disturbed children in a room with equipment and allow them to play constructively or destructively. Slavson (1951) was the permissive psychiatrist who envisioned the group as a secondary family. The group members, through their play, refreshments, and outings, became important to each other, and they gained insights through the group activity. This was known as *activity group therapy.*

In addition to making the therapist's time more effective, since he can meet with several people at once, group therapy helps the patient to realize that he is *not alone* in his problem, that others have similar feelings of guilt, anxiety, or hostility. During the session the participant can explore his attitudes and feelings by interacting with other people and not merely with the therapist. Often patients reassure and support one another.

Frequently group and individual therapy are combined. The group process, though not as intensive, facilitates individual therapy, and the individual sessions allow the patient to explore further some of the insights that have grown out of his relationship with the group. Because group therapy helps to remove the feeling of isolation, it can reduce anxiety and guilt. It also serves as an arena in which to develop social interactions, which are often acutely important for the disturbed individual (Coffey, 1966).

A group of patients who are soon to be dismissed from the hospital, for example, may meet periodically to discuss some of the problems they will face when they leave. These may include relations with their families, their contemporaries, various persons on the job, and problems in the various roles they will have to play in these relationships. One such group discussed what they might tell people who ask where they have been; they worked out how they might discuss their hospital experience and what it meant to them. Another dealt with dependence on some member of their family, which was a problem for them before they entered the hospital.

Some of the themes that Winder and Hersko (1958) found that tend to recur in group sessions, in order of frequency, are hostility to authority, hostility to peers, warmth for authority figures, warmth for peers, expression of need for help, fear of losing self-control, responsibility, jealousy, and recognition of dependency.

Procedurally the patient meets with a small group of people whose situations are somewhat similar to his. The leader creates a permissive atmosphere and makes clear the purpose of the session, the open discussion of their feelings and attitudes. Hopefully this will assist them in working through some of the specific difficulties they are experiencing. By controlling the group climate, the leader reduces defensiveness and creates openness of discussion.

Although the leader of the therapeutic group maintains a permissive, open attitude, it is his responsibility to see that the patients work through the conflicts they are discussing, guiding them gently toward coping responses rather than defensive ones. He tries to manipulate the session so that it will support the patients emotionally rather than be traumatic. He has usually selected the group to exclude individuals who are not ready for the frank interchange or who are so hostile that they will disturb other members of the group. The emphasis is on reducing anxiety and increasing communication, insightfulness, problem solving, and coping.

Psychodrama and Role Playing

A special form of group therapy is *psychodrama* (Moreno, 1946). In this approach several members of the group act out a real situation that is anxiety producing to one of the group members, perhaps a traumatic situation from his past. In reliving this role the patient obtains a certain amount of emotional release and catharsis and may be ready to learn more appropriate ways of responding in a similar situation (Figure 13–1). The drama is planned and supervised by the professional worker, with the audience consisting of patients and therapists. The situation and experience may be defined, but the patient spontaneously plays the role. Some patient members of the audience may be too shy and inhibited to become actors in psychodrama, but by observing others and entering into a later discussion they might gradually become comfortable enough to play a role in the drama.

Role playing is less formal and simpler than psychodrama yet related; actually it is a technique derived from psychodrama. It may deal with any situation that is troublesome to the individual. The boy who is shy about phoning a girl for a date may volunteer or be selected to play this date-getting role before a small group. A girl plays the role of the reluctant coed. He is told he need not be himself, he can play the role of

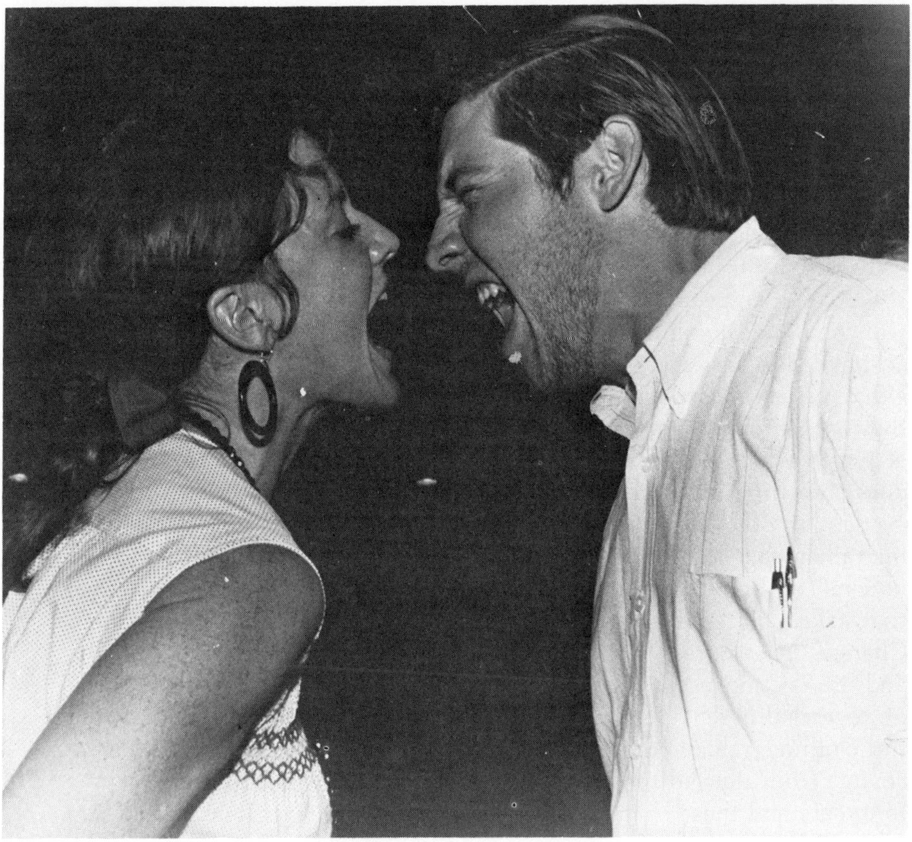

Photo courtesy of *Columbia Missourian*

Figure 13–1 Emotional Release Through Psychodrama.

someone he knows or would like to be. Any practice he gets in this role should have value in meeting the real situation. Role-playing skits may be created for any situation, such as an interview for a job or supervision of an employee. It may be used to understand a person in a different subculture or ethnic group by first observing him and then assuming his feelings, attitudes, and impulses in a role. Police in a training session have played the role of the innocent black suspect they stopped on the street. One of the role players acts out a tough, belligerent policeman while another takes the role of a frightened, innocent victim. The possibilities of the use of role playing for training in social skills are very broad.

Transactional Analysis (TA)

Transactional analysis is a relatively recent approach to group therapy which has received a great deal of popular attention through a book by

T. A. Harris (1967) titled *I'M OK—YOU'RE OK*. The basic theory and practice of transactional analysis is presented in some detail here because it represents a simplified example of a therapeutic system used in group situations. The man generally credited with originating TA is Eric Berne (1964), although one can readily see evidence of the thinking of a number of other psychological theorists in this approach.

The term "transaction" refers to the basic unit of social intercourse. When any two people are together, it is assumed that sooner or later one will communicate, either verbally or otherwise, to the other and thereby acknowledge his presence. This is called the *transactional stimulus*. Whatever response is made by the other to this communication is called the *transactional response*. TA is simply a way of examining the transaction in which one person does something to the other, and the other does something in return. Another feature of TA is that it attempts to systematize the information derived from the analysis of transactions into a language that means the same to everyone using it.

Some of Berne's ideas for TA emerged as he observed the change that takes place in a given person in the course of a conversation. Changes in gestures, facial expression, voice tone, vocabulary, posture, and the like suggest that each person is actually made up psychologically of several different people. Although the skin and bone structure and the clothing remain the same, something inside the person seems to change from time to time. In the process of sorting out and attempting to understand these changes, Berne concluded that everyone is made up essentially of three different "psychological realities," a Parent, a Child, and an Adult.

The Parent consists of an enormous collection of stimuli related to the child's parents, including virtually everything that he saw his parents do and say during roughly the first five years of his life. Because as a young child the person cannot modify perceptions or interpret events which may not mean exactly what they appear, the data relevant to the parent are taken in without any editing process. Thus, the Parent within the individual consists of all the warnings and rules that were laid down for the child by his parents and which he saw them live by. These may have been communicated verbally or on the basis of voice tone, facial expressions, muscular rigidity, and the like. Included in this set of stimuli are the literally thousands of times that the very young child was told not to do something and all of the expressions of displeasure and shame that parents communicated about the child's behavior. The parents' expressions of pleasure and pride in the young child are also part of the Parent. This Parent plays a very powerful role in every individual's life because just as the child would die if he didn't have a parent in the physical sense, the psychologically internalized Parent also protects the individual against a variety of dangers that could be very damaging if it did not exist.

An important Parent problem arises from inconsistency in the communications that have been received. Parents who say one thing but do another confuse and frighten their child to such a degree that he must defend by turning off the recording. A further complication is the fact that Parent data are received from both a mother and a father. If the communications they send out are harmonious, the effect is a relatively pleasant, easily understood one. When their communications are not harmonious, the effect is unpleasant for the child and, again, he must avoid listening if he can.

A good deal of Parent communication is represented in one's current life situation as information on how to do a variety of things. Parent data, incidentally, may be received from a variety of sources other than the biological parents or the child's caretakers. Television, for example, through the adults depicted in the stories observed by the very young child are seen to teach a concept of life akin to what actual parents may convey.

At the same time that experiences with parent figures are recording a body of data that go toward making up the Parent, another body of data is being assimilated. This comes from the child's internal responses to what is happening to him. Again, the significant aspect of the psychological entity called the Child is created during the first five years of life when relatively little language is available to help understand early experiences critically, so that most of what is recorded are feelings. And in this realm, we must keep in mind that the youngster is very small, dependent, clumsy, and incapable of interpreting and understanding what is happening to him in the light of a body of past experience. Thus much that is recorded in the Child is negative information about himself. Many of the messages that he receives indicate that he has been incapable of doing something, that he has done something badly, that it's his fault, that he is weak, and the like. In the language of TA the youngster must conclude about himself, "I'M NOT OK." This conclusion is inevitable in the situation of childhood even when parents are well meaning and essentially "good" parents.

There is a positive side to the Child aspects of the individual. Within the Child is found creativity, the impulse to explore and learn about the immediate surroundings, and the strong, unparalleled feelings of having made discoveries. Many of these are cherished experiences such as "the first drinking from the garden hose, the first stroking of the soft kitten, the first sure hold on mother's nipple, the first time the lights go on in response to his flicking the switch, the first submarine chase of the bar of soap, the repetitious going back to do these glorious things again and again," (Harris, 1967).

The third psychological reality within each individual is called the Adult. This entity begins to emerge at about the age of 10 months when the child is changing from being helpless and capable only of responding to the stimulation of those around him to becoming independent and capable of self-direction. Acquiring this capability gives the youngster a chance to learn *for himself* what is real in the environment around him, and how it differs from what he has been taught up to now in his Parent and what he has felt in his Child. In this first year of life the Adult is a fragile entity because the capacity to explore and sample reality may be easily diverted by commands from the Parent, but despite this most people continue to mature and to acquire their own firsthand impressions of reality. The Adult in every individual is that aspect of the psyche which arrives at decisions by combining information from the Parent, the Child, and his own firsthand experience. One of the Adult's most important functions is to examine critically the data gathered in the Parent and to validate or reject them, and to do the same with the feelings that reside in the Child.

Harris emphasizes that validating Parent data through the personal experience of the Adult does not necessarily erase the Child's NOT–OK feelings. That is, the youngster who feels put down by treatment that he received at the hands of his mother may later come to understand why she had to treat him as she did and that she was correct in doing so. Still, this does not erase the fact that in certain situations he felt NOT–OK. On the other hand, NOT–OK feelings may come to play a relatively less significant role in the present situation because the youngster can in a sense "turn them off" once having understood how they developed.

Another significant aspect of TA is the description of four *life positions* thought to characterize each individual based on the kinds of experiences that he has had in growing up. These four positions are (1) I'M NOT OK—YOU'RE OK; (2) I'M NOT OK—YOU'RE NOT OK; (3) I'M OK—YOU'RE NOT OK; (4) I'M OK—YOU'RE OK. Of these four, the universal position in which virtually everyone starts out in early childhood is the first, I'M NOT OK—YOU'RE OK. Even those who look back upon their childhood as a happy time are thought by transactional analysts to have started out with the feeling I'M NOT OK—YOU'RE OK. This is because experience in the first year of life inevitably conveys to the baby the sense of his own helplessness and weakness which must result in the feeling I'M NOT OK. On the other hand, the youngster's caretakers during this period are inevitably viewed as strong figures capable of providing many important gratifications. This creates the feeling YOU'RE OK. Thus by the end of the first year of life, virtually everyone has adopted the I'M NOT OK—YOU'RE OK position and most people will retain it throughout their lifetime.

There are two ways in which the I'M NOT OK—YOU'RE OK position may influence the lifelong course of a person's behavior. In the first he lives out a role which confirms the NOT OK. This results in a life of *withdrawal,* because if one feels that he is NOT OK, he's not comfortable with other people whom he regards as being OK. What pleasures such individuals attain must come through *fantasy* and a life of wishing. Another variation of this approach might involve behavior that is sufficiently upsetting to others to cause them to react negatively as a means of proving again and again that he is NOT OK. More commonly, this position is lived out according to a "counterscript." Here certain attitudes are borrowed from the Parent which indicate that you can be OK, *if.* Under such circumstances the individual becomes ingratiating to others and attempts to associate himself with friends who themselves have a big Parent, since the bigger the Parent, the bigger are the reinforcements that he can provide. Thus such a person lives a life of *seeking approval* from those around him who are looked upon as important. Neither approach to this position makes a person happy or gives him a sense of lasting worth because no matter what he does he continues to carry around within him the feeling that he is NOT OK.

All positions other than I'M NOT OK—YOU'RE OK develop in most people after the first year of life and are really alterations of that original universal stance. The second position, I'M NOT OK—YOU'RE NOT OK, occurs in those individuals whose parents become cold and unreinforcing as soon as the youngster gives evidence that he is not completely helpless. This occurs some time after the first year of life when some parents may abruptly change their behavior toward the child. The "babying" days are over, few displays of affection and warmth are allowed, and punishments tend to come more frequently and are more severe. All of the first year's comforts are lost, and the child can only conclude resentfully I'M NOT OK—YOU'RE NOT OK. A person who assumes this position tends to give up hope and often enters a state of extreme withdrawal with the intention of merely getting through life as uneventfully as possible. Not uncommonly such an individual ends up in a mental institution. Harris believes that under extreme life circumstances I'M NOT OK—YOU'RE NOT OK may be the initial position for a given individual depending upon how harsh his parents are. In such cases, the result is an autistic child, one who seems to be "psychologically unborn."

The third position is I'M OK—YOU'RE NOT OK. The switch from I'M NOT OK—YOU'RE OK to this third position is made possible under circumstances where the parents are so brutal to the child that he must assume that the parent is NOT OK. On the other hand, from what does the I'M OK feeling derive? This is seen to arise in the youngster who is treated so brutally by outsiders that his only source of comfort must come from within. His only sense of pleasure in life comes when he is left alone to lick his own wounds. Such a youngster seems to learn that, "I'll be all right if only others leave me alone." He shrinks from his brutal parents whenever they appear and is left to conclude I'M OK—YOU'RE NOT OK. Harris feels that the outcome of such a position is often criminal psychopathic behavior. The antisocial behavior displayed by such an individual is felt to be justified because of the terrible harm that has been inflicted upon him by others.

The fourth and most hopeful of the positions is I'M OK—YOU'RE OK. Qualitatively this position differs from the first three in that the first three are carried on at an exclusively feeling level. They were assumed very early in life when language was not available for modifying, understanding, or tempering these positions and went on to exercise an unconscious influence over all later behavior. The fourth position, I'M OK—YOU'RE OK, is arrived at consciously on the basis of considerable thought. The goal of all transactional analyses is to bring people to an I'M OK—YOU'RE OK position. To attain such a position a person needs to be exposed to the kinds of childhood predicaments which resulted in one of the first three positions and the demonstration of how a person's current behavior tends to cause these earlier positions to persist. Underlying this approach is the faith that man can choose to change. In this respect the transactional analyst holds a view similar to those of the humanists. Transactional analysts argue that although cause-and-effect relationships and strict determinism do apply in the case of the inanimate, such concepts are not sufficient to understand human behavior. The reason for this is that man is capable of anticipating a future so that he is not guided entirely by what happened to him in the past. A significant force in his life is what he hopes for in his future.

In TA the basic therapeutic technique is the analysis of the transaction that takes place between one person who produces a stimulus and another who responds to it and whose response then becomes a new stimulus for the first person. The goal of each analysis is to determine the part of each person—Parent, Adult, or Child—that is responsible for issuing each stimulus or response. Sets of verbal as well as gestural cues are identified by the transactional analyst as reflecting Parent, Child, and Adult responses. To a certain extent, such cues are seen to be universal but to some extent a particular parent may be reflected in certain idiosyncratic mannerisms. For example, common Parent mannerisms include furrowing the brow, pursing the lips, showing a horrified look, foot tapping, or placing the hands on the hips. A specific father, however, may have had the habit of clearing his throat just prior to scolding his child for bad behavior. The person who displays such a mannerism has no doubt adopted it from his experience with his own father. Verbal expressions that reflect the parent are such phrases as "I am going to put a stop to this once and for all," "I can't for the life of me," and the use of the words "always" or "never." Many adjectives that evaluate behavior, either critically or supportively, reflect judgments that one person makes about another and often are thought to originate in the Parent. Examples are such words as lazy, sweet, disgusting, shocking, and the like.

Because the Child's first responses to his external world were largely nonverbal, most of the obvious clues of the Child are to be found in some sort of physical expression. The quivering lip, the whiny voice, pouting, expressions of delight, laughter, squirming, and giggling are all examples of Child responses. Most obvious Child responses on a verbal level involve the use of baby talk and certain phrases such as "I wish," "I want," and an excessive use of superlatives. Another special group of words associated with children are seen to reflect the Adult operating within the Child. These words are what, why, where, and the like, all of which are in the service of exploring and satisfying curiosity about the world around one.

Clues to the presence of the Adult within the individual are reflected physically in the manner in which the person listens. His facial expression should indicate that he is taking in stimuli that are around him. This state is thought to be associated with continual movement of the face and eyes with eye blinks about every 3 to 5 seconds. Failure to move signifies that the individual is not listening. The language of the Adult includes, in addition to why, what, and where, other words such as in what way, how much, true, false, and the like. All reflect the Adult's processing and evaluation of information that is coming in to him.

The treatment goal in TA is to make every person an expert at analyzing his own transactions. Harris describes his initial contact with the patient as involving a period of approximately a half hour in which the patient acquaints him with his problem and another half hour in which the patient is introduced by the therapist to the idea of Parent, Child, and Adult. Also included in this first interview is a discussion of a treatment "contract." The term "contract" is used to indicate that the therapist will attempt to teach something to the patient who will come with the intention of learning something. It does not signify a guarantee of a cure. It simply fixes a set of mutual expectations. Treatment will be aimed at dealing specifically with the symptoms that are presented by teaching the patient to analyze his everyday transactions. Cure will result from the freeing of the Adult within the individual, so that his own creativity can lead to new behavioral options and so that he won't have to remain limited the way he was in the past.

Obviously TA can be carried out on a one-to-one basis. However, Harris feels that it operates most effectively in groups. The group setting makes possible a mutual confrontation concerning the ways in which people are appealing to their own Parent and Child rather than to the realities. Also the group setting is much more like the one in which people are likely to live outside of treatment than the one-to-one therapy relationship. These advantages are seen to make TA a faster process when carried out in a group.

RESEARCH ON GROUP THERAPY

It is difficult to control the variables in group therapy without interfering with the spontaneous, dynamic nature of the group. Research, then, has been conducted mainly on the outcome of group therapy. Two hundred institutions were questioned by Corsini (1957) on what they considered the *most suitable kinds of patients* for group therapy. The most suitable patients were tabulated in this order: psychoneurotics, nonpsychotics, passive individuals, and psychosomatics. The poorer prospects were psychopaths, organics, and persons with the following characteristics: character disorders, active delusions, bizarre behavior, hostility, hyperactivity, and senility.

One study of the *outcome* of group therapy was conducted by Powdermaker and Frank (1953) with 104 men in a Veterans Administration hospital. Half of the patients received group therapy and the other half did not. The outcome, in terms of physicians' judgments, indicated that 61 percent of those who had *both individual and group therapy* improved and 52 percent of those who had only individual therapy improved; group therapy stimulated purposeful activity and verbal communication. Even though there are no hard data on the effectiveness of group therapy, it has increased greatly in use, is generally *well accepted* in therapeutic institutions, and the use of groups for improved personal adjustment has been explored in various forms with "normals."

FAMILY THERAPY

Patients often live in a family, and their problem behavior can be seen to reflect the stresses, conflicts, and adverse relationships between the patient and other family members. There is, thus, an increasing tendency to treat the family as a whole because they are all involved in some way in the behavior of the referred member. In the process of therapy the patterns of interaction in the family are noted; the way the patient is controlled by the others and how he uses his problem behavior to gain power over the family is explored. The therapist remains an open-minded observer and refuses to take sides in the family struggles. His major role is to help the whole family—to help them to see objectively the factors that cause their difficulties and to work out better ways of relating with each other. By his objectivity and emphasis on the feelings of all the family he serves as a model for better interaction among the members. The therapist may achieve the goal in various ways, such as by observing the members of the family in various combinations, and by using various techniques to arouse behavior. He usually, however, encourages intense communication and interaction and expression of feelings between members of the family (Haley, 1963).

Summary

1. The helping professions include professionals of many kinds, all of whom work to maximize the adjustment of the emotionally disturbed. Their emphases vary usually in keeping with special features of their training.
2. Certain common conditions characterize most forms of psychotherapy and counseling. These include lowering the patient's anxiety level, establishing a strong personal relationship, verbal or nonverbal communication, and commitment on the part of the patient. Seven different therapeutic goals have been identified, all or some of which may be striven for by a given counselor.
3. Many types of psychotherapy have been described including insight, client centered, behavior modification, emotive, and group therapy.
4. Insight therapy probes the patient's remote past in an effort to understand and bring under conscious control the deep-lying motives for behavior. One of the best-known forms of insight therapy is psychoanalysis.
5. Client-centered therapy is described as giving the client the initiative to explore his feelings in a warm, accepting, empathetic atmosphere. The process assists clients to achieve personal understanding and make decisions.
6. Behavior therapy is the use of basic learning principles, like extinction and counterconditioning, to shape behavior in more socially desirable directions. Examples of its use with self-destructive children by means of punishment are discussed. The "token economy" hospital ward treatment plan is another example of behavior modification. Behavior that is moving toward desirable goals is immediately reinforced by giving the patient a token that, with other tokens, can be exchanged later for desired objects or services. Systematic desensitization has been used to reduce fears such as fear of public speaking. It consists of the teaching of deep relaxation and the gradual exposure of the client to feared objects during relaxation. Imitation has also been used in modifying behavior. Finally, self-control has been placed in the behavior therapy model with success.
7. Emotive therapies are based on the theory that distressing psychological symptoms can be relieved by expressing powerful emotions that have been inhibited through life. Their various forms all stress the release of affect.

8. Groups have long been known to influence human development; now they are used therapeutically. There are many different kinds of groups, but they have certain elements in common. The leader is fairly permissive and encourages members of the group to interact freely and to discuss problems that concern them. Feelings are expressed readily. Members of the group may confront or support each other. Insights and understanding are encouraged.
9. Transactional Analysis (TA) is a currently popular form of group treatment that presumes that every person is made up of three different "psychological realities" which engender certain feelings about oneself and others. The treatment process attempts to expose these self-feelings and to help alter them.
10. The group method often includes the immediate family of a disturbed individual in a session. The therapist observes the conflicts and stressful interrelations between the patient and various family members. Insights and suggestions for altered interactions emerge.

Words to Remember

Anxiety
Behavior Therapy
Client-Centered Therapy
Clinical Psychologist
Counterconditioning Technique
Free Association
Gestalt Therapy
Insight Therapy
Nondirective Therapy
Psychiatric Nurse
Psychiatric Social Worker
Psychiatrist
Neuropsychiatrist
Primal Therapy
Psychodrama
Rational-Emotive Therapy
Repression
Role Playing
Self-Control
Self-Disclosure
Systematic Desensitization
Token Economy
Transactional Analysis
Transference

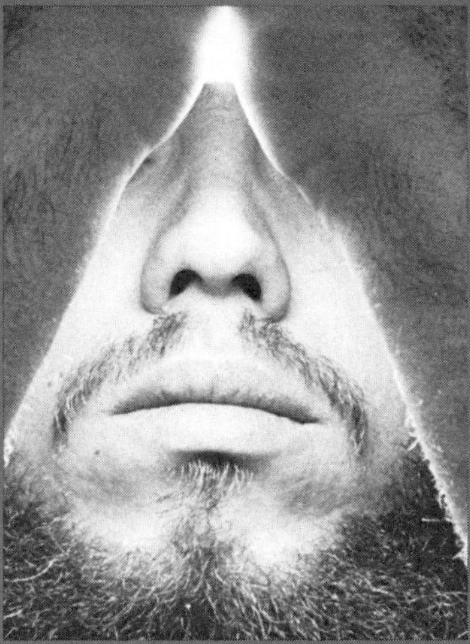

14. Maximizing Human Potentials

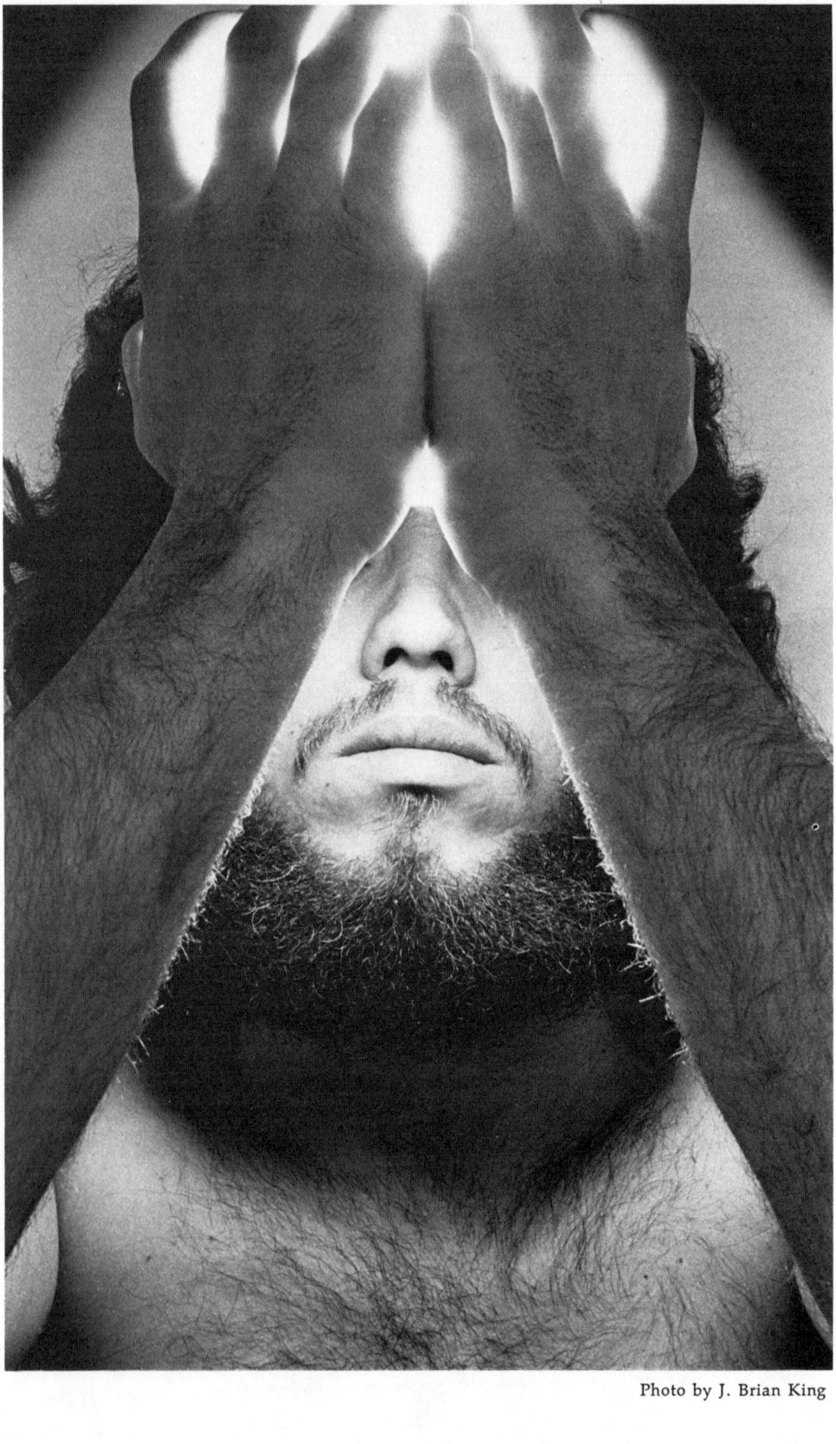

Photo by J. Brian King

Objectives

After studying this chapter the reader should be able to:

1. Describe the major objectives and techniques used in modern encounter or human potential groups.
2. Discuss the positive and negative features of encounter group experience.

The past 20 to 30 years have seen the rise of a number of movements dedicated to enhancing the adjustment of the "normal" personality. These movements have attracted relatively well-educated, affluent, middle-class individuals who are bored and dissatisfied with the routine of life as laid out for them by society. They therefore seek experiences and a life-style that promise to provide a richer existence than they assume they can have otherwise. Many such movements have been associated with group processes known variously as T-groups, sensitivity groups, or encounter groups. Such experiences are ordinarily grafted onto the everyday life of the individual. For some, an even more extreme approach to maximizing individual potentials involves the adoption of a totally different life-style from that of the larger society. This chapter will be devoted to an examination of both approaches.

Group Experiences

The various contemporary group movements all have their origins in a workshop held in 1946 in New Britain, Connecticut, by the Massachusetts Institute of Technology Research Center for Group Dynamics. It brought together a group of local leaders who were in positions to facilitate understanding of, and compliance with, the Fair Employment Practices Act. The participants included teachers, businessmen, social workers, and interested citizens. In this workshop three small groups were formed of 10 members and a leader. Each group then discussed the practical problems that had to be faced at home around the issues relevant to the workshop topic. In addition to discussion, members of the groups engaged in some role playing in order to highlight certain aspects of the problems and to rehearse ways of solving them. Research observers were attached to each group to look into the issue of the here and now interaction between individual group members. These researchers met together in the evenings and discussed the observations of group processes they had made and notes they had taken during daytime group sessions.

Hearing of this, some participants asked for permission to attend these meetings. Almost without thinking, the research group leader agreed, though many of his colleagues expected him to refuse. The research group then proceeded as though the participants were not present. No one predicted the consequences of this series of events. In effect, the discussions of the specific behaviors of individual group members had "an electric effect both on the participants and on the training leaders" (Benne, 1964, p. 82). Instead of remaining passive listeners during these conferences, group participants entered enthusiastically into the discussion. One might deny, for example, that an observer's report was accurate, only to have another defend it stoutly. Participants even joined in attempting to analyze and interpret what had taken place in a group session. Before long the word spread and all group participants began attending the evening research sessions which were lasting as long as three hours. Through the discussion that was taking place at these sessions, participants began to feel that they were developing some very important understanding of themselves as well as of the group in which they were participating. The training and research staff also became aware that the evening meetings were educating participants about their own behavior and the way it affects the behavior of the group. This research group activity became, in effect, the forerunner of the modern T-group.

Despite the very powerful and meaningful effect of the "here and now" discussion of behavior of individual group members, no immediate thought was given to the idea of eliminating the initial group procedure oriented around specific content. A second workshop was planned for the summer of 1947 to be held in Bethel, Maine. At this workshop, it was intended that a great many educative functions would be served. Participants would be taught many systematic concepts concerning group phenomena: they would learn about the skills necessary to be an effective change agent; they would be taught many of the group variables that would assist them in recognizing the criteria for group development, and the like. These training functions required the group leader to spend a good deal of time instructing participants in several concrete content areas. He soon became aware that this interfered with his capacity to help participants learn about themselves and their input into the ongoing life of the group. When these obstacles were recognized, a third stage in the evolution of the modern T-group came about with a move toward exclusive emphasis on the here and now. The group became a vehicle through which the individual could gain insight into how he was regarded by others and the way in which he functioned in a group.

From these accidental and relatively modest beginnings of the T-group, there ensued over the fifties and sixties a rapid expansion of the group movement. One writer (Massarik, 1972), giving only a partial listing of the variety of different groups in existence in recent years, includes 39 different types. Common to virtually all of the different group approaches developed in recent years is a search for deep inner understanding. Concern with the "here and now" reactions of others to the individual and the image that a given individual conveys to those around him as occurs in the T-group, seems only to whet the appetite of many for better personal understanding. Subsequent developments in the group movement have involved pushing deeper for inner understanding and for the liberation of feelings heretofore buried.

Back (1972) has characterized the popular spread of interest in groups as a social movement having religious as well as therapeutic undertones. Basically it has provided for many participants "a consistent world view and some of the emotional aspects and controls of religious ritual" (p. 19). Similarly, although T-groups started from a scientific base, newer group developments have disassociated themselves from scientific procedures and from most attempts to evaluate their consequences. Back sees the new group developments as a social movement appealing to a well-educated, reasonably affluent, middle- to upper-middle-class public who are bored with everyday life and are either disenchanted with or skeptical about traditional religion. For such individuals the group seems to offer a way to reach deep into themselves to find undiscovered well-springs of feeling, creativity, sensitivity, and perceptiveness that can enrich the course of their existence.

To attempt to catalog and describe the various different types of group approaches now in use would be impossible. Even within a single general classification of a group approach, one can find a myriad of different techniques used and new ones developing every day. The best that can be done is to describe various techniques that have characterized different aspects of the group movement in an effort to convey some sense of how its leaders have gone about attempting to achieve the purposes it strives for.

THE ENCOUNTER GROUP

The nature of the encounter group may vary quite widely, depending on the leader. At one extreme, there is the one in which virtually all the interaction is verbal; at the other, one in which physical contact plays a prominent if not the predominant role. The approaches of Rogers (1969) and Schutz (1967) provide a clearly visible contrast along this dimension. In Rogers' groups most of the interaction is verbal. The leader sees himself as a facilitator who makes it clear to the group at the outset that they must decide for themselves what direction they will take. The granting of this unusual freedom generally results in a period of confusion followed by some effort at developing an organizational structure for coping with the need to assume personal responsibility. During this period someone may suggest establishing an agenda, and frequently such a proposal is ignored by some and supported by others. Most commonly the idea is ignored, and there is more casting around among the group for a means of proceeding. Eventually a suggestion such as "why not simply introduce ourselves to each other" is made, and this can prompt several hours of discussion about who will lead the group, what its purpose should be, and who its members are. During such a discussion, considerable frustration may be directed toward the leader who is offering few cues to how they should proceed and what is expected of them.

In the initial stages of the group described by Rogers (1969) a certain amount of resistance commonly appears against revealing overly personal material. When one member begins to do so, the group ambivalence may be revealed in another member or members suggesting that the individual may be going too far in opening himself up and that he is somehow being seduced by the group atmosphere. Despite such attempts to shut off the flow of feeling, such emotions do find expression, and the business executive may well talk about his frustrations at work, the housewife may complain about her husband's lack of consideration, and the like. For the most part these early expressions of feeling focus on situations outside the group or those that have occurred in the remote past. The reluctance to deal with feelings that are being aroused at the moment by other group members still remains.

When here and now feelings do appear, Rogers (1969) indicates that they are generally negative feelings, expressions of dissatisfaction toward the leader, or an attack on another member for taking some particular stand. Rogers (1969) speculates that negative feelings are more likely to appear early because they are a good means to test the degree to which the group is a free and open situation, and, furthermore, an attack on another group member can at its worst only provoke some sort of retaliation which most people feel they are capable of managing. If a member expressed warm positive feelings, he would always run the risk of being rejected, and this might be devastating. Rogers finds that following negative expressions of feeling, often one or another group member begins to reveal himself in important ways. Apparently enough trust has developed that at least some group members feel that whatever they talk about will be accepted in an understanding way. Thus a man may speak of the impossibility of his marital situation because of his inability to communicate with his wife, or a successful scientist may speak of the degree to which he has buried himself in his job as a means of fostering an isolated existence that he is finding more and more painful.

Eventually group members can begin to talk about the feelings that other members arouse in them at the moment. Rogers (1969) is struck by the degree to which the group members in any encounter group can be accepting and helpful when their fellow members reveal painful material. Indeed, as sessions continue, group members become more and more sensitive to and rejecting of a façade, or the defenses that each is apt to erect against self revelation. As Rogers describes it, "gently at times, almost savagely at others, the group demands that the individual be himself, that his current feelings not be hidden and that he remove the mask of ordinary social intercourse" (Rogers, 1969, p. 31).

In this atmosphere of very free expression and interaction, each group member quickly gets to know how the others feel about them. The woman who goes out of her way to help finds that some group members resent her acting like an intrusive mother. The man who weighs his words carefully and speaks very precisely finds that others see him as stuffy. At times these impressions are conveyed through confrontation in which one group member actually "tells off" another.

Rogers (1969) describes many dividends resulting from participation in the encounter group. Group members help each other both within and outside the group to assimilate new and painful self-perceptions. The group aspect of the interaction forces people together into far closer and more direct contact than they ordinarily have with others in everyday life. The experience of being able to expose intensely important private feelings brings one very close to the people who hear and accept these feelings. Not uncommonly important behavior changes take place within the group such as a softening of voice tone and development of spontaneity. Members of the group may become more thoughtful and considerate of each other and helpful in ways that reveal considerable sensitivity. Rogers (1969) feels that the most fundamental change to come about in the encounter group is in the attitude of the participant toward himself. Secondary to this are changes in his close interpersonal relationships. Thus, he is likely to be more open and spontaneous with his wife, his children, and his close friends.

Rogers (1969) points out that the kind of intensive group experience that he promotes entails some risks. A minor problem is that in many cases behavior changes that take place as a result of the group are not long lasting. More serious is the fact that some individuals may become quite involved in self-exploration, only to be left when the group ends with many problems that have not been worked through completely. Far more serious is the fact that occasionally an already borderline individual suffers a psychotic break as a result of a group experience. It is Rogers' feeling that when the group process has been proceeding in a very positive fashion the danger of lasting serious psychological damage to any group member is low. However, he admits that a great deal more needs to be known about this problem.

Other problems may arise as the result of group experiences. For example, if one member of a married couple engages in the group, and he or she makes strides toward flexibility and growth, this change may threaten the spouse who has not participated. Associated with this problem is the fact that many positive and warm feelings normally develop between group members, and inevitably these will occur between male and female members. Some such feelings will often have a sexual component that can be upsetting to participants and threaten existing marriages, if the feelings are not dealt with satisfactorily.

While acknowledging all of these potential dangers, Rogers justifies his approach nonetheless. As he puts it, "in groups as elsewhere in life, all significant learning is to some degree painful and involves turbulence within the individual and within the system. I see no way of avoiding this if there is to be constructive change" (Rogers, 1969, p. 61).

Schutz (1967) engages in a brand of encounter group which seems vastly different from the highly verbal interaction described by Rogers and as such helps to convey the degree of diversity to be found in this field. The basic goals toward which Schutz strives are no different from those of Rogers. Schutz sees the fulfillment of personal potential as leading to feelings of joy, the ultimate in a sense of aliveness, self satisfaction, and successful dealings with other people. For Schutz, the obstacles to achieving this state reside in social organizations that stifle creativity and force people into a lockstep way of life. Hypocrisy and superficiality are seen to be imposed by society and to result in interpersonal relationships that are merely tolerable rather than sources of genuine happiness. In his encounter groups, Schutz uses a wide variety of techniques designed to release human potentials and to sweep away the inhibitions that have blocked their expression.

To a great extent, Schutz's techniques are related to his idea that three basic interpersonal needs characterize mankind. The first of these needs is called *inclusion.* This term refers to the need to feel significant in the eyes of others, to receive the interest and attention of other people. An aspect of inclusion is the feeling that one has a unique identity as a person. One feature of this singular identity is the wish to be understood which carries with it the idea that others are interested enough in you to find out about your special characteristics. Inclusion is distinguished from the second major need identified by Schutz, which is *control.* Inclusion differs from control in that it involves the desire to be prominent, whereas control refers to the need to dominate.

Behavior associated with control involves making decisions concerned with power and the holding of authority, as well as the converse need to be controlled by others. When two people argue, the one who is concerned about inclusion simply wants to participate in the argument. The person who is concerned about control is primarily interested in winning the argument. The inclusion person may actually prefer to lose the argument. Associated with the need for control is rebellion and other behavior directed toward establishing one's independence. Such actions reflect an unwillingness to allow others to be in control. Acceptance of the control of others is reflected in overcompliance and submission. Another distinction between the need for control and the need for inclusion is that one can be a controlling person without necessarily being prominent. The person who operates as "the power behind the throne" is having his control needs quite well satisfied, despite the fact that he is not especially prominent. By contrast, the adolescent who plays the clown among his peers is displaying a prominent need to be included, even though he has very little power. The important distinction between behavior directed toward control and that involved with *affection,* the third of Schutz's basic needs, is that control deals with power relations rather than with emotional closeness.

Behavior associated with the need for affection concerns personal emotions between two people, particularly the emotions of love and hate. According to Schutz, affection can only occur between pairs of people at any one time, whereas the need for inclusion or control may occur in pairs or between a single individual and a whole group of people. In groups, behavior motivated by affection is characterized by the expression of friendship toward other individuals. Some avoid close ties with any single group member but are superficially friendly with a number of people in the group and are popular. Thus popularity in itself may not involve affection. Instead, it may be more closely associated with the need for inclusion. Schutz differentiates further between the three needs in the following way: The student who fails to win an invitation from the fraternity that he aspires to has his inclusion needs frustrated; when he is failed in a course by his professor, his control needs are frustrated; and when his girl friend rejects him, it is primarily his needs for affection that are denied.

The stages through which groups pass in their organization and eventual development are seen by Schutz to be a function of these three sets of needs. The first to be important in a group setting are the needs for inclusion, since all group members are in the process of deciding whether they wish to, or are opposed to forming a group. The introverted person may insist that he wishes to maintain his privacy and avoid becoming involved with other people, despite the fact that at an unconscious level he would like to have their attention. The extraverted person will actively seek out others and will consciously want them to seek him out. Both fear that they will be ignored but will react to this anxiety in their own characteristic way. Schutz has designed several techniques that he uses in encounter groups to highlight issues around contact and inclusion.

One such technique involves having all group members sit very closely together, either on the floor or on chairs, and to close their eyes for approximately a five-minute period during which they are encouraged to "feel their space." This involves stretching their hands out and feeling for all the space in front, behind, above and beside them. Inevitably they touch those group members close to them. Following this activity a discussion is held around the feelings that have been aroused by this exercise. Some group members have been wary of intruding onto the space of others; others may feel angry at the fact that those beside them have intruded into their own space. Thus the possibility for opening up discussion around many aspects of aloneness and need for contact is high.

Another technique described by Schutz dealing with the need for inclusion involves the bestowing of new names on group members. When group members have not known each other before the group began, Schutz feels a valuable opportunity is presented for avoiding dealing with individuals on the basis of expectations aroused by past experiences. There is the further opportunity for the group member to assume an entirely new identity, and taking a new name is one way of fostering this. Once such new names are taken, they are used for the life of the group. Various means can be used for assigning names. They can be assigned randomly. In some cases an individual may stand before the group who suggest possible names for him, until one is hit upon that satisfies both him and the other group members. Another way is to have the group member choose his own name in keeping with his particular aspirations. At times a member will try to change his name during the life of the group or even to go back to his own real name. An example of how the process of name changing worked out in a particular group involved a "dowdy-looking, middle-aged, plump school psychologist" whose own name was Henrietta. When she asked the group to assign her a name which was just the opposite of the way she looked, since she was not happy with herself, the group settled on "Bubbles." The name seemed to free her up somewhat, although she remained rigid and formal to the point that one group member said that he felt like shaking her. With encouragement, he actually did so with the result that Bubbles began to radiate feeling in a way that had never been typical of her in the past.

In any group it is common for feelings such as alienation, isolation, or not belonging to be aroused in some members. When these become evident, Schutz suggests a procedure that he calls *breaking in* as a means of dealing with such feelings. Those group members who are seen to be "in" are asked to stand in a circle with their arms interlocked. The person who feels alienated is then encouraged to try to break physically through their locked arms into the circle by any means and the others are encouraged to try to keep him out. Following this exercise, the feelings that the person had as he tried to break in as well as the feelings of those who were banded together to keep him out are discussed.

As an example of the breaking in approach, Schutz describes a group in which one girl felt that five or six members tended to dominate discussions because they knew each other fairly well and were familiar with the group techniques. She was, therefore, asked to designate those group members who she felt were dominating the meetings, and they formed a circle which she was asked to break into. Following a few weak attempts, she picked out the strongest male member of the group and attempted to break his grip on his partner. After several minutes of a futile effort, she gave up, saying that she really didn't care to push her way into this group, in any case. Some members of the audience reacted to this performance with considerable anger. One berated her for her casualness and described the kicking and clawing that he would have engaged in to force his way in. Another said he would have attempted to find weak spots in the circle and to intrude through such an opening. He proposed tickling members of the circle until he found one who was vulnerable and who could be forced to release his grip. Further discussion revealed how the solution attempted by the first girl and those proposed by the other group members were typical of the way each had dealt with important aspects of their own life situations.

Once inclusion needs have been resolved, the next set of needs that seem to take a prominent position in the group are those involved with control. A differentiation of roles begins to take place within the group and invariably these are associated with struggles for power, competitiveness, and the like. Some individuals abdicate all pretense of assuming control and are termed by Schutz as "abdicrats." They avoid responsibility for decisions and are content to have someone else take charge. Such an individual is thought to question his own capacity for behaving as a responsible adult, so he is content to avoid situations that will display his weakness. On the other hand, other group members are "autocrats" seeking to establish a power hierarchy in which they are at the top. For those individuals who are comfortable with their control needs, either type of role is possible depending on the situation and what seems most appropriate. Several nonverbal techniques are advocated by Schutz for dealing with control needs.

One approach that Schutz advocates is an exercise called *pushing*. In this procedure two people face each other and clasp hands palm to palm with fingers intertwind. At a signal they begin to push each other in an attempt to make the other give ground. Schutz describes the case of one group member who played an extremely subservient role to the group leader, so much so that it became one of the group objectives to help this person come to feel more as a peer to the leader. It was suggested by one member that this person push with the leader as a means of attempting to achieve peership. The person refused until the group helped him recall the unhappiness he had suffered in his family because he felt like an unwanted child. He had felt worthless and insignificant much of his life. When encouraged to fantasy about this childhood situation, he was able to work up considerable emotion including crying and a feeling of anguish. As soon as he had finished this fantasy, he decided that he wanted to push with the leader and spent about five minutes doing so. The exercise ended in a spontaneous embrace between the two, and from then on this particular group member was able to relate to the leader as an equal.

Another exercise associated with control needs that Schutz (1967) recommends is called *breaking out*. In this procedure the group members form a circle with arms interlocked. One person stands within the circle and must try to break out of the group in any way he can. Group members try their best to prevent this from happening. This technique is used with group members who feel that they are being held back by one or another individual such as a spouse who ties them down. Schutz describes the example of a 24-year-old female group member who was very overcontrolled. She spoke in a very low and controlled voice tone, being careful that her thoughts were always logical and well organized. Her face showed little expression and she moved stiffly and gracelessly. A fantasy of hers depicted her father entering her body and tying down all of her organs with steel straps. This fantasy, along with other recollections of actual childhood events, pointed up the important role her father played in making her feel constricted.

She was encouraged to participate in psychodrama where she confronted another group member playing her father and spilled many of the feelings that she had never been able to express to him directly. At the point of declaring herself independent of him, however, she weakened and began to behave in a somewhat childish manner. At this point it was felt that she needed to do something more in order to gain the strength and confidence that she would need to deal openly with her father, and someone suggested that she participate in a breaking out situation. She did so and started out by furiously attempting to break out of the circle by pounding on people so energetically that when the group held fast she fell to the floor exhausted and gave up. The group insisted, however, that she continue to try, and ultimately she did attack the circle vigorously enough to smash through. Following this episode, she returned to the psychodrama and physically attacked the group member who was portraying her father, pushed him to the floor, and with her knee on his chest declared that he would never again hold her back. Ultimately she is described as having become a much happier person, who appeared more feminine and could be much more informal than ever before with people.

Because the needs for affection are associated with the building of strong emotional ties, these become predominant in the later phases of group development, after inclusion and control needs have been dealt with. Those who display too little affection avoid getting very close to others and may actually speak of not wanting to be "emotionally involved." Such individuals seem to harbor an unconscious wish for truly affectionate relationships but are afraid that no one can love them. At the opposite extreme are those individuals who make overt efforts to become very close to others. Needing very strongly to be loved, they seem to fantasy that although past experiences with affection have not worked out well, if they only try again, matters may turn out more favorably. Such individuals constantly seek approval, and relate in a very personal, ingratiating way. Those who are comfortable with their needs for affection find no difficulty in close personal relationships. They can be intense with others when appropriate and can also maintain a proper distance when that seems more appropriate. Such individuals want to be liked but can accept situations where they are not particularly liked. They don't take the latter situation as evidence that they are entirely unlovable.

One technique that Schutz recommends for dealing with affectional needs is called *rock and roll.* This approach is designed to deal with one of the basic issues in the matter of affection, the feeling that one can trust others. In this approach the person who doubts that others are trustworthy stands in the middle of a group that has formed a circle around him. He closes his eyes, attempts to relax all of his muscles, and tries to allow himself to be given over to the group members who pass him around the circle from person to person. In the beginning, the person engaging in this exercise is commonly quite stiff and controlled, but as he is passed around he begins to relax and it's possible for the group members to pick him up and hold him at chest level. He is then gently swayed back and forth with as little noise as possible. Gradually he is lowered to the floor and all hands are removed from his body very gently and tenderly. One female group member who participated in this exercise likened the experience to making love or giving birth to a child because of the feelings of "release and rapture" that seem to follow it. Following the meeting in which she engaged in this procedure, she described feeling very much in love without necessarily being able to attach the feeling to any particular individual.

Comparison of Rogers' (1969) approach in his conduct of encounter groups and that of Schutz reveals the wide variation that is possible in such groups. There seems to be little that is standard about the techniques that are used. Rogers relies virtually entirely on verbalization, whereas Schutz' groups apparently depend heavily upon various types of physical exercises. What they share are the common goals of attempting to reach deep inside the individual to liberate feelings that have presumably been bottled up for years and that have exercised an adverse affect on behavior. Rogers and Schutz vary with respect to the types of techniques they use to achieve these goals. Other approaches attempt to reach similar goals more effectively by varying the time spent in a given group session. The most dramatic of such variations are practiced in *marathon groups.*

Marathon groups were introduced by Frederick Stoller and George Bach (Stoller, 1968) in an effort to develop very intensive interactions within a relatively brief period of time. It was felt that this intensity could be achieved if group members were kept together over a period of a few days rather than for a few hours at a time. After experimenting with many different approaches, Stoller and Bach settled on the use of weekends for the marathon. Generally, the preferred setting for conducting a marathon is a private residence. Group members can relax better in a homey atmosphere, and this fosters being as open as possible. The formality of an office is seen to impede such necessary openness. When marathons are set up, a time schedule is always specified beforehand. Stoller prefers to begin his sessions around 8 P.M. on Friday evening and to terminate at 6 P.M. on Sunday evening. Except for two eight-hour breaks between 2 A.M. and 10 A.M. on Saturday and Sunday mornings, group members remain together even during meals so that all of the waking hours are devoted to the session. Some marathon group leaders prefer to have their groups active throughout 24-hour periods without allowing a break for sleep.

The fundamental ground rule in the marathon group is that all group members remain together throughout the entire session. They are, of course, allowed to walk around to exercise or take short breaks to attend to their physical needs, but they must commit themselves to staying with the group the entire period. Violations of this fundamental rule are taken as symptoms of the way in which the member characteristically copes with crises. Another basic rule in the marathon group is that all members be as honest and as direct as possible in expressing their personal feelings about other group members. Stoller discourages the use of structuring techniques such as psychodrama or role playing because he feels that they dilute the authenticity of the interaction among members.

The role of the leader in the marathon group is to set forth the ground rules, act as a timekeeper, and to keep the focus on the goals of the session. Beyond these functions, he is free to participate as any other group member expressing his own feelings and reactions. At times he may specify that a follow-up session will be held and decides when and where such sessions will take place and what the specific arrangements will be. Stoller recommends that a single follow-up session be held approximately 6 weeks after the marathon weekend.

A variation on the typical marathon group described by Bindrim (1969) involves nude interactions between group members. The idea for such a procedure was introduced by Abraham Maslow, who felt that the process of becoming emotionally open might be speeded up and intensified if the group members were without their clothes. It was felt that encouraging body contact between unclothed men and women without permitting sexual expression might lead quickly to an emotional closeness and a sense of "intensified personal identity."

Bindrim (1969) described a marathon that took place in a nudist camp equipped with a swimming pool and a Jacuzzi bath large enough to accommodate the entire group. The group consisted of 10 men and 10 women, most of whom were married to each other. As in other marathons, all group members were required to remain together for the entire period and to take part in all activities that had been scheduled. Participants were free to remove their clothes or not, no alcohol or drugs were permitted, overt sex acts were not permitted, and only first names could be used. The duration of the marathon was from 9 P.M. on Friday until 3 P.M. on Sunday, with a six-hour sleep period each night.

At the group's beginning, members got together clothed and talked about how they felt about being nude together. Following an hour's discussion, they went to the communal bath where they had the option of either bathing in the nude or not. All chose to bathe nude and the session was followed by a final meeting for the day in which individual members were invited to stand in front of the room where a projector shone colored lights over their bodies.

The next day was begun with a discussion of the impressions garnered the day before. Group members talked about how they felt about their own bodies, and what feelings had been aroused in seeing other group members without their clothes on. This was followed by more bathing and a one-hour session with a dance therapist. On Sunday morning a one-hour period was held during which "meditation with sensory saturation" took place. Many participants singled this out as the most moving experience of the entire weekend. This exercise involved having opposite-sexed couples sit facing each other close up. In the background a prelude to a Wagnerian opera played as all group members, with their eyes closed, touched, tasted, and smelled objects that each had been instructed to bring before the exercise in anticipation of this experience. For example, one member touched a piece of velvet, tasted a chocolate, and smelled a rose. This exercise is said to have produced a state not unlike a drug high during which members were asked to fantasy the time in their life when they felt the most free and the most joyful. Following this, group members touched fingertips with their partners and gazed quietly into each other's eyes. After 20 minutes of "eye-centered meditation," the group discussed the feelings that had been engendered by these experiences.

Bindrim (1969) feels that the nude marathon provides warmth and tactile contact for adults who need such experiences almost as much as the infant does. In the ordinary standoffish world of society, contact needs among adults inevitably go unsatisfied. Thus the nude marathon offers "tenderly sensual" experiences in the absence of sexual gratification as a way of winning genuine acceptance and warmth from one's fellows. It is expected that self-acceptance, which is the ultimate goal of the group procedure, will naturally follow the experience of being accepted by others.

REACTIONS TO THE GROUP MOVEMENT

As noted earlier, Back (1972) sees the group movement in the United States as being very similar to a new religion. He feels that it appeals to a relatively well-educated, affluent, largely middle-class person who has become disenchanted with existing religions and is casting around for some other faith that would help to give his life direction. The group movement is particularly attractive to such an individual because it seems to have been rooted in a scientific base, which is reassuring to the well educated, but, at the same time, it has abandoned that scientific base sufficiently to take on much of the fervor and spirit of a religion.

Back asserts further that the modern-day group movement has won particular acceptance and enthusiasm in the United States because of certain special conditions of life in this country. He points out that in other countries where T-groups are practiced, such as Great Britain, efforts have been made to stick closely to a scientific base and to avoid the emotionalism and the sensationalism that has characterized the movement in this country. At Tavistock, a prominent clinic in England, T-groups are used to deal only with specific problems of clients who are deemed to be particularly suited for the procedure. The program remains in the hands of highly trained professionals, and the lay public probably knows very little of sensitivity training in general. In many other foreign countries outside England the current group movement has been confined to academic and professional settings. For example, efforts to introduce encounter groups in Sweden failed because the Swedes could not be as informal as seemed necessary in the conduct of the groups. They simply were not comfortable being on a first-name basis with each other or being spontaneous enough to interrupt another speaker, as is required in the American version of the T-group.

Back (1972) feels that the special appeal of the group movement in the United States derives from a particular set of social conditions which have existed in this country for the past 20 years. Many Americans are dissatisfied in an affluent society; they feel insecure about their life-style and the goals toward which they strive; and they find their interpersonal relationships unsatisfying. The extensive and enthusiastic spread of the sensitivity group movement is seen by Back to have occurred because these conditions and feelings exist and he points to several reasons for their existence. First, American society is mobile. The country is large and from its earliest history the idea of seeking new frontiers, new worlds to conquer, has been fostered. In recent years many blacks have migrated from the South into urban areas in the North, but for the most part it is the well-educated, middle-class person who has been particularly mobile. In some cases the moves have been from the city to the suburbs, but in many others there have been moves between states, and certain areas of the country have burgeoned because they have special attractions. Back (1972) points out that it is just in such growing population centers—for example, in the West and particularly California—that the primary centers for encounter groups have developed. In a sense, he sees the encounter group as having replaced the "lonely hearts club" for those who are new to a community and feel they are without roots.

A second condition that Back sees as fostering the encounter group movement is the fact that American society is particularly affluent. This means that people have no concerns about subsistence needs. Few go hungry or without comfortable shelter, and a spectacular amount of money is spent on luxuries such as television sets, automobiles, trailers, boats, travel, and the like. Many people find that despite the many satisfactions available to them, they still suffer boredom, a sense of worthlessness, and a feeling of joylessness. Something more seems to be needed. For many the excitement of personal exploration has become that something more.

Still another condition in American society that has fostered the widespread development of the group movement has been the tendency to turn toward science and away from religion for the ultimate truth. In earlier times, one of religion's functions was to provide a basis for understanding the world. As scientific knowledge advanced, it took the place of religion in providing such understanding and thereby diminished the value of religion for the individual. In the past few decades society has come to rely very heavily on secular, scientific knowledge and to reject religion as the source of important truths. On the other hand, religion also served another important human need aside from the desire for understanding. Religion justified the very intense emotional expression that seems to be necessary if man is to exist comfortably. In effect, then, what today's society needed was some new institution that was acceptable to those who place their faith in science and rationality, but which, at the same time, permitted an intense emotional experience such as would have been gained through the practice of religious rituals in the past. Back (1972) feels that sensitivity training has provided just such an emotional outlet.

Apart from the whys and wherefores of the current group movement, many express very positive personal reactions to encounter groups. Gibb (1972), for example, a sympathizer with the movement, describes the effect that encounter groups have had on him personally. He feels that through such groups he has learned to trust in himself, the people around him, and the processes of nature. As such, he is more at home with his own impulses and inner feelings, the dimension on which he has achieved his greatest growth. Second, he feels that participation in groups has made him a more open person who can communicate more deeply with the people around him. He can reveal himself to a greater extent than he could before and can permit the feelings and perceptions of others to reach him. Third, he feels that the group experience has helped him to move in the direction of greater self-determination. He now has the capacity to find out what he's like and what he wants to be and can therefore approximate more closely being the kind of person that he seeks to become. Finally, he has accepted a sense of interdependence such that in his daily life he recognizes his dependence upon others and theirs on him.

Blanchard (1972) points to still other benefits of the group experience by contrasting the modern group to psychotherapy. He sees psychotherapy as being aimed at helping a person become better adapted to the society in which he lives, better able to satisfy his needs within the confines of a reality that is presented to him by society. The major value of the encounter movement for Blanchard is, on the other hand, that it operates as a subversive force with respect to the *status quo*. It challenges existing social structures and does not lock the individual into the limits they impose. Thus it provides an opportunity for one's true self to gain the utmost in expression.

Koch (1972), on the other hand, has examined the image of man which he feels is implicit in the encounter group movement and is horrified by it. To Koch, the group movement says, in effect, that to have private feelings is not healthy, that "total psychic transparency" is therapeutic and potentially growth releasing. Furthermore it assumes that man is an undifferentiated mass living in a social space inhabited by a large number of others who are similarly undifferentiated. This, Koch feels, threatens man's essential human dignity.

As an illustration of this point, Koch describes a symposium he attended at which Bindrim (1969) discussed the nude marathon group. In this discussion Bindrim is said to have enthusiastically described a new therapeutic technique of his own invention that he called "crotch eyeballing." In this technique a group member is "spread-eagled" by two other group members while the rest of the group stares for a long interval at the person's crotch. This is thought to be therapeutic because the crotch is regarded by Bindrim as the site of three types of serious "hang-ups" for most individuals: (1) those associated with the problems of the toilet-training period; (2) those associated with guilt over masturbation; and (3) those associated with all of the problems of sexuality. Somehow, crotch eyeballing is supposed to remedy all of these problems. For Koch, such techniques along with a variety of others that characterize the human potential movement are a threat to human dignity. It is a conception that robs a man of his own private inner life. Koch has been critical of behaviorism because, from a scientific point of view, it denies the existence of an inner life. Still, behaviorism permits the individual to maintain the illusion that he has one nonetheless. Those in the human potential movement, however, hold that to have a private inner life is not healthy.

Another type of criticism rendered toward the encounter movement is that some of its promoters and group leaders lack a sense of personal responsibility toward those who become group members. The reader may question how one might find the responsible group leader. A partial guide to this is an inquiry into his professional qualifications and his membership in recognized national professional organizations. See the discussion of "The Helping Professions," Chapter 13, pages 373–375. The philosophy of the movement places great stress on the here and now. This characterizes the content of encounter group sessions, and it is also true of the relationships that are established within the group. Groups are generally made up of strangers coming together for a weekend or several days or, at times, only a few hours, who have never seen each other before, who have had no choice in whom they will meet with, and will very likely never see each other again. Back (1972) acknowledges that one of the encounter group's most impressive features is the degree to which people can display deep feeling for each other in the short time that they interact. Both genuine affection as well as intense aggression may be aroused, but it all ends when the group ends. Likewise the group leader, whose job it has been to promote intensity, sees his job as finished as soon as the group ends.

In more traditional psychotherapeutic approaches, the group leader or the therapist who has guided or has been a companion to the client through a change process accepts the *responsibility* of standing behind the client after change has taken place in order to be available to help, if any problems with aspects of the new style arise. This is not the case in the encounter group. The leader's responsibility ends with the final session. Furthermore, the encounter group leader disavows all responsibility for what occurs to individual group members even during the ongoing session. Back (1972, p. 215) asserts that this disavowal of responsibility is well characterized by a statement of Perls, the founder of Gestalt Therapy: "Sir, if you want to go crazy, commit suicide, improve, get turned on, or get an experience that will change your life, that is up to you. You came here out of your own free will." Back also quotes a statement by William Schutz which further elaborates the leader's disavowal of responsibility for the group member. At a New York workshop Schutz is said to have stated,

> I'd like to say first that, whatever happens, you are responsible for yourself. That is, if during the course of these things you want to become physically injured, then you can do that if you want to; if you want to bow to group pressure, you can do that. If you want to not bow to group pressure, you can also do that. I want you to understand clearly at the outset that you are responsible for whatever happens to you here (Back, 1972, p. 226).

The failure of some encounter group leader to accept responsibility for the long-range effects of his group procedure poses many serious dangers for potential consumers. No attempt is made to screen out, even in a very gross way, subjects who may be attempting to use the group inappropriately or whose current adjustment is so tenuous as to make participation a serious danger to them and upsetting for others. No efforts are made to *follow up* those who have undergone a profound emotional experience and may be struggling with its aftereffects. No concern is displayed even for those who suffer very serious and prolonged disorders as the result of participation in an encounter group.

The encounter grouper's response to many of these criticisms takes many forms. A critical scientific tone is assumed with respect to the failure to screen prospective group members. The technical difficulties of making accurate predictions concerning the likely vulnerability of a prospective group member are described. Allusions are made to the past failure of traditional psychiatric diagnostic procedures to predict behavior accurately. With respect to the concern that encounter groups cause serious psychological harm to some group members, instances of such negative effects are minimized (Blanchard, 1972; Gibb, 1972).

The issue, of course, of what potential harm may occur as the result of encounter group experiences is an extraordinarily significant one and, unfortunately, the question of how frequently and to what extent encounter groups result in negative experience for its participants is as yet unresolved. To be sure, many reports have been made of the occurrence of serious psychological disturbance as a result of encounter groups leading to such dramatic outcomes as suicide, prolonged psychotic illness, and even physical injury. However, careful study of the frequency of occurrence of such disorder has not been done, and proponents of encounter groups deny that such negative outcomes occur often. It is probably true that when dramatically negative behaviors are provoked by a group experience, they are likely to create so significant an impression that their incidence and significance become greatly magnified. On the other hand, many other more subtle negative outcomes are possible in encounter groups which the leaders of such groups, since they do no follow-up with their subjects, are not in a position to learn about. Thus instances in which a person has not become psychotic but has suffered the serious disruption of many aspects of his life situation and has endured considerable unhappiness as a result of the group experience may be going unnoticed.

What this points to is the need for systematic research evaluating the outcome of encounter groups. The stated object of the group is to elicit very deep and intense feelings which have been defended against by most people for a long time. It is not unreasonable to expect that in the release of such emotion some individuals will become seriously troubled, at least temporarily. Therefore, it would not seem unreasonable to ask that proponents of encounter groups take a careful look at the effects of their techniques on differing types of individuals. To be sure, some studies have been done to assess negative outcomes of encounter groups. Reddy (1972) has surveyed several of these and reports extraordinarily low rates of seriously negative outcomes. On the other hand, most of these studies have not involved systematic follow-up, and have focused on the incidence of very serious and dramatic negative consequences such as the occurrence of psychosis or suicide.

Bebout and Gordon (1972) have done an extensive study in an attempt to assess the value of the encounter group experience for its participants. They were concerned with the outcomes in 150 nonprofessionally led groups comprising a total of about 1100 group members. Their findings are that encounter groups seem to have relatively little effect on problems that its members are encountering in school, or in enhancing their work productivity. On the other hand, various self-report measures indicate that participants see themselves as having changed in such areas as self-reliance and self-awareness. In this study, the groups were tested at the beginning of the encounter experience and again at a 6-month follow-up. For the various measures used by Bebout and Gordon only about one-third of their originally tested group responded to the follow-up questionnaire, and a large percentage of these had postive remarks to make about the group experience. In the first 28-month period of the project, only 4 serious disturbances were known to occur in group participants.

The significance of the findings of Bebout and Gordon's study is very difficult to assess, given the relatively low rate of response on follow-up. Although responses to follow-up questionnaires invariably result in a low return rate, one cannot help but suspect that those who do take the time to respond to questions about the value of an encounter experience would be those who had been the most enthusiastic, whereas those who have experienced difficulty as the result of the experience would be less likely to respond.

Lieberman, Yalom, and Miles (1972) have reported another study evaluating the impact of encounter groups on its participants. Their concern was with both the effectiveness of such groups and the risks entailed in participating. In their study, Lieberman et al. included a group of subjects, each of whom took part in one of 18 groups in which 10 different approaches were used, as well as a control group of subjects matched to the group participants but not experiencing an encounter group. Several pencil-and-paper measures were used to assess change. Some of these were filled out by group participants who described their general attitudes toward encounter groups and their functioning, some were filled out by group leaders who used rating scales to describe the kind of change taking place in their group participants, and each participant was asked to name several people in his social network who were also approached to make ratings about the individual's behavior. Measures were taken at the beginning of each encounter group and again at a follow-up period 6 to 8 months after the group's conclusion.

The preliminary findings of the study indicate that clients feel satisfied with the group at its conclusion. The reports of their friends, however, indicate that subjects in the experimental and control groups appear just about the same with respect to positive changes and that more negative changes are described in experimental group subjects than in controls. The most significant change reported by group participants is in their feeling of self-esteem. The most distressing findings of this study involve the negative outcomes found in the follow-up. About 7.5 percent of participants in encounter groups showed some kind of negative outcome ranging from severe to moderate (e.g., psychotic episode, severe depression, lowered self-esteem, distrust of others). Equally disturbing is the fact that those who seemed best able to predict group casualties were fellow group members rather than the group leaders. Furthermore casualties in the group were not well identified during the life of the group but only on follow-up later on. Those individuals who seemed to be most vulnerable psychologically were persons who were banking very heavily on growing as the result of the encounter experience, particularly if they were in groups where the leaders conveyed the impression that they could provide the wished-for salvation.

Clearly much more research on encounter groups is necessary before their true worth and dangers can be assessed. Whether such efforts will actually be made by those who are most strongly supportive of the movement is doubtful. Their enthusiasm seems to be based on a faith in the worth of what they are doing. It is paradoxical, however, that in the process of seeking to promote optimal growth in their fellow man, proponents of encounter groups may well be endangering his individuality as well as his psychological stability.

Another modern movement aimed at enhancing the growth of the individual has involved the development of alternate life-styles which in effect are mini-societies set up within the framework of the larger society. The aim of these societies seems to be quite similar to that of the encounter movement, and Blanchard (1972) sees them as logical extensions of encounter groups.

The Commune Movement

The commune represents an attempt to establish an alternative life situation in which it is possible to satisfy man's needs and fulfill his potentials more effectively than occurs in the usual society. The dream of creating such an ideal or utopian situation is probably as old as civilized man. Man's conception of an afterlife in some heavenly realm probably bore the seeds for later concrete attempts to create ideal living situations on earth. Attempts to create utopian living situations date back to the second century B.C. and at different times in man's history have appeared in various parts of the world. In the United States, the nineteenth century saw the establishment of a large number of societies designed to provide an ideal life for man here on earth.

Modern utopian communities seem to be emerging in response to many of the same kinds of pressures that provoked development of the nineteenth-century communal societies. Broad social movements are appearing, organized around issues that are somewhat similar to both periods: women, blacks, and even temperance, although in this case it is abstinence from drugs rather than alcohol that is emphasized. Both periods saw dissatisfaction with the evils of the capitalistic system. In both periods anarchists who resented any form of social organization and spiritualists who were acting in accordance with the will of their messiah appeared. Both periods too are characterized by a concern for individual fulfillment (Figure 14–1).

One major difference between the nineteenth- and twentieth-century utopian movements is that in the nineteenth-century traditional religious ideals generally formed the guiding purpose behind the new society. In the twentieth century the guiding motives are expressed in psychological terms emphasizing "personal growth" or the opportunity for a person to "do his own thing." Thus, the striving for a psychological ideal for the twentieth-century utopian seems to have become the equivalent of the religious ideals of the nineteenth-century utopian. This difference in guiding purpose has resulted in some important practical differences in the nature of the societies that have resulted.

In the nineteenth century much concern was expressed for social reform and the bringing about of economic and political change which would enhance the welfare of the entire community. In the twentieth century the utopian is concerned with his own personal growth rather

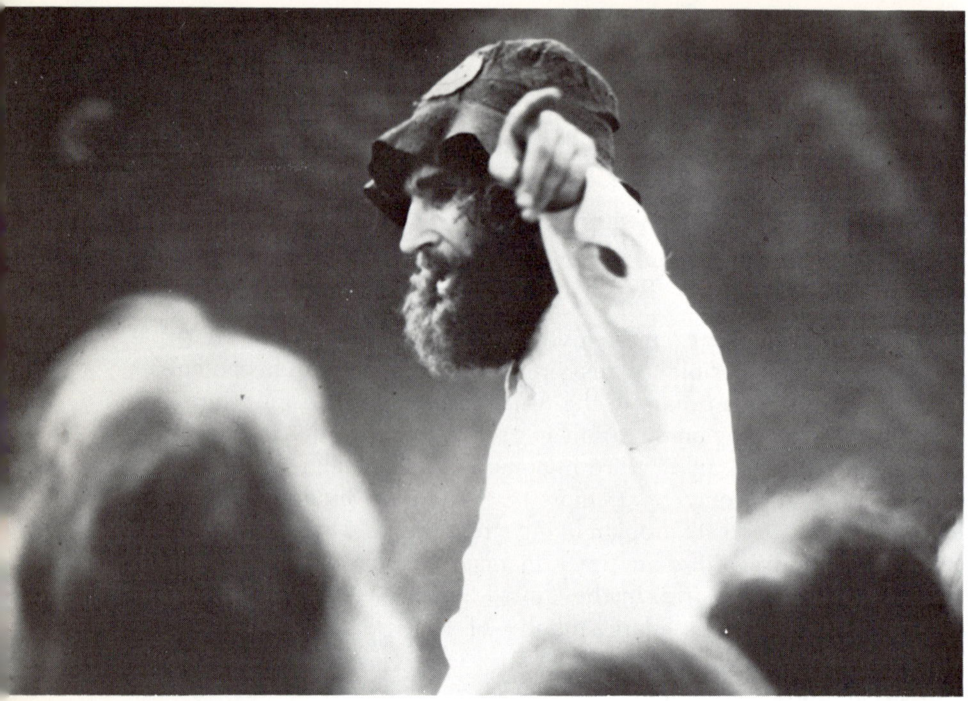

Photo by J. Brian King

Figure 14–1 On to Utopia.

than with social ideals. As a result many of the modern-day communes are not utopian in character. Rather, their living situations involve shared property, and close interpersonal relationships, but no common ideology. In many respects they involve collections of people who live as an extended family rather than as members of a utopian society. As such, behavior in such communities is not guided by a long-range vision of an ideal way of life, but instead by the intuitive feelings of the moment. Therefore, the successful community is one in which the "vibes" are good rather than one in which the group is cohesive and enduring. Furthermore many look upon the modern commune as a temporary living situation, a way station in life that is necessary for the moment but is not expected to be a permanent social structure.

Many modern commune members look back to a romanticized past full of nostalgia for simple, smalltown life. The crafts of rural societies, natural foods, and the dress, hairstyles, and even tools of an earlier, less complex age are glorified (Figure 14–2). Associated with this romanticized nostalgia is a longing for a return to the feeling of innocence and simplicity characterizing a childhood free of obligations.

Whether today's communes are concerned with setting up a long-standing utopian society or a temporary family, they all face certain

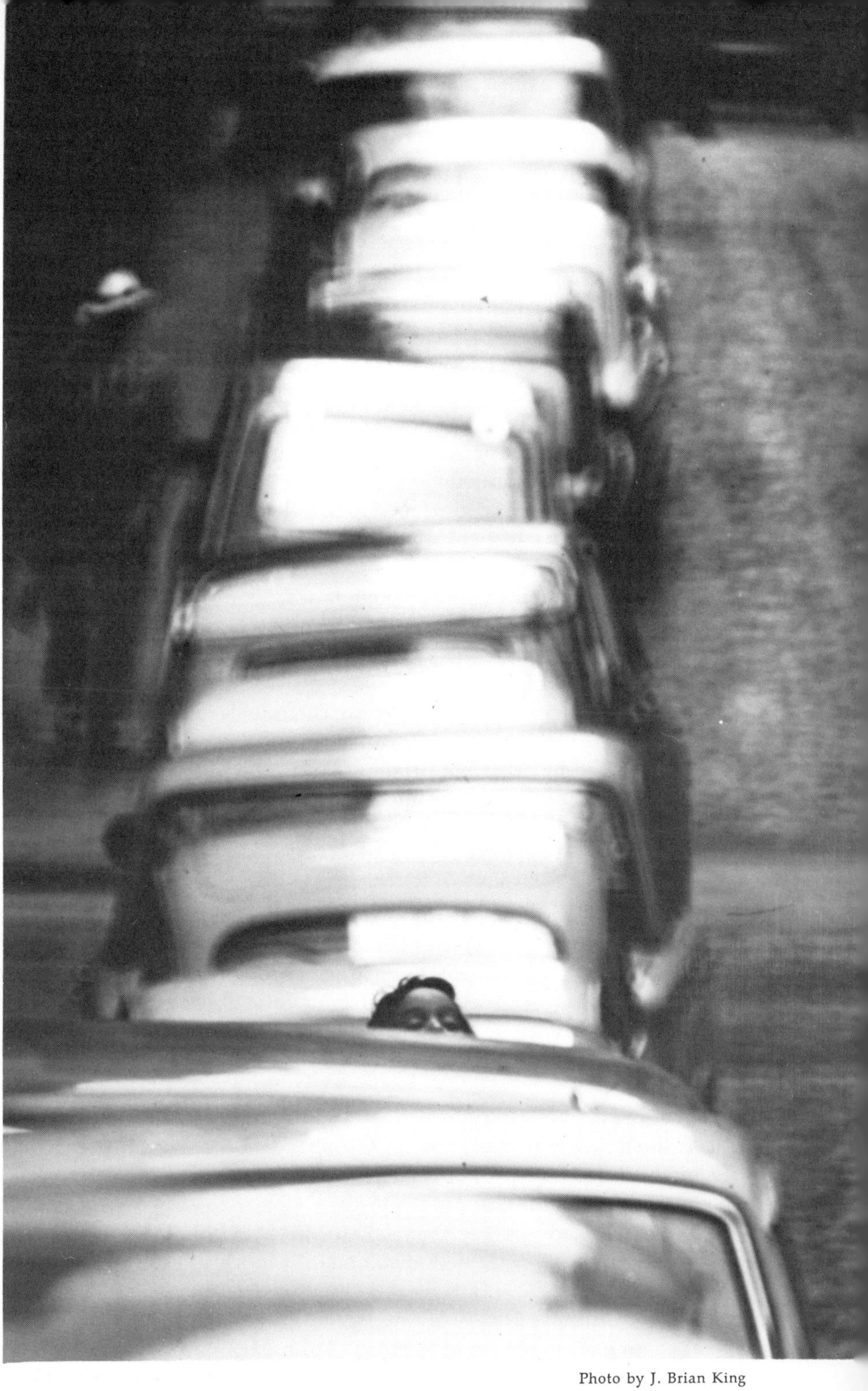

Photo by J. Brian King

Figure 14–2 Utopia—Escape from a Mechanized Society.

common problems with respect to establishing a stable group. One major problem is to clearly mark out the group's boundaries and to prevent the outside society from intruding and diluting the group's character. This problem is a more difficult one to deal with in modern times than it was in the nineteenth century. In the nineteenth century a group of people could go out into a remote, isolated area that would be difficult for the outsider to reach. People's technological needs were minimal, so there was relatively little need to maintain contact with the outside world. Whether in the choice of a career or of a life-style, the nineteenth-century person had fewer options than modern man. In modern times, it is difficult to prevent the environment from intruding through group borders. Communication is instant. People are unwilling to do without the advanced technology of the time. Thus small groups find it difficult to become entirely self-sufficient. Any distinctive set of beliefs is constantly threatened by the influx of new ideas and stimuli. To deal with this problem of creating firm group boundaries, many modern communes have settled on either an affirmative or negative set of guiding principles. Negative principles define the group by what it rejects; affirmative principles define it by what it accepts.

Kanter (1972) has classified modern communes into two groups on the basis of affirmative and negative principles. Communes having boundaries based on negative principles are called "retreat" communes. These are characterized as being small, having anarchistic views of organization, and as dissolving readily. Most of these are rural groups involving youthful members. The major goals of such communes are the establishment of interpersonal relationships, and they tend to admit members very readily, are permissive about life in the society, and are temporary in nature. Communes characterized by affirmative boundaries hold some form of service as an ideal and through this activity interact broadly with the wider society. Their boundaries are held firm by their mission. These groups are found either in urban or rural areas, and generally have a strong core of members which holds the community together.

Retreat communes are typically set up in remote areas benefiting very little from technological advances. Group members often live without plumbing or electricity. These groups are poorly organized, reject work schedules, and even the necessity to earn money to support the group. Their material needs are typically taken care of by relatives, welfare, or whatever is brought in by new members. As much as possible, the outside world is ignored. Defined as they are by what they reject, and turning its back on those forces of the larger society that create order, the retreat commune cannot hope to have a strong, committed, stable group. It is not surprising, therefore, that groups of this sort provide a satisfying experience for some individuals for a limited period of time, but they simply fail to endure.

Service communes, on the other hand, are established on the basis of affirmative principles dedicated to meeting some special need of society. Therefore, rather than avoiding the larger society, such a group often seeks out involvement with other people and, therefore, must settle in large urban areas. The service communes are also different from the retreat communes in that they set up firm boundaries that encourage group coherence and considerable commitment on the part of the members. Although it is too soon to make a judgment about their capacity to endure, service communes seem to be demonstrating that they are capable of lasting over a long period of time.

Many service communes emphasize education such as those nineteenth-century utopian communities that eventuated in colleges like Oberlin and Antioch. Some modern-day service communes have emerged from the human potential movement and look upon themselves as "growth centers" or centers emphasizing the study of human relations. Some teach the Zen macrobiotic life-style, care for the mentally handicapped, or attempt to rehabilitate drug addicts. Two types of membership characterize the service communes: (1) a core group deeply committed to the community and holding major responsibility for its teaching functions; and (2) a transient group with limited involvement which is expected to move in and out of the society.

The idea of creating a new, better way of life or a utopian community is an appealing alternative to the notion that people suffer from various problems because they are "sick." Instead, this idea assumes that the individual can grow up to be a happier, more productive, more efficient, more fulfilled person if he lives in a society that promotes such ends. Thus the individual's problems are seen to stem from society's defects, an idea held by most people involved in the encounter movement. However, instead of focusing on the individual to change him directly, alternative life-styles attempt to change the social institutions within which he must function.

The prospect of being able to start fresh with a group of people dedicated to creating a new form of social organization which will maximize their satisfaction of important needs and minimize the problems that society ordinarily creates for the individual is extraordinarily attractive. Unfortunately the experience of literally hundreds of such attempts both in the nineteenth and twentieth centuries in this country indicates that this approach is not an easy one to carry off. Utopian communities have proved difficult to create and even more difficult to sustain. Simply to have them endure requires enormous dedication, involvement and subordination of personal needs that many find unappealing. Furthermore, even the longest lived and most successful communes in the nineteenth century seemed to satisfy most of their members for only limited periods of time.

Despite the discouraging history of efforts to establish alternative life-styles in the past, some observers of the current scene are optimistic. Fairfield (1971), for example, sees considerable value in twentieth-century communes. He does not feel that the criterion of the success of such ventures ought to be their longevity or capacity to survive. Instead, he looks to the feelings they produce in their individual members—the sense of aliveness that is provided, the greater self-awareness—as the proper test of the commune's worth. From this point of view, Fairfield regards the present-day American commune as being a very successful one. It has been a leader in a revolution aimed at taking people out of "a private, intolerable, grasping, solitary self toward the cooperative, sharing, loving, universal self."

Fairfield also feels that many of the basic ideals that guide the commune movement are extraordinarily valuable for the society at large. These include encouragement to return to what is basic and essential in life. This may involve removing man from a polluted, crowded, unhappy city and taking him back to a more natural habitat where he can breathe fresh air and till the soil. Also held out is the ideal of shared human relationships which promise escape from the alienation felt by many in modern society (Figure 14–3). In encouraging self-actualization and self-exploration the commune movement also provides an example for the rest of society of how to live a better life. Nonetheless Fairfield recognizes that the commune movement in recent years has encountered many problems in establishing stable communities. He attributes this to the fact that utopians who are inevitably products of a competitive, overly intellectualized society are themselves too "cerebral." He points out that having ideas or ideals may be meaningless and often personally harmful. As an illustration, Fairfield describes a party he attended where he noticed a friend sitting dejectedly in a corner despite the fact that around him a variety of activities were taking place: demonstrations in hatha yoga, animated conversations, wild dancing, and a great variety of delicious food being served, good drinks being consumed, and even fireworks. When the friend was asked why he was blue, he replied, "Sure, it's a good party, I guess. But we're not getting any closer to the community we want this way!" Fairfield's concern is that this person was convinced that the community had to be in a particular place engaging in a particular kind of behavior and that he was simply unable to enjoy the pleasures of the moment because he was permitting his ideals to stand in the way of his appreciation of the unplanned, unexpected pleasure.

Fairfield's example is intended to illustrate that one can feel a sense of community even in the middle of a "really great party." On the other

Figure 14–3 The Constraints of Straight Society.

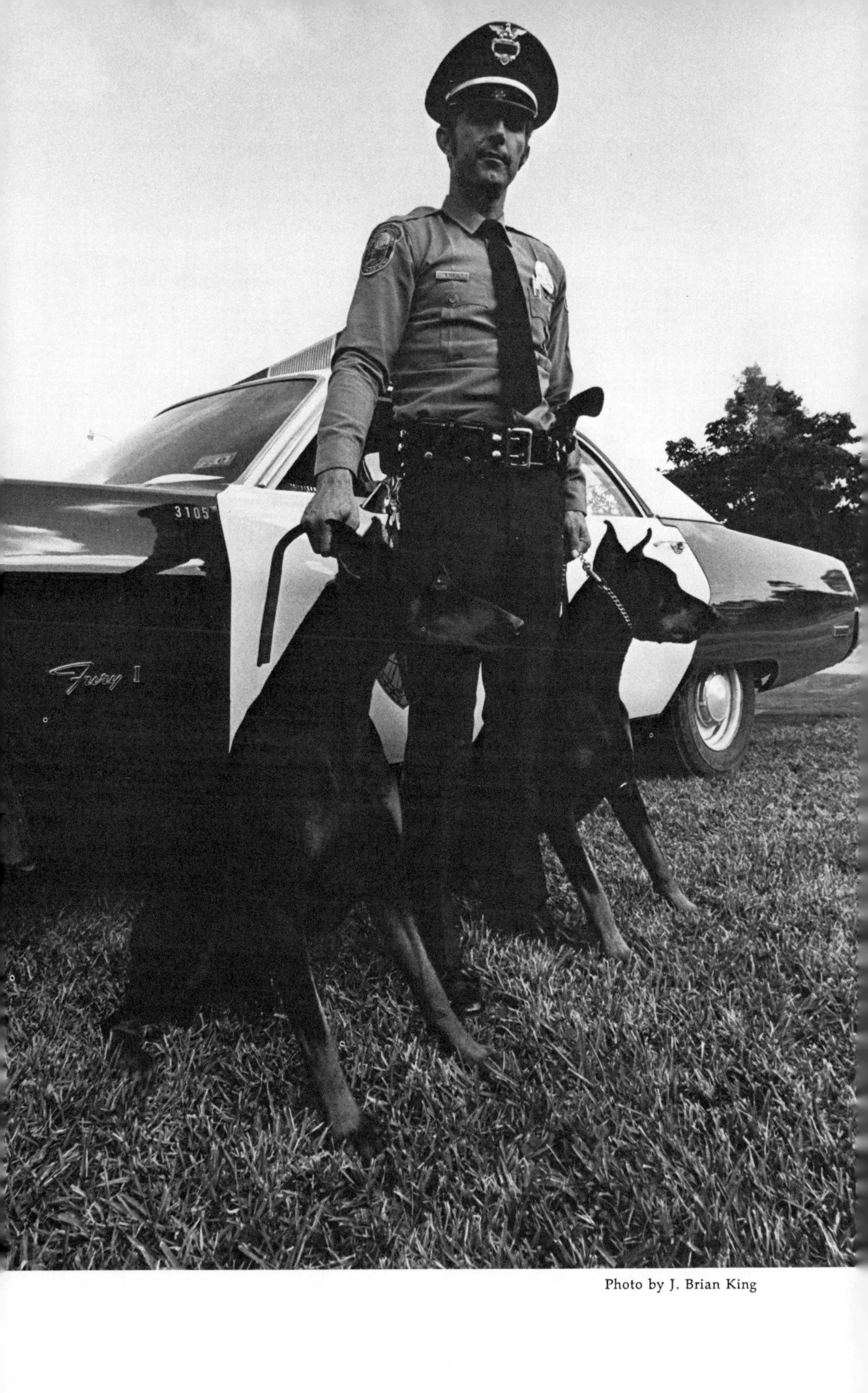

Photo by J. Brian King

hand, one can hardly help sympathizing with the sad friend who may have needed someone to talk to seriously and meaningfully more than the kicks that he could experience at the party. The admittedly transitory nature of many modern communes suggests that like Fairfield's party they are quite limited in what they can provide. They may supply a temporary lift that serves certain people at certain times in their lives. It is difficult to see, however, how they can provide a sense of intimacy, a feeling that one is understood at a very basic level, and serve as an arena in which self-actualization can occur.

Given the obvious problems that have been observed in establishing enduring utopian social organizations in the past and the limited needs that modern communes seem to satisfy, particularly those that are inevitably transitory in nature, it is easy to become pessimistic about our capacity for creating alternative life-styles capable of fulfilling the high ideals sought by many of their originators. Sarason (1973) expresses such pessimism and feels that we simply don't know enough about how to create a social organization that will be more satisfying than those that have evolved in the larger society and that will endure over long periods. This is because social relationships are extraordinarily complex, and a great deal more must be learned about them before man will be in a position to design an optimal living situation. Sarason's own strategy is to attempt to understand first the problems involved in creating the mini-social organizations that make up an entire society.

Meditation

Relaxation is known to reduce anxiety. Various methods of producing relaxation are gaining increased regular usage in intellectual circles. The Eastern world has for centuries practiced various methods of altering states of consciousness. These are now being recognized not only by avant garde groups but also by scientists. Transcendental meditation is one of these methods designed to produce relaxation and tranquility of thought and body and it has been the target of research. Benson and Wallace (1972) have found that meditating subjects have lower metabolic rates, are more relaxed and less anxious. There are numerous recorded cases of drug users who turned to meditation for experiences they previously obtained through the use of drugs.

Transcendental meditation consists of saying a mantra (a sound such as OM) subvocally over and over while sitting in a relaxed position for about 20 minutes twice a day. Numerous thoughts arise in the consciousness of the subject while he continually favors the mantra. This kind of relaxed concentration can lead to states described by subjects as emptiness, clearness, voidness, or pure awareness. This is a pleasant and very relaxed state of being with aftereffects of freshness and enhanced perception of oneself and the world. Ornstein and Naranjo (1971) discuss in detail the nature and effect of this and other kinds of meditation.

Summary

1. In the past 20 or 30 years a number of movements devoted to enhancing the adjustment of the normal personality have arisen. These include various types of group experiences as well as alternative life-styles.
2. Modern encounter or human potential groups have sprung from experience with analysis of the here and now interactions taking place in T-groups. They stress release of deep wellsprings of feeling as a means of providing self awareness.
3. The techniques used in encounter groups to promote affective expression are many and varied, ranging from entirely verbal approaches to the use of physical exercises.
4. Manipulation of the time spent in the group is another technique for promoting affective expression. This gave rise to *marathon groups,* some of which are conducted with nude members, a tactic also thought to promote psychological openness.
5. Some criticisms of the human potential movement are based on the concern that its fundamental philosophy in essence robs man of his privacy and his dignity. Others focus on the group leader's failure to accept responsibility for the fate of participants who suffer adverse reactions as the result of the group experience. Still others are concerned that serious negative consequences result from group participation in a high percentage of cases.
6. Relatively little adequate research has been done to assess carefully the outcome of encounter group experience. What has been done suggests that participants often report feeling greater self-esteem but that little behavior change occurs. A recent study reports that 7.5 percent of participants suffer moderate to serious psychological damage.
7. The modern-day commune movement represents an attempt to create living situations that are more conducive to self-actualization than is ordinary society. Modern communes may be classified with respect to their emphasis on "retreat" or service. The "retreat" commune is characterized by the rejection of certain aspects of society, while the service commune is characterized by a mission to serve society in some positive way.
8. Virtually all alternative life-styles or utopian societies have failed to endure or to make possible the personal satisfactions they set out to provide. Modern communes, particularly of the "retreat" variety, are

especially fragile and seem at most to serve the need of some individuals for a temporary way station in life.

9. Transcendental meditation is one of the methods of relaxation and enhancing perception of oneself and the world.

Words to Remember

Affection	Inclusion
Commune	Marathon Group
Control	T-Group
Encounter Group	Transcendental Meditation

15. Adjustment in Perspective

Objectives

After studying this chapter the reader should be able to:

1. Define *adjustment.*
2. List three basic concepts that govern soundness of growth.
3. Discuss the interactions between society and the individual with regard to personal soundness.
4. List general guidelines for improving your own mental hygiene.

Several years ago, one of the authors talked with a young man who was holding a promising position in one of the television networks in New York City. He was from a relatively affluent Manhattan family—his father was a medical specialist practicing in the city. The young man had earned a degree from a reputable eastern state university. His part of the conversation ran something like this:

"You're a psychologist? I met a member of your profession when I was in college. He was in the Dean's office. He called me into his office when I was a freshman, picked up a card from his desk and said, 'I see you're not doing well.' That was news to me! I was under the impression I was doing very well—better than at any time I could remember. My tennis game was better than ever; I had just been pledged to one of the best fraternities on campus; I had just made some very good friends, and most of the fellows I was meeting were among the most impressive I'd ever known; I was dating some really lovely girls! Furthermore, I had discovered what I needed to do to get grades, was passing all my courses, and doing quite well in some. What was he talking about? He went on talking as I sat there. He mentioned two courses in which I had done poorly on the first exam—but these shocks had taught me to study more effectively and I had pulled up my grades in those courses to a passing mark.

"I surely was not impressed with your colleague! I let him talk. He at no time encouraged me to talk, nor did he try to find out what I was really like. I got out of that office as soon as I could!"

Let us take this statement at its face value and assume (with good reason to believe it) that the young man's report of his interview was fairly accurate. He had since graduated and, moving along well in the television industry, seemed to be mature in attitude, to be getting along well with others, and happy. The anecdote of the dean's nonstop and one-sided evaluation of this student introduces us to the *complexity* of the concept of adjustment and to the pitfalls that one risks in judging others unless one is in command of broad and deep sources of information. It also suggests the difficulty of appraising an individual without knowing his view of life and without sufficient indirect and direct objective observation.

Without dwelling further on the behavior of the interviewer, the anecdote may be used as a starting point for a discussion of the various aspects of adjustment. This young man made clear in our casual encounter how he evaluated his adjustment at the time of his appointment with the dean. He had first examined the aspects of his life in which he was striving, using a *social conformity* view of adjustment and possibly also a *statistical* view. Thus he compared himself to members of a group he admired and found himself to be at least on a par with them. The fact his early low grades quickly motivated him to improve them implies the operation of the *tension-reduction* aspect of adjustment. His satisfaction with his behavior at this time suggests also the *self-satisfaction* concept of adjustment. In evaluating his status he concentrated on the social, play, and academic aspects of his life, while the dean focused on the narrow, grade-measured academic aspect. Whether either was considering still other aspects of adjustment is not clear in the anecdote.

These other aspects of adjustment, using the Sechrest and Wallace (1967) analysis, are the *medical,* which emphasizes emotional health; the *legal and ethical,* which relates to moral and legal behavior; the *positive striving,* which involves self-esteem, and one's unique potential and mastery of the environment, or the *engineering* concept of optimal functioning in terms of structure.

We need to know much more about this young man to understand him. We don't know enough about his self-concept, his frustrations and conflicts, his values, his long-term goals, and his personal needs, all of which we have discussed generally and impersonally in the previous chapters.

Our Approach to Adjustment

Our approach to adjustment has been broad. It has implicitly taken into consideration the *complex and individual nature* of adjustment. We have recognized that the various views of adjustment overlap, and that the concept is fraught with individually perceived *values.* Moreover, we recognize that problems of individual adjustment may peak in a specific area of endeavor and at specific times in life. We have, in this book, pivoted on the uniqueness of each individual and have included a number of cases to illustrate this uniqueness, not only of individuals, but of the problems they encounter and their ways of facing them. Underlying the specific and individual adjustments, however, we saw *positive striving* toward individual goals. Some of the cases previously presented may be reread now to give more meaning to the general overview that is to follow.

In order to examine the various areas of individual adjustment we have reviewed the concepts and facts in some important general areas of psychology, such as learning, frustration, conflict, and self-concept. Facts and generalizations on some important content aspects of adjustment, such as vocational, marital, sexual, social, and personal have also been included. We now look in perspective at the person and the interaction of his personality-structured dynamics with his environment.

Emphasis on Growth Toward Positive Striving

JAHODA'S VIEWS ON PSYCHOLOGICAL SOUNDNESS

Some writers are concerned that the term *adjustment* implies *conformity* to restricted social norms and values and favors stability in contrast to movement toward new goals. The term *adjustment* applies more aptly to specific events that produce tension that can be reduced by certain responses and, as suggested above, presents problems, whereas it used to refer to the "whole" person. Jahoda (1958) surveyed most of the writing in this area and rejected the ideal of man as one who is adjusting *passively* to stresses in order to be comfortable and free of symptoms and of socially disapproved habits. "Positively striving" seemed to her a better description of the psychologically healthy and sound individual. She suggests three interacting basic features of positive mental health:

1. active *mastery* of one's environment;
2. a unified and *integrated personality*—no one aspect functioning at the expense of another;
3. accurate *perception* of one's self and the world.

The concept of *striving* or growth toward personal goals is important. Jahoda widens the perspective of striving toward growth goals. She shows the equal importance of unity and *integration* of the many aspects of life's interactions. Also, she points to the importance of accuracy and realism of *perception* of one's self and the world while one is striving.

ERIKSON'S GROWTH CRISES AND DEVELOPED TRAITS

Erikson (1959), for one, accepts these features of positive striving and relates them to his emphasis on growth through successive developmental crises toward a psychologically healthy adult personality. We have referred to Erikson's crises at the various stages of development and to the positive traits that are developed at each crisis stage. The positive traits result in increased capacity to master life's difficulties. The crises at successive stages each present a polarity between pathology at one extreme and health at the other. At the early oral stage, for example, *trust* in the adult to feed him and trust in himself and in the responses of his body to life's urges can develop in the child. These simple trusts are in contrast to overoptimism or overpessimism in respect to feeding by adults, which leads to distrust. At the anal (in psychoanalytic parlance) stage, when toilet training becomes important, the child struggles with shame, and either self-doubt or a sense of autonomy can result. At a later stage he can develop management skills through rules and effective behavior or guilt, which hampers freedom and initiative. In a healthy development he is controlled by conscience, but he is not guilt-ridden because of the pressures of that conscience. The other traits that may be developed at successive stages are industry versus inferiority, identity versus role confusion (at adolescence), generativity versus self-absorption (middle age), and finally, integrity versus despair (old age).

The identity versus role confusion stage has interested psychological writers more actively than the others. The youth's world is broader than the child's, with many ways of perceiving and behaving. He may be confused about who he is and what he can become, or, conversely, he may have achieved an integrated view of who he is and what he can become.

WHITE'S MULTIPLE PATHS

White (1966), in his *Lives in Progress,* pointed to the obvious fact that there are multiple ways of living. He does not believe that one can list traits that inevitably produce mental health regardless of the temperament, aptitudes, or circumstances of the individual; no one trait pattern is seen to be equally productive of mental health in a surgeon, a composer of music, a personnel manager, a bookkeeper, and a scenery-shifter on a motion-picture lot. Individuals lead happy and useful lives in many diverse ways. White's book stresses individuality and all the ways in which an individual can differ from another individual and thereby develop differently. No one is free to develop in every direction that a single list of hypothetical "healthy" traits might suggest. White's emphasis is on individuals developing in their own special ways toward becoming effective persons. Studies on psychologically sound individuals support his general position.

We have chosen the position that positive striving is a factor of personal adjustment, with an emphasis on soundness or relative stability, knowing that we are dealing with a complex variable that is difficult but not impossible to assess. By *soundness* we mean a pattern of traits—relative stability instead of unresolved conflict and autonomy of dependency, for example. It is broader than the view that sees reduction of tensions as a characteristic of adjustment, and it can better encompass the observation of the total person.

Studies of Soundness and Positive Striving

More is usually found in psychological textbooks on maladjustment than on adjustment, but some researchers have sought to describe persons of unusual soundness, positive striving, or mental health; others have focused on creativity. Striving toward life goals can be shaped in a manner to produce soundness or pathology. To these sound or "healthy" patterns we now turn.

CHARACTERISTICS OF ASTRONAUTS

Lazarus (1969) has reviewed and commented on several kinds of studies of individuals who give evidence of soundness. Seven astronauts were described in detail by Korchin and Ruff (1964). They are seen as rigidly selected individuals who have the ability to function effectively under conditions of stress. Perceptual and motor efficiency and mood were studied under normal nonstressful conditions and under the stress of simulated flight. No differences in efficiency were evident under the two conditions. In mood, the astronauts generally described themselves as friendly, energetic, and clear-thinking, rather than as aggressive, jittery, and depressed. After simulated flight there was a slight tendency to describe themselves as less energetic and clear-thinking than usual, but as more anxious and more friendly. Their anxiety was directed toward the success of the flight rather than toward fear of injury or death. They seemed to have gained through training mastery of the necessary skills and ability to handle critical situations in a problem-solving manner. They expressed the judgment that it is better to keep busy than to worry.

The seven men were selected from 69 military jet test pilots. They were between 32 and 37 years of age, married, and with children; came from middle- or upper-class families, from farms or small towns; enjoyed sports and outdoor living; had graduated from college in engineering; were ambitious, intelligent, confident, persevering, and realistic, with a high degree of control over their feelings and emotions; had firm identities—knew who they were and where they were going; had grown up in stable communities and had identified with a competent father or father surrogate. Their development had progressed smoothly, with few crises. Their exceptional ability was bolstered by success in mastering situations with their skills, and these successes had produced high self-esteem. These men, much in the public eye, represent one kind of sound, striving personality.

Lazarus (1969), in reporting the study, pointed out that the astronauts apparently were not observed for such traits as altruism and love, spontaneity, spiritual experience, intimacy, or creativity versus conformity—some of the characteristics mentioned by Maslow (1954) in describing his self-actualizing personalities. Whether or not the astronauts have these characteristics is not known, nor does the study compare them empirically with a group of other men. Lazarus rightly raises the question of whether the astronauts were actually exposed to subjective threat. No evidence is offered to reveal how these men would have handled threats to their self-esteem, bereavement, or the degrading experiences suffered in an enemy prison camp. We see here men of unusual aptitudes and stable upbringing who experienced relatively few serious crises in their lives and were able to function exceptionally well in their fields as young adults.

STUDENTS OF OUTSTANDING COMPETENCE

Silber, Hamburg, Coelho, Murphy, and Rosenberg (1961) studied high school students who were planning to go on to college. The researchers began with volunteers who were in the upper half of their class academically. From these, they selected students who received the most favorable teacher ratings for motivation, industry, initiative, influence and leadership, concern for others, responsibility, and emotional stability. These selected students were interviewed, and students who seemed overly troubled, who admitted neurotic symptoms, or with whom the interviewer had difficulty establishing rapport were dropped. The remaining six boys and nine girls were interviewed weekly in the last part of their senior year.

These highly selected students were satisfied with their scholastic achievement and were not at all anxious about their intellectual ability. Each had a strong wish to be what they called "well rounded"—that is, they had developed a variety of interests. They enjoyed close, warm friendships, in which they experienced mutual satisfaction. These students belonged to groups that were social or religious, although they were not among the most popular people in the school. They were oriented toward problem solving and welcomed new experiences rather than fearing them as threats. The typical self-image they projected seemed to be of a capable person who *coped with his environment realistically*. They had worries, but they used them to lead to ways of dealing with critical situations; and they shared their problems with others who were coping with similar ones.

A similar study was conducted by Coelho, Hamburg, and Murphy (1963). Nine girls and five boys were chosen in a manner similar to that in the Silber et al. study (1961). These subjects were studied in college to observe their reactions to the actual situation rather than their anticipation of these experiences. The experimenters selected students who were realistic in their problem solving, who organized their time well, and who did not dislike study. The students elected a wide range of courses without expecting to excel in all of them. On campus, they related well to upperclassmen and faculty. They too had good self-esteem and dealt with their problems in a way that allowed them to maintain this positive view of themselves. They seemed to be adaptive rather than rigid, and blunted their disappointments by balancing them with successes in friendships and college activities. They actively sought situations that promised success.

GRINKER'S HOMOCLITES

A psychiatrist (Grinker, 1962) who spent most of his time with emotionally maladjusted people was impressed with the soundness of a group of students who showed no previous evidence of maladjustment, whom he observed during the college training of YMCA workers. He called these "normal," "just plain guys," who seemed emotionally sound, *homoclites.* This is a neutral word, the opposite of the Greek word *heteroclite,* which means "deviating from the common rule." The fathers of these homoclites were in the laborer, semiskilled, and white-collar classes, earning a satisfactory living. The homoclites had IQ's ranging from 88 to 113—average, 110. Their grades in the first year of college were slightly better than C (the school average was C+). As students they had a clear idea of what they were training for—a secure, respectable job that they liked. While none had a history of disabling or handicapping illness, some exhibited a few symptoms of emotional disturbance, such as suspicion, unhappiness, and fear. In general these individuals were able to control their symptoms, so they did not interfere with their work. The homoclites' attitudes toward themselves were good and their attitudes toward the future were positive. Their relationships with parents, friends, and teachers were warm, and their hopes were to do well and to be liked. None of them showed strong desires to raise their standard of living above that of their parents. They were not outstandingly competent or creative, but they were realistic in their striving toward satisfaction of their goals.

The homoclites were not noticeably visible in their communities. They lived simply but comfortably, enjoyed their children, and retired eventually on modest pensions. This is one version of the healthy and satisfied individual who has modest needs and plans and accomplishes them.

THE CREATIVE PERSON WITH SOUNDNESS

A different approach to personal soundness was that of Barron (1963). Barron was alert to characteristics such as creativity, originality, independence of judgment, and the ability to enjoy life's complexities and ambiguities. His emphasis was *not* primarily on conformity to cultural norms.

In Barron's study 80 graduate students in various fields from an outstanding university were selected randomly from a larger sample. All were rated for soundness on a 9-point scale by members of their departments and were then divided into groups of 10 who lived together for two 24-hour days. Among the living groups were several staff psychologists who also rated them. In addition to the Department Ratings and Staff Ratings, items from their personal histories and test scores were also obtained.

Personal soundness was defined as soundness, balance, and degree of maturity the individual shows in relation to other people. The 80 students were divided into two groups on the basis of high and low soundness. The subjects with higher soundness ratings had developmental histories indicating a low incidence of serious illness or training problems in childhood. Their home environment was stable, and their parents were successful, were respected by the subjects, and served as good models. In these respects these subjects resembled the astronauts.

There were, however, some marked individual exceptions to this general stable trend in background. Those subjects who rated low in soundness came from homes in which more overt parental conflict was found than in the homes of high-rated subjects; more of the mothers were the dominant figure in the family, and there was evidence that more of them were considered seductive. Also it seemed that the conditions in childhood were not as important as the *way of responding to these conditions.*

The ratings from the professors in the students' departments correlated significantly with those from the psychological assessment staff. Still considerable disagreement was found between the two sets of ratings on certain individuals. Both rating groups found the more sound students efficient and well integrated in pursuit of their goals—*adaptable.* The highly rated students were judged, on the bases of performance in class and grades to be better organized, persistent, and resourceful—integrated in contrast to low-rated students, who were more often seen to be unstable, confused, undependable, dissatisfied, and defensive. The psychological assessors also observed some attractive but less goal-oriented characteristics in the high-rated student: friendliness, lack of affectation, naturalness, fairmindedness, tolerance, and goodnaturedness. Test scores indicated greater equanimity, self-confidence, objectivity, and virility among the students with high soundness ratings. In perceptual tests the high-rated students were more realistic and less easily confused by surrounding context than the low-rated students; they also showed more self-insight. The data rather well support the characteristics of soundness and mental health attributed earlier to Jahoda.

Barron (1963) points out that the high-soundness subjects were not without irregularities and complexities that were obscured in the group data. This finding led him to state that soundness is a *way of reacting to problems,* not an absence of them. Like other people, the high-soundness subjects suffered fears, unrealizable desires, self-condemnations, and tensions. There were some cases of pseudosoundness in the high-soundness group whose balance was precarious. Sound subjects with problems were people who "bear with their anxieties, hew to a stable course, and maintain some sense of the ultimate worthwhileness of their lives" (p. 65).

Barron (1968), in commenting later on this study, stated that it is healthy to be well behaved and cool and collected, "but there are times when it is a mark of greater health to be able to upset one's own balance and to seek a new order of selfhood" (p. 19). In the Barron study we see a kind of soundness and mental health that may be found in the bright, achieving, creative, and atypical person at the highest level of education.

Psychological Processes and Personal Soundness

FRUSTRATION, CONFLICT, ANXIETY, DEFENSE MECHANISMS, AND RATIONAL COPING

Turning from the characteristics of the individual to the psychological processes underlying them, we now examine those which may influence his maladjustment or his growth toward personal soundness. This approach enables us to look at specific daily experiences and behavior that induce temporary or permanent maladjustment or disequilibrium.

We have seen in earlier chapters that the *frustration* of ongoing motivated behavior, particularly that which is high in intensity or has high priority for the individual, is deeply disturbing. The ways in which he copes with this frustration are important for him. If his approach encourages exploration of various methods to remove or surmount the block to his needs and he finally discovers a satisfactory compromise, he has engaged in adaptive activity or problem-solving behavior. Through such efforts he may have learned a method of attack he can use in the future and thus have increased his self-confidence. For example, a freshman who wants to stay in school and make satisfactory grades fails his first exams in several courses. The experience of failing several courses is deeply disturbing to him, since it threatens to force him to leave college. His failure may be so traumatic that he represses it and turns to diversions (staring at TV, drinking, play, sex), which may create new problems; that is, the loss of study time will further damage his grades. On the other hand, he may talk over his situation with an older student or an adviser, at the same time reviewing his exam papers to understand why he failed, and come to some realizations, such as that he hadn't learned the most important concepts well enough. He may even get information at a counseling center about his aptitudes and interests and how to use them best. The latter methods obviously will either help him to meet his needs or lead to knowledge about how well he can meet them. Any permanent digressions from a problem-solving, coping attitude are less likely to lead to an adjustment or to the development of traits that generate effective striving or soundness.

From one standpoint the freshman's experience may also be an example of *conflict*—possibly between his needs and failures or between his self-concept and ideal self. When deep-seated conflicts occur, *anxiety* usually results, a very disturbing consequence often leading abruptly to a *defense mechanism.* This is an unconscious means of temporarily reducing the anxiety but is not necessarily a true solution to the problems.

Frustrations that recur in a person who lacks adequate satisfaction of important needs detract from soundness and stability. Deep-seated, unresolved conflicts disturb self-esteem and make him especially vulnerable to anxiety, and defense mechanisms which are usually incompatible with realistic compromise solutions. One of the more usual defense mechanisms is repression—the unconscious obliteration or denial of the experience that led to the anxiety. Obliteration may keep the individual from becoming overwhelmed by negative feelings and self-rejection, but it does little to help him solve his problems. Indeed it increases his helplessness, ignorance, and lack of control.

In almost all the cases examined, the individuals had learned to cope—to turn to other resources. Essentially they were striving positively. People differ in the capacity to move toward problem solving, rational coping, or facing issues. They differ in the extent to which they have in the past built habits of confrontation and also in the extent to which they have been confronted by difficult problems before they had learned ways to deal with them. People's circumstances and personalities, for example, may or may not encourage them to move toward those in the helping professions, such as counselors, who can aid in reducing their anxiety and guide them in rational coping or in problem solving. Some processes can help us deal with conflicts and anxiety while others lead to further disintegration.

PROCESSES THAT LEAD TO "NORMALITY" OR ABNORMALITY

Previously we have stated that the problems an individual faces do not seem to be as important as his method of handling them. Allport (1961) identified sound and emotionally healthy individuals on the basis of the predominant methods they use in meeting the frustrations, conflicts, and anxieties that are inevitable in every life. He calls those methods that lead to growth *anabolic,* which means "building up," and those which lead to "tearing down" and distintegration, *catabolic* (Figure 15–1). Allport points out that although a given individual may use both kinds of mechanisms, the important factor is which processes predominate—anabolic or catabolic. For example, a person who constantly confronts reality may also indulge in some fantasy and still show growth. Below are lists of the two kinds of mechanisms, those that promote abnormality and those that encourage positive growth:

Catabolic Processes	**Anabolic Processes**
Escape or withdrawal (including fantasy)	Confrontation (or, if you prefer, "reality testing")
Regression or dissociation	Availability of knowledge to consciousness
Other ego defenses, including rationalization, reaction formation, projection, displacement	Self-insight, with its attendant humor
Impulsiveness (uncontrolled)	Integrative action of nervous system
Restriction of thinking to concrete level	Ability to think abstractly
Fixation of personality at a juvenile level	Continuous individuation (without arrested or fixated development)
All forms of rigidification	Functional autonomy of motives
	Frustration tolerance

Development of Traits That Facilitate Positive Striving

Erikson (1963) has pointed to the need to build, during life's development, certain traits that will help one to weather crises and teach him the techniques to deal with them. At various critical stages the individual will develop traits favorable or unfavorable to effective growth to normality. They are, in order of acquisition during childhood: trust, autonomy, initiative, industry, identity, intimacy (generativity and integrity at adulthood). These traits represent the development of anabolic processes and make it possible, under the right conditions, for other anabolic processes

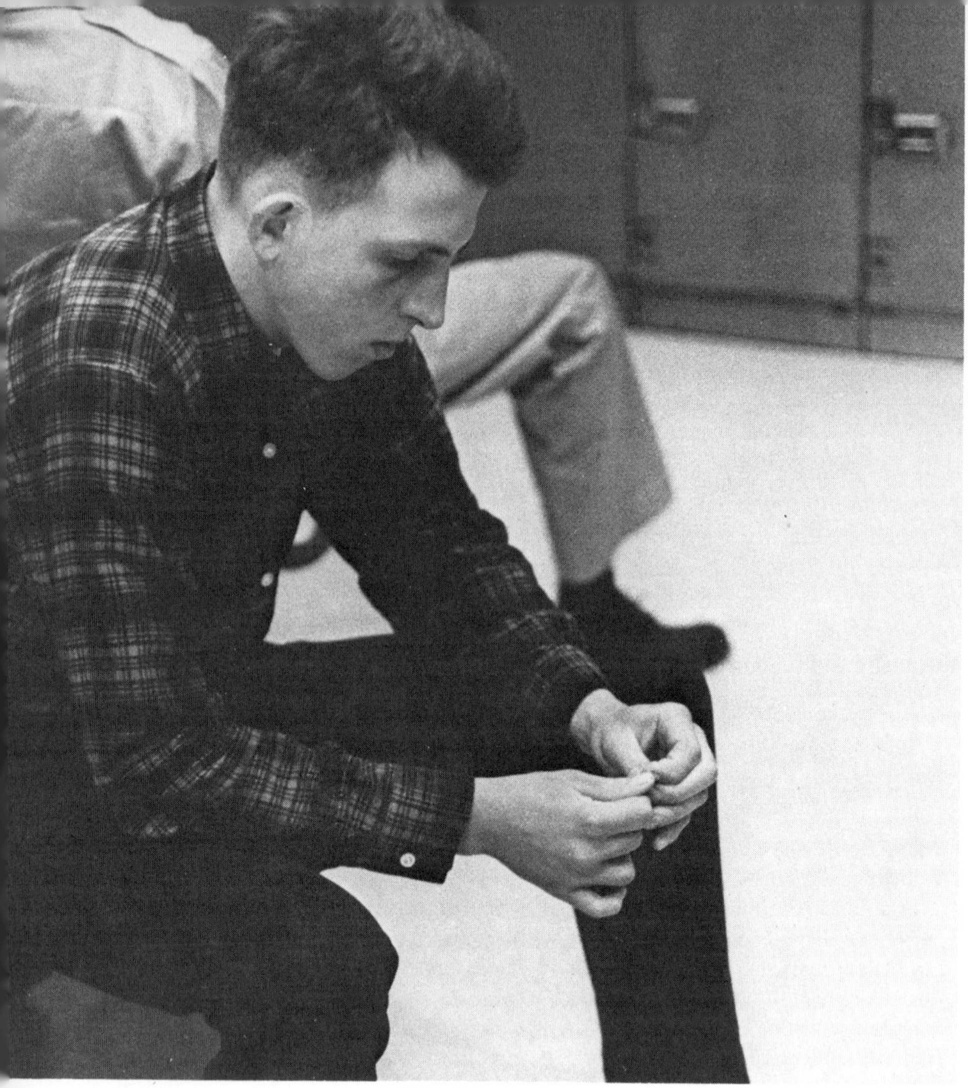

Photo by J. Brian King

Figure 15–1 Withdrawal—A Catabolic Mechanism.

to operate. They represent the accumulation of skills and attitudes that produce tolerance of frustration and anxiety.

One of Erikson's concepts that has impressed counselors as being important is *identity*. The youth who, through factors in his development, has come to see himself realistically, who knows what he is and represents and what he is not, what he can do well and what he cannot do well, and who has some clear and feasible plans for the future, has identity. One who is confused and in conflict about himself, others, and his future, is experiencing an identity crisis. Again, we see the process of positive striving toward personal development of effectiveness, despite difficulties and deviations.

EGO STRENGTH

A concept that is frequently used to indicate a high degree of frustration and anxiety tolerance, personal control of behavior, and the capacity to endure and rally from setbacks is *ego strength.* Barron (1968) devised an ego strength scale empirically by comparing patients who profited most by psychotherapy and those who profited least. The results of the study give us a more specific meaning of the concept. Those receiving higher scores in ego strength showed better physical functioning, more spontaneity and capacity to share emotional experiences, were non-fundamentalistic in religion, more realistic, exhibited a greater feeling of personal adequacy and greater physical courage.

In discussing the processes of inner strength, values must be added as a possible source of inner reference, as a stabilizing force for the individual. The strong individual knows what he believes, how he views events in the world, and what he can accept and reject. If his values are, in the main, open to change and are ego-autonomous rather than rigid, he will be more adaptable. The empirical factors in ego strength found in Barron's studies indicate the importance of realistic, functional, and modifiable values.

Society and Personal Soundness

THE SANE SOCIETY

We have looked at personal soundness in terms of psychological processes within the individual. We have considered *catabolic* processes, such as withdrawal and escape, depression, fixations at juvenile levels, and rigid responses, as well as *anabolic* processes, such as confrontation, availability of knowledge, self-insight, and processes that are associated with ego strength (Figure 15–2). How much are these individual processes related to the social forces in the society in which the individual develops? We have evidence that certain kinds of criminal and mental disorders, suicide, and alienation are found more frequently in low social-economic neighborhoods than in middle- and upper-class areas. The lower-class neighborhoods do not provide a predominance of acceptable social models or other anabolic influences, such as conditions favorable to enhancing personal identity or ego strength.

There is a convincingly large literature that shows a disproportionately high rate of schizophrenia among the lowest social class in cities throughout much of the Western world. It is not at present clear to what extent the conditions of life on the lowest social level are conducive to the development of schizophrenia or to what extent schizophrenia leads to a decline in social position (Kohn, 1970). Many problems of experimental

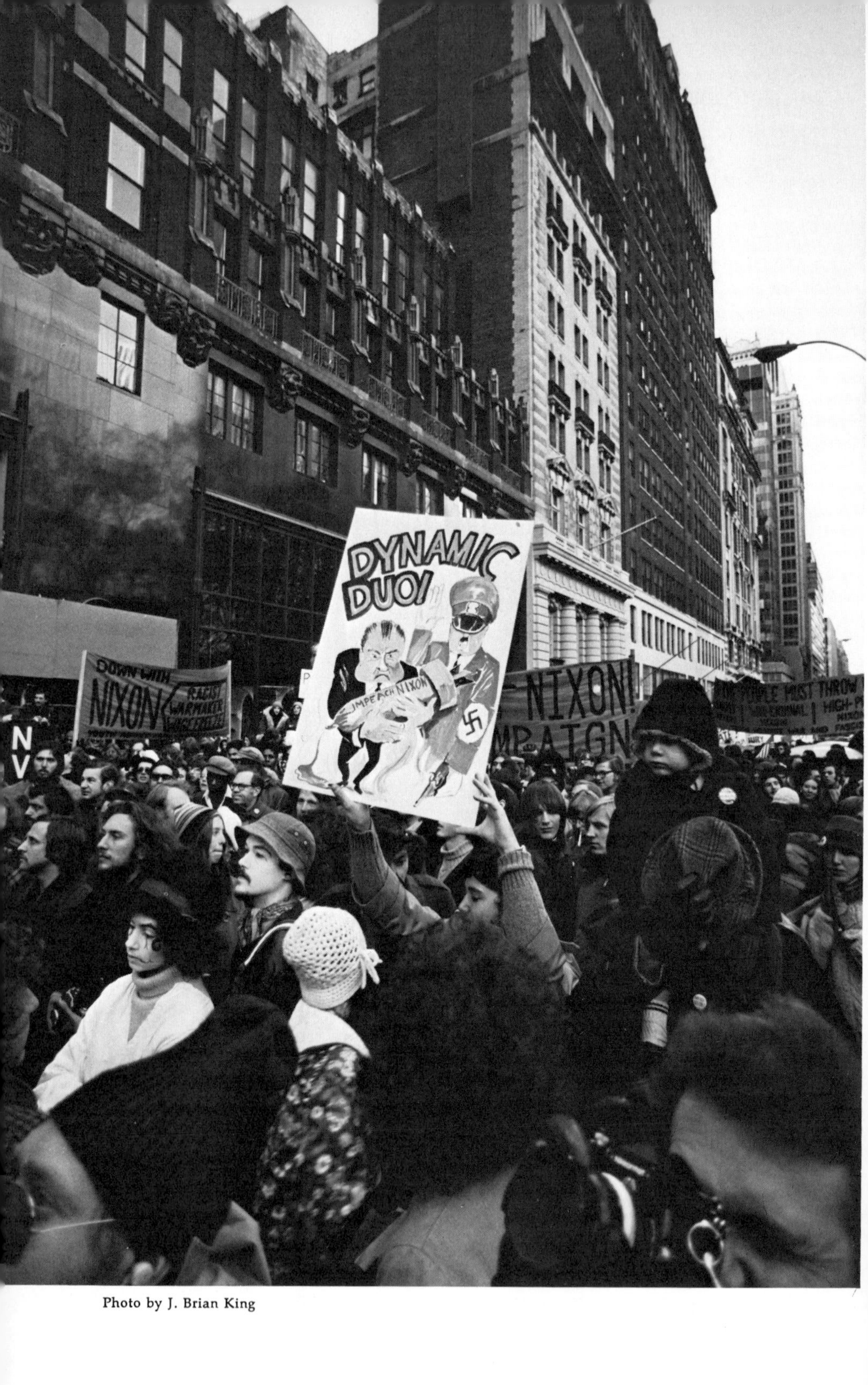

Photo by J. Brian King

design and sampling need to be solved to reach precise conclusions on this matter (Mishler & Scotch, 1970).

We accept in general the idea that some of our subcultures do not promote soundness; in fact, many of the adults in these subcultures are models for psychopathology. Some of the frustrating and conflicting conditions in these subcultures foster aggression and defense mechanisms. All subcultures, however, are related to the nature of the larger society which produces them and allows the unsound conditions to exist.

This discussion raises the question of the roots of stable and unstable, sound or unsound subcultures and societies. The question is clearly faced by Fromm (1955), who sees in Western society some questionable signs, that is, national delusions of grandeur or divine mission (save the world from communism), delusions of persecution, arrogant destructiveness in war, sadistic fantasies and violence on television screens, distorted perceptions in which, for example, great surpluses of food mean economic disaster. He might have added corporate "successes" that create environmental pollution, ecological destruction, and health hazards for citizens. To Fromm, a sane society is one that satisfies the needs of man, as seen objectively. It is one that prevents the deprivations and frustrations that produce breakdowns, delinquency, and war. He rejects the rationalization of those who profit by the status quo that man can adapt to any culture. Rather, he takes the position that certain universal conditions of mental health are valid for the whole human race. He points to the necessity for social change if man is to survive.

Murphy (1939) takes a similar position. He declares that if man is to be molded to society, society must be molded to man. Writing in a similar vein, Frank (1936), in an article on "Society as the Patient," suggests that the idea that our problems of crime, mental disorders, family disorganization, juvenile delinquency, and prostitution are the results of rebels or depraved individuals who threaten society and therefore must be punished gives many people a comfortable feeling. It allows them to retain the belief that we live in an orderly society. A differing viewpoint holds that the ills of a society are related to its cultural traditions, and that these can be reconstructed by man to better serve his present needs. As an alternative to the frequent emphasis on more laws to force the misbehaving person to act in a more orderly way, let us examine the culture that produces this disorderliness.

We know that culture (the solutions to societal problems that are passed on to the new generation) differs in different societies. Customs, traditions, and mores flow from values that are defended strongly by society's members (especially the older, rigid, prestigious, and prosperous

Figure 15–2 A Social Protest—Anabolic or Catabolic?

members). The position of Fromm and Frank implies that, whereas some aspects of our cultural heritage are valuable—valid knowledge of a technical or humanistic kind—some of them are relics from an earlier time. Such superannuated practices or attitudes are not only inappropriate for today's problems but actually harmful. A society based on valid thinking and intelligence needs to modify its behavior in terms of knowledge that is currently valid, particularly when existing conditions produce so much human pathology.

PROBLEMS IN CHANGING SOCIAL CONDITIONS

Some factors hamper social changes and some facilitate changes that help the greater number in society. Rigidity, such as is found in the authoritarian personality, is a potent force in inhibiting change. Stagner (1965) has suggested four psychological mechanisms that prevent attempts to deal with the social changes that are needed in a healthy society: (1) persistence in striving for culturally established goals like family security and business success; (2) need to retain the presently structured framework rather than upsetting established ways of behaving and adapting to new, strange ones (the anxiety that can be aroused by change away from the familiar); (3) the pull of the familiar and its positive attraction; (4) the various unconscious defense mechanisms aroused by anxiety. Denial of danger, rationalization of the situation, fantasy, and temporary isolation are mentioned as forces that prevent realistic action for change. Stagner observes that a society's inability to perceive conditions that lead to social disaster is a tragedy similar to individual psychosis.

These hazards to formation of open problem-solving attitudes toward serious contemporary issues need to be recognized today when we face so many serious global problems. Among them are the availability of the hydrogen bomb to a number of nations, the shrinking supplies of vital energy, human malnutrition in various parts of the world, burgeoning world population, economic problems such as inflation and inadequate distribution of the world's goods, rapid development of technologies, abrupt changes in values and standards, and the resulting conflicts and confusion among different cultures and subcultures concerning these changes. Contemporary man has many problems to face and needs to cooperate and marshal all the rational and humanistict resources he can muster.

SOME BASIC CONFLICTS INTRINSIC TO OUR SOCIETY

What are some of the conflicts into which a child is born in the Western world? To what extent are the mental conflicts we experience

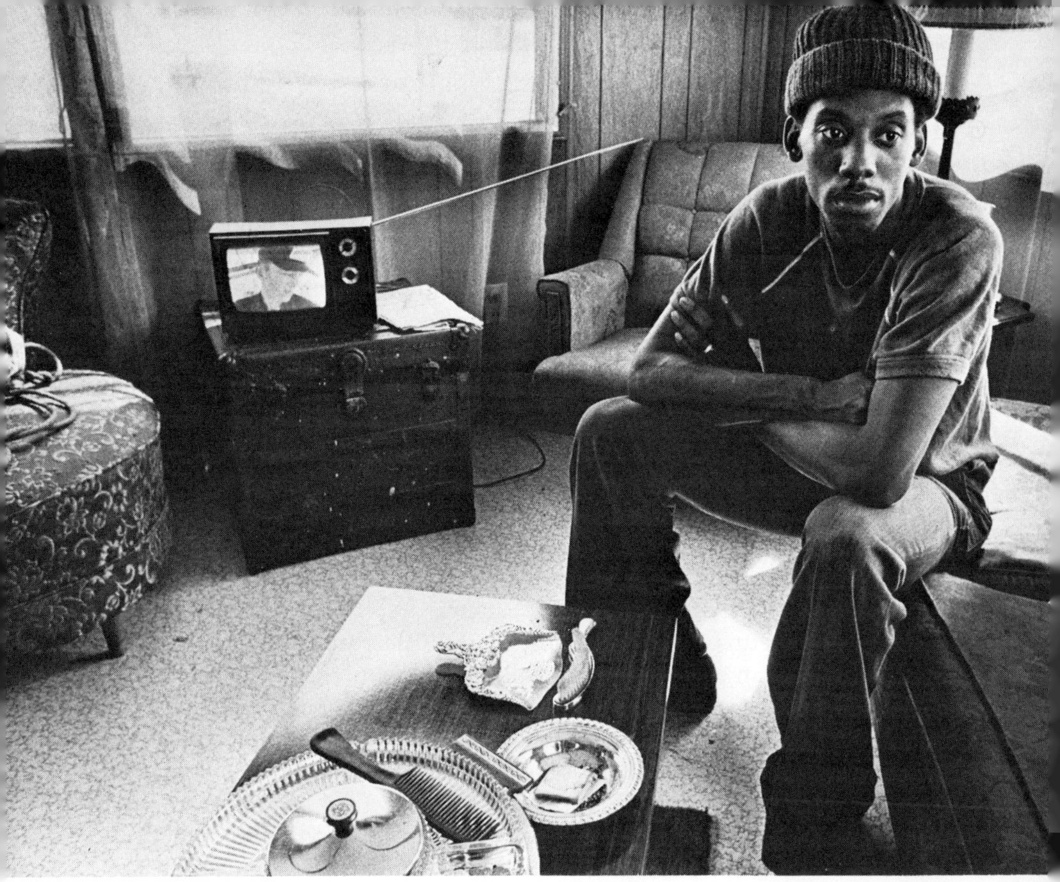

Photo by Kent Mueller

Figure 15–3 How Free Is He?

a result of clashes between incompatible standards in our society? To what extent are they due to circumstances brought about by society that prevent us from reaching our ideals? Some of these conflicts were evident in our earlier discussion of values. One outstanding psychiatric writer has called attention to three conflicts intrinsic to our Western civilized society:

1. It has been suggested that our advertisement-created desires for new commodities—cars, refrigerators, clothes, gadgets—conflict with our present abilities to buy them (Horney, 1937). Advertising and some movies and television programs are to an extent responsible for the dissatisfaction individuals feel with their appearance, since these media, unlike some modern art, tend not to depict people and the world as they really are but rather to select exceptional models who are the extreme of beauty, symmetry, color blending, and so forth. These ideal models are incompatible with the many variations in physique, complexion, facial features, and dress found in realistic living and which are so interesting to the true artist. The kind of homes, cars, and recreational areas that

serve as backgrounds for the advertisements and plays are for the most part unattainable by the majority of Americans.

2. There is the conflict between competitive success and brotherly love. Similarly, individualism frequently conflicts with the welfare of the group as a whole, but we are taught to respect both. Competitiveness is taught to the child even before he enters school. He must stand up for his rights but on the same day is told to share his toys with playmates. In the American social structure, even in the schools, much more emphasis seems to be placed on competition than on cooperation, yet many believe that the survival of human groups strongly depends on cooperation.

3. There is the conflict between continual mouthings about the freedom of the individual and daily experiences of limitations of that freedom. Anyone who has lived in the more backward sections of the American South or in ghettos anywhere knows how little real freedom the dark-skinned American enjoys, be he black, Puerto Rican, Chicano, or Indian (Figure 15–3). He is "kept in his place" by subtle or open threats, including death. The North cannot be pleased about its position. It is a rare suburb in which a black professional is encouraged to buy property. The freedom for all to rise to any heights by sheer hard work and honesty has been questioned by many. The delusion that *any* American can move from rags to riches is still taught by many parents, despite the fact that it is rare for the people of some neighborhoods or communities to attain such success. Registrations in state universities before the passage of the GI Bill showed relatively few individuals from the slums or from lower-middle economic and educational groups. As one author suggests, ambition and hard work are not sufficient to guarantee economic security, not to mention outstanding success (Klein, 1944). Despite this fact, children are taught this delusion, only to have it conflict later with reality. The disabilities that are ignored in our declarations of freedom are not limited to social and economic lacks. The child of low intelligence, for example, cannot hope to attain as an adult the equal of his peers of high intelligence.

In Western society we assume other conflicts that lengthen this list. Judaeo-Christian ideals frequently conflict with Western materialism. This is probably one of the deepest conflicts inherited by American children. Every Sunday they are taught and they recite lessons in nonaggression, brotherhood, self-effacement, importance of inner development, and purposiveness in the universe, yet some time before the day ends they have also been taught to fight for their rights, beat the other fellow to it, "the Lord helps him who helps himself," put up a good front, and other lessons of competitive aggression. Some aspects of the teachings of Jesus seem to conflict with the more rigid forms of organized religion. Jesus' emphasis on the simple life, the unimportance of property, antagonism toward ritual that kills spirit, the supremacy of brotherhood whenever it conflicts with any other allegiances, certainly are incompatible with modern practices of various sects. There are the existing elaborate cathedrals, the Jim-Crow practices among various churches, congregations that promote class consciousness among their members, and the gross materialism exhibited in the pomp and ceremony of many churches. Many clergymen and religious groups, however, are clearly conscious of these conflicts and are attempting to resolve them in favor of the ideals from which they sprung. Of all institutions, the church is outstanding for the examples shown by some of its leaders, especially the younger ones, in their attempts to solve some of the causes of mental discord.

We have referred previously to our conflicting attitudes toward sex in the United States. Sex is blatantly and publicly exploited in advertising, moving pictures, novels, and songs, whereas individual overt sexual behavior that violates the codes leads to social derogation (Ellis, 1951).

On the positive side, one critical writer, after reviewing much that has been written about contemporary America, sees among our many culture conflicts a *motivation and capacity for growth, a plastic strength* that has and can further shape us into a great civilization (Lerner, 1957).

SOCIAL CONDITIONS INIMICAL TO A WHOLESOME SOCIETY

We mentioned briefly the disabilities suffered by the child who grows up in a deprived neighborhood and the effect these have on healthy personal development. Anthropologists who have studied various primitive cultures have reported that they find relatively infrequent neurotic signs in those cultures that have few *repressive taboos* associated with strong drives (Malinowsky, 1927). Many of the psychological casualties of World War II have been attributed in part to the training of English-speaking people in repression of aggression and disapproval of the expression of fear. Serious guilt resulted when men so reared had to participate in warfare (Chisholm, 1944). Sherman and Sherman (1934) compared cultures in mountain communities of varying degrees of isolation and complexity and found that neurotic symptoms increased with *complexity* of social organization. Benedict (1934) points out that the extreme gratification of the ego in our society, which allows arrogant individualism, would be considered egomania in other societies. It must be remembered, in discussing these generalizations, that cultures cannot be transplanted from one society to another. Any suggestions about our own society are merely hypotheses that must be tested before being accepted as established conclusions.

Emphasis on nationalism, extolling the virtues of our way of life to the discredit of differing cultures, conflicts violently with the serious need

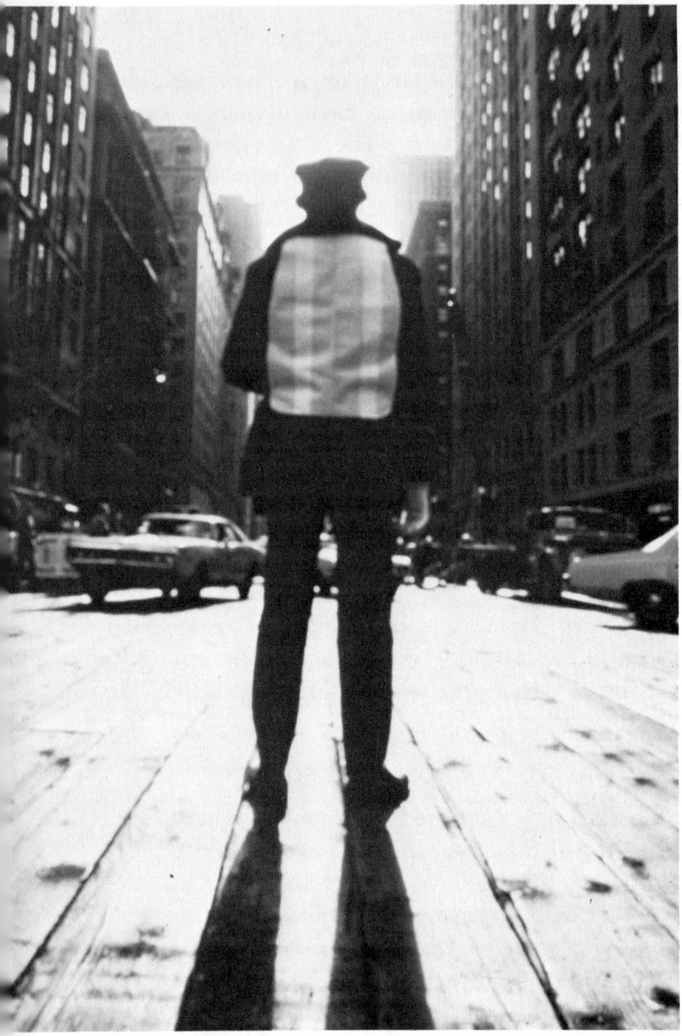

Figure 15–4 Defenders of the Status Quo.

Photo by J. Brian King

for internationalism and the efforts for peace so strongly advocated by present-day youth. Nationalism is especially inappropriate in a world that has been unified technologically by rapid communication and transportation. Several outstanding psychologists (May, 1943; Murphy, 1947; Tolman, 1942) all express concern about this issue and its effect on peace. There are many conflicts among the motives of man, but these conflicts are promoted, in the main, by the insularity of cultures.

There is a natural conflict between society's emphasis on the *status quo* and the need for change dictated by new inventions and new skills. Sometimes this conflict is between youth and older generations (Figure 15–4). The fast American tempo of living and our escapes into sensational experience related to our competitive culture and our urban frustrations conflict with the need for meditation, calm, and serenity advocated by health authorities and religionists (Jung, 1936).

In addition to these conflicts intrinsic to our society are those that are inevitable when our differing subcultures are at odds. There are the convictions of the small businessman, the farmer, organized labor, intellectuals, big business, the clergy, the aged, the young—all disagreeing on some points. These *culture conflicts* are illustrated by the incompatibility of the ideas that woman's place is in the kitchen and the fact that some of the greatest professional careers have been those of women; the exaltation of efficiency and the opposing admonition to be less machinelike and more human; parents may emphasize thrift while advertisements urge the satisfactions of instant spending on ready credit.

The question may be raised whether our national and international culture sufficiently emphasizes vehicles for the resolution of conflict and the integration of the various subcultures. The modern church, the United Nations, the free press, forum groups, and cultural interchange between groups and nations are all movements in that direction.

CHARACTERISTICS OF A SOCIETY CONDUCIVE TO MENTAL HEALTH

Both Fromm and Frank emphasize the importance of shaping a society that allows the satisfaction of human needs, which includes the reduction of disabling frustrations, conflicts, and anxieties. A relatively ideal society, from a mental hygiene standpoint, is one that will provide for the *development of mature, well-integrated, or unified individuals* who can meet the demands of their motivation without unhealthy conflict. This society produces *sociality, motivation* within the limits of the personality, *adaptability,* and *unity.* Furthermore, it encourages *interest in the basic realities* of the present world but looks to the world of tomorrow (Symonds, 1946). No thoughtful person advocates the abolition of all conflict. Those conflicts that can be resolved without being destructive to the individual are stimulating to him. The goal of those who wish a healthy society is the control of conflict, so that it may be effectively *assimilated* by the individual.

HIGH MORALE IN A HEALTHY SOCIETY

One possible index of a healthy society is high morale, which reflects security. The attitudes that accompany good morale are the antitheses of conflict, discouragement, inertia, apathy, or surrender. Positive morale signifies zest, faith in the fundamental purposes of the group, belief in and loyalty to the leaders. With high morale are found confidence in the group and oneself, perseverance, and a good spirit toward work and hardship. The attitude of the British after Dunkirk and during the darkest hours that nation ever knew, when they sustained hardships, frustration, and losses and showed faith in a cause that was their way of life is an example of high morale.

Morale is always implemented by the knowledge that those around us have a similar attitude, that we and our fellows feel the same about the crisis we are facing. The group shows zest when there are *common strivings*. A leader who is knowledgeable and can gain respect is essential to group morale. Faith in man and his eventual survival has been recognized as another valuable factor (Raines & Kolb, 1943; Boring, 1945). Additional boosters of morale consist of satisfaction of physical needs, of a sense that we are contributing to the common cause, are moving toward victory (goals), and are "in the know," even though the news may not be good. Recreation has also been found to assist in maintaining morale (Boring, 1945). In industry, being a part of the firm or a team, knowing that he has status, that he is as important as the profit, makes a measurable difference in the worker's production. Nothing lowers individual morale more than holding a job that carries a stigma, that does not tap one's abilities and interests, or that is supervised by someone who is not respected. Group morale falls when security with regard to job status and permanence is jeopardized (Miller & Form, 1951). Low morale, as well as personal problems and social stability, reflects itself in such behavior as absenteeism (Mayo & Lombard, 1944) and poor punctuality (Dudycha, 1936).

In a democratic atmosphere the individual develops, with fewer restrictions, into a more creative person. Morale in a community or a nation is in some ways similar to that in an effective organization, army, or industry. In a free, ideal democracy, achieving morale may at first seem more difficult than in a state in which there is a single party, a controlled press, low literacy, a ruling group, and a submissive population. On the contrary, a free state will encourage the development of more creative and individual attitudes and less stereotyped behavior. But there are common purposes amid the different personalities, and these must be emphasized without jeopardizing individual development. Favoring the development of morale in a democracy is the opportunity for the individual to feel that he can participate in the group destiny, knowledge about the state of the nation, and the stronger assurance of civil liberties. This morale is endangered when the theoretical freedoms of speech and worship and freedom from want and fear are not realized in actuality and when the people's elected representatives are agents of pressure groups rather than of their constituency.

If man is to have any society at all, to say nothing of a healthy society, the forces presently at work must be moving toward the *prevention and redirection of man's destructive tendencies*—war and violence. In 1945 the American psychologists issued a statement endorsed by 99 percent of the profession who responded to a communication about it (Murphy, 1945). In it appeared the assertion that war can be avoided by educating for peace in the coming generation. Furthermore, "the frustrations and conflicting interests which lie at the root of aggressive wars can be reduced and redirected by social engineering. . . . Men can realize their ambitions within the framework of human cooperation and can direct their aggressions against those natural obstacles that thwart them in the attainment of their goals" (p. 455).

In addition, the "white man must be freed of his concept of the 'white man's burden.' The English-speaking peoples are only a tenth of the world's population; those of white skin only a third. . . . The time has come for a more equal participation of all branches of the human family in a plan for collective security." The statement continues: "Disrespect for the common man is characteristic of fascism and of all forms of tyranny. The man in the street does not claim to understand the complexities of economics and politics but he is clear as to the general directions in which he wishes to progress. His will can be studied (by adaptations of the public-opinion poll). His expressed aspirations should even now be a major guide to policy" (pp. 456–457).

To summarize, a societal structure that permits the optimal development of a socialized personality through the satisfaction of basic motives and the prevention of irreconcilable conflicts is desirable. This culture is one that does not jeopardize his self-esteem or integrity but promotes the conditions that allow him to *realize his intrinsic dignity*.

INDIVIDUAL MENTAL HYGIENE

Man, throughout the millennia of his existence, has survived many threats to his being. All of us have confronted problems and difficulties and have adjusted to them, sometimes beneficially, sometimes destructively. Most of us have developed traits and resources to deal with predicaments in the future and some have been able to assist their fellows. The struggle of man to meet his basic needs and adapt to or change his environment is a normal biological process and necessity. Most of us need little professional help, but all of us can be aided in our adjustment by knowledge accumulated by students of man's development.

Mental hygienists have attempted to formulate simple generalizations and they have stated them in pamphlets and psychological textbooks so that individuals may reflect on them, pass them on to others, and attempt to use them in their own lives. It is obvious that mental health cannot be improved by health drills, but rather by *an atmosphere, a way of life, personal morale, self-understanding, and creativity.*

Lives and circumstances differ, and traits that may lead to soundness in one person in one area of endeavor may not be appropriate for another who is living a quite different kind of life. Some psychological conditions, like severe conflict and anxiety for which the individual has not been prepared, are, however, stressful for most people.

At this point you have read much of this book, particularly the ideas discussed in this chapter, and you are in a position to work out specific guidelines that may improve your own mental health. You might consider the following areas of psychological functioning as you work out your plans:

1. Physical well-being.
2. Satisfaction of your many needs in the manner that is best for you. These needs may involve relationships with people (including affection), work, recreation, etc.
3. Severe frustrations, conflicts, anxieties, and self-defeating defense mechanisms. Try to understand them and find ways of dealing with the conditions that produce them.
4. Formulate meaningful and realistic goals and values.
5. Find the best ways to cope with crises and with strong emotions.

You have read suggestions in the text, but your guidelines will be related to the specific events in your life.

Summary

1. Personal adjustment to the environment is a complex and individual phenomenon, and any evaluation of a given individual entails broad and intensive study.
2. Adjustment may be regarded in many ways, including social conformity, the statistical view, and aspects like tension reduction, self-satisfaction, medical, legal, ethical, and positive striving.
3. The concept of adjustment is value laden; sometimes it has implied conformity to social norms, and it is better applied to specific behaviors than to the whole person.
4. In using concepts that apply to persons rather than to specific areas of behavior, such as mental health or soundness of growth, three interacting basic features of effective human striving are suggested: (1) mastery of environment, (2) integrated personality, (3) accurate perception of self and world.

5. Using the above characteristics of soundness or positive growth and the realization that growth will be different as background and circumstances differ, several studies with different kinds of people are critically considered: (a) astronauts, (b) students with outstanding competence, (c) homoclites or "just plain guys," and (d) sound, creative persons.
6. Psychological *processes* are discussed in terms of soundness of personality. Severe frustration, conflict and anxiety, and self-defeating defense mechanisms are seen as hazards to sound development. The *catabolic* processes can be counteracted by a predominance of *anabolic* processes, such as confrontation, knowledge, self-insight, continuous individuation and identity, frustration tolerance and anxiety tolerance, and well-developed ego responses. These are seen as developing in stages through childhood by Erikson.
7. Ego strength (frustration or anxiety tolerance and the capacity to meet problems effectively) has been studied empirically and involves (1) good physical functioning, (2) spontaneity and ability to share emotions, (3) conventional religion and permissive morality, (4) good contact with reality, (5) feelings of personal adequacy, (6) courage and lack of fear.
8. Some psychologists have raised a question about the soundness or sanity of *cultures and subcultures* insofar as they allow the broad satisfaction of human needs, promote more sound personalities, and reduce human social pathology.
9. With society's role in personal soundness, conflicts within our society are examined. Among these conflicts are mass-media-created multiple desires and models not readily obtainable by many viewers; undue emphasis on competition, in conflict with need for cooperation for survival; verbalizations about freedom, despite many realistic limitations, particularly in lower economic and minority groups; sex stimulation by mass media conflicting with societal taboos.
10. Characteristics of a society conducive to mental health are also considered. Among desirable characteristics are those that promote mature, well-integrated individuals who are adaptable and realistic. Such a society hypothetically produces high morale through common striving, peace, recreation, education, and basic freedoms.
11. The reader now can write his own mental hygiene guidelines. They might well include: (1) physical well-being, (2) broad satisfaction of needs, (3) reduction of frustration, conflict, and anxiety by becoming aware of them and by dealing with the conditions that caused them, (4) formulation of realistic goals and values, and (5) discovery of ways to cope with crises, including strong emotions. The specific daily events that lead to soundness under your life circumstance can now be explicated by you from an understanding of these processes.

Words To Remember

Adjustment	Repression
Anxiety	Role
Identity	Self-Disclosure
Integrated Personality	Values

References

Achenbach, T., & Zigler, E. (1963). "Social competence and self-image disparity in psychiatric and nonpsychiatric patients." *J. Abnorm. Soc. Psychol.* **67:** 197–205.

Adams, C. R. (1951). *Preparing for Marriage.* New York: Dutton.

Aldrich, M. G. (1942). "An exploratory study of social guidance at the college level." *Educ. Psychol. Measmt.* **2:**209–216.

Alexander, F. (1950). *Psychosomatic Medicine.* New York: Norton.

Alexander, F., & Szasz, T. S. (1952). "The psychosomatic approach in medicine." In F. Alexander and H. Ross (Eds.), *Dynamic Psychiatry.* Chicago: University of Chicago Press.

Allport, G. (1961). *Pattern and Growth in Personality.* New York: Holt, Rinehart and Winston.

Anastasi, A. (1964). *Fields of Applied Psychology.* New York: McGraw-Hill.

Anon. (1942). *Alcoholics Anonymous.* New York: Alcoholics Anonymous Publishing Company.

Anon. (1968). "Alcoholism compounded." *Science News.* **10:** 94–95.

Anthony, E. J. (1970). "Childhood psychosis." In P. Mussen (Ed.), *Carmichael's Manual of Child Psychology.* New York: Wiley.

Arbuckle, D. S. (1953). *Student Personnel Services in Higher Education.* New York: McGraw-Hill.

Arnstein, H. S. (1964). *What to Tell Your Child About Birth, Illness, Death, Divorce, and Other Family Crises.* Indianapolis: Bobbs-Merrill.

Aronfreed, J. (1968). *Conduct and Conscience: The Socialization of Internalized Control over Behavior.* New York: Academic Press.

Asch, S. E. (1956). "Studies of independence and submission to group pressure: A minority of one against a unanimous majority." *Psychol. Monogr.* **70**(416).

Atkinson, J. W. (1964). *An Introduction to Motivation.* New York: Van Nostrand Reinhold.

Atthowe, J. M., & Krasner, L. (1968), "A preliminary report on the application of contingent reinforcement procedures (token economy) on a 'chronic' psychiatric ward." *J. Abnorm. Soc. Psychol.* **73:**37–43.

Axline, V. M. (1947), *Play Therapy*. Boston: Houghton Mifflin.

Ayllon, T., & Azrin, N. H. (1965), "The measurement and reinforcement of psychotics." *J. Exper. Anal. Behav.* **8**:357–383.

Azrin, N. (1967). "Pain and aggression." *Psychol. Today.* **1**:27–33.

Back, K. W. (1972). *Beyond Words.* New York: Russell Sage Foundation.

Bailey, C. J., & Miller, N. E. (1952). "The effect of sodium amytal on an approach avoidance conflict in cats." *J. Comp. Physiol. Psychol.* **45**:205–208.

Bakan, D. (1966). *The Duality of Human Existence.* Skokie, Ill.: Rand McNally.

Baker, H. J., & Traphagen, V. *The Diagnosis and Treatment of Behavior-Problem Children.* New York: Macmillan, 1935.

Baker, L. G., Jr (1968). "The personal and social adjustment of the never-married woman." *J. Marr. Fam.* **30**(3):473–479.

Bandura, A. (1969). *Principles of Behavior Modification.* New York: Holt, Rinehart and Winston.

Bandura, A., Blanchard, E., & Ritter, B. (1969). "The relative efficacy of desensitization and modeling approaches for inducing behavioral, affective, and attitudinal changes." *J. Pers. Soc. Psychol.* **13**:177–199.

Bandura, A., Grusec, J. E., & Menlove, F. L. (1967). "Vicarious extinction of avoidance behavior." *J. Pers. Soc. Psychol.* **5**:16–23.

Bandura, A., Ross, D., & Ross, S. A. (1963). "Imitation of film-mediated aggressive models." *J. Abnorm. Soc. Psychol.* **6**:3–11.

Barron, F. (1963). *Creativity and Psychological Health.* New York: Van Nostrand Reinhold.

Barron, F. (1968). *Creativity and Personal Freedom.* New York: Van Nostrand Reinhold.

Bateson, G., Jackson, D. D., Haley, J., & Weakland, J. (1956). "Toward a theory of schizophrenia." *Behav. Sci.* **1**:251–264.

Bebout, J., & Gordon, B. (1972). "The value of encounter." In L. N. Solomon and B. Berzon (Eds.), *New Perspectives on Encounter Groups.* San Francisco: Jossey-Bass.

Beck, A. T. (1967). *Depression.* New York: Harper & Row.

Becker, J. (1960). "Achievement-related characteristics of manic-depressives." *J. Abnorm. Soc. Psychol.* **60**:334–339.

Becker, J., Spielberger, C. D., & Parker, J. B. (1963). "Value achievement and authoritarian attitudes in psychiatric patients." *J. Clin. Psychol.* **19**:57–61.

Belbin, R. M. (1972). "Retirement strategy in an evolving society." In F. M. Carp (Ed.). *Retirement.* New York: Behavioral Publications.

Beller, E. K. (1955). "Dependency and independence in young children." *J. Genet. Psychol.* **87**:25–35.

Benedict, R. (1934). "Anthropology and the abnormal." *J. Genet. Psychol.* **10**:59–82.

Benne, K. D. (1964). "History of the T-Group in the laboratory setting." In L. P. Bradford, J. R. Gibb, and K. D. Benne (Eds.), *T-Group Theory and Laboratory Method.* New York: Wiley.

Bennett, E. M., & Cohen, L. R. (1959). "Men and women: Personality patterns and contrasts." *Genet. Psychol Monogr.* **59**:101–155.

Benson, H., & Wallace R. K. (1972). In T. J. Taylor (Ed.), *Altered States of Awareness.* San Francisco: W. H. Freeman.

Benson, P. (1955). "The common interests myth in marriage." *Social Problems.* **3**:27–34.
Berger, S. M. (1962). "Conditioning through vicarious instigation." *Psychol. Rev.* **69**:450–466.
Berkowitz, L. (1968). "Impulse, aggression, and the gun." *Psychol. Today.* **2**:19–22.
Berlyne, D. E. (1966). "Curiosity and exploration." *Science.* **153**:25–33.
Berne, E. (1964). *Games People Play.* New York: Grove Press.
Bettelheim, B. (1943). "Individual and mass behavior in extreme situations." *J. Abnorm. Soc. Psychol.* **38**:417–452.
Bindrim, P. (1969). "Nudity as a quick grab for intimacy in group therapy." *Psychol. Today.* **3**:24–28.
Blanchard, W. H. (1972). "Encounter group and society." In L. N. Solomon and B. Berzon (Eds.), *New Perspectives on Encounter Groups.* San Francisco: Jossey-Bass.
Blane, H. (1968). *The Personality of the Alcoholic: Guises of Dependency.* New York: Harper & Row.
Blau, P. M. (1962). "Patterns of choice in interpersonal relations." *Amer. Sociol. Rev.* **27**:41–55.
Blood, R. D., Jr., & Wolfe, D. (1960). *The Dynamics of Married Living.* New York: Free Press.
Blum, R. (1964). *Utopiates: The Use and Users of LSD-25.* New York: Atherton Press.
Blum, R. H. (1966). "Drugs and personal values." Paper read at NASPA Drug Education Conference, Washington, November 1966.
Bordin, E. S. (1946). "Diagnosis in counseling and psychotherapy." *Educ. Psychol. Measmt.* **6**:169–184.
Boring, E. G. (1945). "Psychology for the armed services." *Infantry Journal,* chap. 16 & **17**:118–120; 183–185.
Bossard, J. H. S., & Ball, E. S. (1957). *One Marriage: Guidance on Interfaith Marriage.* New York: Ronald Press.
Brady, J. V. (1958). "Ulcers in 'executive' monkeys." *Sci. Amer.* **199**:95–100.
Brayfield, A. H. (1968). "Human resources development." *Amer. Psychologist.* **23**:(7)479–482.
Bronfenbrenner, U. (1960). "Freudian theories of identification and their derivatives." *Child Dev.* **31**:15–40.
Brophy, A. L. (1959). "Self, role, and satisfaction." *Genet. Psychol. Monogr.* **59**:263–308.
Brown, C. (1937). "A social activities survey." *J. Higher Educ.* **8**:257–265.
Brown, R. (1965). *Social Psychology.* New York: Free Press.
Burgess, E. W., & Cottrell, L. S., Jr. (1939). *Predicting Failure in Marriage.* Englewood Cliffs, N.J.: Prentice-Hall.
Burgess, E. W., & Wallin, P. (1953). *Engagement and Marriage.* Philadelphia: Lippincott.
Burma, J. H. (1947). "Student attitudes toward participation in organizations." *Sociol. Soc. Res.* **32**:625–629.
Butler, R. N. (1972). "A life-cycle perspective: Public policies for later life." In F. M. Carp (Ed.), *Retirement.* New York: Behavioral Publications.

Byrne, D. (1966). *An Introduction to Personality: A Research Approach.* Englewood Cliffs, N.J.: Prentice-Hall.

Byrne, D., & Blaylock, B. (1963). "Similarity and assumed similarity of attitudes between husbands and wives." *J. Abnorm. Soc. Psychol.* **67**:636–640.

Carp, F. M. (1972). "Retirement as a transitional life stage." In F. M. Carp (Ed.), *Retirement.* New York: Behavioral Publications.

Catanzaro, R. J. (1967). "Understanding the alcoholic." In F. McKinney (Ed.), *Psychology in Action.* New York: Macmillan, Inc.

Cavanaugh, J. O. (1942). "The relation of recreation to personality adjustment." *J. Soc. Psychol.* **15**:63–74.

Chisholm, G. B. (1944). "Some factors in the high rate of n. p. casualties." *Bull. Menninger Clin.* **8**:36–38.

Christensen, H. T. (1960). "Cultural relativism and premarital sex norms." *Amer. Sociol. Rev.* **25**:31–39.

Clark, K. B. (1965). *Dark Ghetto.* New York: Harper & Row.

Clark, K. B., & Clark, M. P. (1947). "Racial identification and preference in Negro children." In T. M. Newcomb and E. L. Hartley (Eds.), *Readings in Social Psychology.* New York: Holt, Rinehart and Winston.

Clark, R. A., & Sensibar, M. R. (1956). "The relationship between symbolic and manifest projections of sexuality with some incidental correlates." *J. Abnorm. Soc. Psychol.* **53**:182–186.

Cleckley, H. M. (1959). "Psychopathic states." In S. Arieti (Ed.), *American Handbook of Psychiatry.* New York: Basic Books.

Coelho, G. V., Hamburg, D. A., & Murphy, E. B. (1963). "Coping strategies in a new learning environment: A study of American college freshmen." *Arch. Psychol.* **9**(5):433–443.

Coffey, H. S. (1966). "Group psychotherapy." In I. A. Berg and L. A. Pennington (Eds.), *An Introduction to Clinical Psychology.* New York: Ronald Press.

Cohen, H. L., Filipczak, J., Bis, J., Cohen, J., Goldiamond, I., & Larkin, P. Case II—Model; *A Contingency Oriented Twenty-Four Hour Learning Environment in a Juvenile Correctional Institution.* Silver Spring, Md.: Institute for Behavioral Research Press, 1968.

Cohen, M. B., Baker, G., Cohen, R. A., Fromm-Reichmann, F., & Weigert, E. V. (1954). "An intensive study of twelve cases of manic-depressive psychosis." *Psychiat.* **17**:103–137.

Cohen, S. (1968). "The cyclic psychedelics." *Amer. J. Psychiat.* **125**:393–394.

Cole, J. O., Jones, R. T., & Klerman, G. L. (1961). "Drug therapy." In E. J. Spiegel (Ed.), *Progress in Neurology and Psychiatry,* Vol. XVI. New York: Grune & Stratton.

Corsini, R. J. (1957). *Methods of Group Psychotherapy.* New York: McGraw-Hill.

Crites, J. O. (1961). "Factor analytic definitions of vocational motivation." *J. Appl. Psychol.* **45**:330–337.

Davitz, J. R. (1952). "The effects of previous training on post-frustration behavior." *J. Abnorm. Soc. Psychol.* **47**:309–315.

Dethier, V. G. (1964). "Microscopic brains." *Science.* **143**:1138–1145.

Dobzhansky, T. (1973). *Genetic Diversity & Human Equality.* New York: Basic Books.

Doidge, W. T., & Holtzman, W. A. (1960). "Implications of homosexuality among Air Force trainees." *J. Consult. Psychol.* **24**:9–13.

Dreikurs, R. (1959). "Early experiments with group psychotherapy." *Amer. J. Psychother.* **13**:882–891.

Dudycha, G. J. (1936). "An objective study of punctuality in relation to personality and achievement." *Arch. Psychol.* **53**(204).

Duvall, E. E., & Hill, R. (1945). *When You Marry.* Lexington, Mass.: Heath.

Dyer, D. T. (1939). "Relation between vocational interests of men in college and their subsequent occupational histories for ten years." *J. Appl. Psychol.* **23**:280–288.

Ehrmann, W. (1959). *Premarital Dating Behavior.* New York: Holt, Rinehart and Winston.

Ellis, A. (1951). *The Folklore of Sex.* New York: Charles Boni.

Ellis, A. (1966). "Psychosexual and marital problems." In I. A. Berg and L. A. Pennington (Eds.), *An Introduction to Clinical Psychology.* New York: Ronald Press.

Ellis, A., & Harper, R. A. (1961). *A Guide to Rational Living.* N. Hollywood, Calif.: Wilshire Book Co.

Engel, B. T., & Shapiro, D. (1971). "The use of biofeedback training in enabling patients to control autonomic functions." In J. Segal (Ed.), *Mental Health Program Reports—5.* Washington, D.C.: U.S. Government Printing Office. Pp. 349–376.

Erikson, E. H. (1959). "Identity and the life cycle." *Psychological Issues.* Monograph No. I.

Erikson, E. H. (1963). *Childhood and Society.* New York: Norton.

Fairfield, R. (1971). *Communes USA: A Personal Tour.* Baltimore: Penguin Books.

Feshbach, S. (1955). "The drive reducing function of fantasy behavior." *J. Abnorm. Soc. Psych.* **50**:3–12.

Feshbach, S. (1956). "The catharsis hypothesis and some consequences of interaction with aggressive and neutral play objects." *J. Pers.* **24**:449–462.

Fiedler, F. E. (1950a). "A comparison of therapeutic relationships in psychoanalytic, non-directive, and Adlerian therapy." *J. Consult. Psychol.* **14**:436–445.

Fiedler, F. E. (1950b). "The concept of an ideal therapeutic relationship." *J. Consult. Psychol.* **14**:239–245.

Fitts, W. H., & Hammer, W. T. (1969). *The Self Concept and Delinquency.* Nashville, Tenn.: Nashville Mental Health Center.

Frank, J. D., & Powdermaker, F. B. (1959). "Group psychotherapy." In S. Arieti (Ed.), *American Handbook of Psychiatry,* Vol. II. New York: Basic Books.

Frank, L. K. (1936). "Society as the patient." *Amer. J. Sociol.* **42**:335–344.

Freud, S. (1966). *New Introductory Lectures on Psychoanalysis.* New York: Norton.

Fromm, E. (1955). *The Sane Society.* New York: Holt, Rinehart and Winston.

Frumkin, F. M. (1954). "Communal interests crucial to marital adjustment." *Ohio Journal of Science.* **54**:107–110.

Funkenstein, D. H., King, S. H., & Drolette, M. E. (1956). *The Mastery of Stress.* Cambridge: Harvard University Press.

Gardner, G. G. (1964). "The psychotherapeutic relationship." *Psychol. Bull.* **61**:426–437.

Gaudet, F. J., Caril, A. R., & Dennegar, L. S. (1950). "Attitudes of veterans towards vocational guidance services." *J. Appl. Psychol.* **34**:347–350.

Geen, R. G., & Berkowitz, L. (1966). "Name-mediated aggressive cue properties." *J. Pers.* **34**:456–465.

Gibb, J. R. (1972). "Meaning of the small group experience." In L. N. Solomon and B. Berzon (Eds.), *New Perspectives on Encounter Groups.* San Francisco: Jossey-Bass.

Gibson, R. W. (1958). "The family background and early life experiences of the manic-depressive patient." *Psychiat.* **21**:71–90.

Ginott, H. G. (1965). *Between Parent and Child: New Solutions to Old Problems.* New York: Macmillan, Inc.

Ginott, H. G. (1969). *Between Parent and Teenager.* New York: Macmillan, Inc.

Ginott, H. G. (1972). *Between Teacher and Child.* New York: Macmillan, Inc.

Glassberg, B. Y. (1965). "Sexual behavior patterns in contemporary youth culture—Implications for later marriage." *J. Marr. Fam.* **27**:190–192.

Glidewell, J. C., & Swallow, C. S. (1969). *The Prevalence of Maladjustment in Elementary Schools: A Report Prepared for the Joint Commission on the Mental Health of Children.* Chicago: University of Chicago Press.

Glynn, E. L. (1970). "Classroom application of self-determined reinforcement." *J. Appl. Behav. Anal.* **3**:123–132.

Goode, W. J. (1956). *After Divorce.* New York: Free Press.

Goodman, P. (1956). *Growing Up Absurd: Problems of Youth in the Organized System.* New York: Random House.

Green, R. (1974). "Children's quest for sexual identity." *Psychol. Today.* **7**:51.

Grier, W. H., & Cobbs, P. M. (1969). *Black Rage.* New York: Bantam.

Griffith, J. (1966). "A study of illicit amphetamine drug traffic in Oklahoma City." *Amer. J. Psychiat.* **123**(5):560–569.

Grinker, R. R. (1962). "Mentally healthy young male (homoclites)." *Arch. Gen. Psychiat.* **6**:405–453.

Grinspoon, L. (1969). "Marijuana." *Sci. Amer.* **221**:17–25.

Hadden, S. B. (1955). "Historic background of group psychotherapy." *Int. J. Group Psychother.* **5**:162–168.

Haggstrom, W. C. (1964). "The power of the poor." In F. Rieseman, J. Cohen, and A. Pearl (Eds.), *Mental Health of the Poor.* New York: Free Press.

Haley, J. (1963). *Strategies of Psychotherapy.* New York: Grune & Stratton.

Hall, C. S., & Lindzey, G. (1957). *Theories of Personality.* New York: Wiley.

Hall, E. T. (1959). *The Silent Language.* New York: Fawcett World Library.

Halliday, J. L. (1953). "Concept of psychosomatic affection." In A. Weider (Ed.), *Contributions Toward Medical Psychology,* Vol. I. New York: Ronald Press.

Halpern, H. M. (1963). *A Parent's Guide to Child Psychotherapy.* New York: A. S. Barnes.

Hand, H. C. (1938). *Campus Activities.* New York: McGraw-Hill.

Harris, T. A. (1967). *I'm OK—You're OK.* New York: Harper & Row.

Harlow, H. (1959). "Love in infant monkeys." *Scientific Amer.* Reprint. San Francisco: W. H. Freeman.

Haughton, E., & Ayllon, T. (1965). "Production and elimination of symptomatic behavior." In L. P. Ullmann and L. Krasner (Eds.), *Case Studies in Behavior Modification.* New York: Holt, Rinehart and Winston.

Havemann, E., & West, P. S. (1952). *They Went to College: The College Graduate in America.* New York: Harcourt Brace Jovanovich.

Havighurst, R. J. (1969). "Suicide and education." In E. S. Scheidman (Ed.), *On the Nature of Suicide.* San Francisco: Jossey-Bass.

Havighurst, R. J., & Albrecht, T. (1953). *Older People.* New York: Longmans, Green.

Havighurst, R. L., Neugarten, B. L., & Tobin, S. S. (1968). "Disengagement and patterns of aging." In B. L. Neugarten (Ed.), *Middle Age and Aging.* Chicago: University of Chicago Press.

Hawley, R. D. (1938). "College training as preparation for life and for living." *Sch. and Soc.* **48**:468–472.

Heston, L. L., & Denney, D. (1968). "Interactions between early life experience and biological factors in schizophrenia." In D. Rosenthal and S. S. Kety (Eds.), *The Transmission of Schizophrenia.* New York: Pergamon Press.

Hilgard, E. R., Atkinson, R. C., & Atkinson, R. L. (1967). *Introduction to Psychology.* New York: Harcourt Brace Jovanovich.

Hilgard, E. R., & Bower, G. (1966). *Theories of Learning.* New York: Appleton-Century-Crofts.

Hoffman, M. L. (1970). "Moral development." In P. Mussen (Ed.), *Carmichael's Manual of Child Psychology.* New York: Wiley.

Holland J. L., & Richards, J. M., Jr. (1965). "Academic and nonacademic accomplishments: Correlated or uncorrelated?" *J. Educ. Psychol.* **56**(4):165–174.

Hollingshead, A. B. (1957). *Two-Factor Index of Social Position.* New Haven, Conn.: Author.

Hollingshead, A. B., & Redlich, F. C. (1958). *Social Class and Mental Illness.* New York: Wiley.

Horney, K. (1937). *The Neurotic Personality of Our Time.* New York: Norton.

Horney, K. (1942). *Self Analysis.* New York: Norton.

Hubel, D. H., & Wiesel, T. N. (1963). "Single-cell responses in striate cortex of kittens deprived of vision in one eye." *J. Neurophysiology.* **26**:1003–1017.

Hull, C. L. (1943). *Principles of Behavior.* New York: Appleton-Century-Crofts.

Huxley, A. (1954). *The Doors of Perception.* New York: Harper & Row.

Irwin, T. (1968). "Attacking alcoholism as a disease." *Today's Health.* **46**(11): 28–29, 87–88.

Isaacs, W., Thomas, J., & Goldiamond (1960). In "Application of operant conditioning to reinstate verbal behavior in psychotics." *Journal of Speech and Hearing Disorders.* **25**:8–12.

Jack, L. M. (1934). "An experimental study of ascendant behavior in preschool children." *Univ. Iowa Studies in Child Welfare.* **9**:7–65.
Jahoda, M. (1958). *Current Conceptions of Positive Mental Health.* New York: Basic Books.
Janov, A. (1970). *The Primal Scream.* New York: Putnam.
Jarvik, M. E. (1967). "The psychopharmacological revolution." *Psychol. Today.* **1**:51–59.
Jason, L., Clarfield, S., & Cowen, E. L. (1973). "Preventive intervention with young disadvantaged children." *Amer. J. of Community Psychol.* **1**:50–61.
Jellinek, E. M. (1960). *The Disease Concept of Alcoholism.* New Haven, Conn.: Hillhouse Press.
Jensen, A. R. 1969). "How much can we boost IQ and scholastic achievement?" *Harvard Educ. Rev.* **31**:1–123.
Jensen, S. E., & Ramsey, R. W. (1963). "Treatment of the chronic alcoholic with lysergic acid diethylamide." *Canadian Psychiat. Assn. J.* **8**:182–188.
Jones, M. C. (1924). "A laboratory study of fear: The case of Peter." *Pedagog. Sem.* **31**:308–315.
Jones, M. C. (1968). "Personality correlates and antecedents of drinking patterns in adult males." *J. Consult. Clin. Psychol.* **32**:2–12.
Josephson, E., & Josephson, M. (Eds.) (1962). *Man Alone: Alienation in Modern Society.* New York: Dell Publishing Co.
Josselyn, I. M. (1948). *Psychosocial Development of Children.* New York: Family Service Association.
Jourard, S. M. (1971). *The Transparent Self.* New York: Van Nostrand Reinhold.
Jourard, S. M., & Remy, R. M. (1955). "Perceived parental attitudes, the self, and security." *J. Consult. Psychol.* **19**:364–366.
Jung, C. G. (1936). *Modern Man in Search of a Soul.* New York: Harcourt Brace Jovanovich.
Jurgensen, C. E. (1949). "What do job applicants want?" *Personnel.* **25**:352–355.
Kallman, F. J. (1953). *Heredity in Health and Mental Disorder.* New York: Norton.
Kanter, R. M. (1972). *Commitment and Community: Communes and Utopias in Sociological Perspective.* Cambridge, Mass.: Harvard University Press.
Kaplan, M. F., & Singer, E. (1963). "Dogmatism and sensory alienation: An empirical investigation." *J. Consult. Psychol.* **27**:486–491.
Keister, M. E. (1937). "The behavior of young children in failure." *Univ. Iowa Studies in Child Welfare.* **14**:29–82.
Kelly, E. L. (1955). "Consistency of the adult personality." *Amer. Psychologist.* **10**:549–681.
Keniston, K. (1966). *Drug Use and Student Values.* Paper read at NASPA Drug Education Conference, Washington.
Kephart, W. (1961). *The Family, Society, and the Individual.* Boston: Houghton Mifflin.
Kimmel, D. C. (1974). *Adulthood and Aging.* New York: Wiley.
King. G. F. (1958). "Differential autonomic responsiveness in the process-

reactive classification of schizophrenia." *J. Abnorm. Soc. Psychol.* **56**:160–164.

Kinsey, A. C., Pomeroy, W. B., Martin, C. E., & Gebhard, P. H. (1953). *Sexual Behavior in the Human Female.* Philadelphia: Saunders.

Kinsey, A. C., Pomeroy, W. B., & Martin, C. E. (1948). *Sexual Behavior in the Human Male.* Philadelphia: Saunders.

Kirkpatrick, C. (1963). *The Family as Process and Institution.* New York: Ronald Press.

Klein, D. B. (1944). *Mental Hygiene.* New York: Holt, Rinehart and Winston.

Knapp, R. R. (1965). "Relationship of a measure of self-actualization to neuroticism and extraversion." *J. Consult. Psychol.* **29**:168–172.

Koch, S. (1972). "An implicit image of man." In L. N. Solomon and B. Berzon (Eds.), *New Perspectives on Encounter Groups.* San Francisco: Jossey-Bass.

Kohn, M. L. (1970). "Social class and schizophrenia: A critical review." In H. Wechsler, L. Solomon, and B. M. Kramer (Eds.), *Social Psychology and Mental Health.* New York: Holt, Rinehart and Winston.

Korchin, S. J., & Ruff, G. E. (1964). "Personality characteristics of the Mercury astronauts." In G. H. Grosser, H. Wechsler, and M. Greenblatt (Eds.), *The Threat of Impending Disaster.* Cambridge, Mass.: MIT Press.

Kroeber, T. C. (1963). "The coping functions of the ego mechanisms." In R. W. White (Ed.), *The Study of Lives.* New York: Atherton Press.

Lacrome, C. W. (1963). "Sex and personality differences in relation to fantasy." *J. Consult. Psychol.* **27**:270–272.

Landis, J. R., & Landis, M. G. (1963). *Building a Successful Marriage.* Englewood Cliffs, N.J.: Prentice-Hall.

Lang, P. J., Lazovik, A. D., & Reynolds, D. J. (1965). "Desensitization, suggestibility, and pseudotherapy." *J. Abnorm. Soc. Psychol.* **70**:395–402.

Lawlis, G., & Rubin, S. (1971). "16-PF study of personality patterns in alcoholics." *Quarterly J. of Studies on Alcohol.* **32**:317–327.

Lazarus, R. S. (1969). *Patterns of Adjustment and Human Effectiveness.* New York: McGraw-Hill.

Lecky, P. (1945). *Self-Consistency: A Theory of Personality.* New York: Island Press.

LeMasters, E. E. (1957). "Parenthood as crisis." *Marr. Fam. Liv.* **19**:352–355.

Lemere, F. (1966). "The danger of amphetamine dependency." *Amer. J. Psychiat.* **123**:569–572.

Lerner, M. (1957). *America as a Civilization.* New York: Simon & Schuster.

Levinger, G., & Senn, D. J. (1967). "Disclosure of feelings in marriage." *Merrill-Palmer Quart.* **13**:237–249.

Lidz, T., Fleck, S., & Cornelison, A. R. (1965). *Schizophrenia and the Family.* New York: International University Press.

Lieberman, M. A., Yalom, I. D., & Miles, M. B. (1972). "Impact on participants." In L. N. Solomon and B. Berzon (Eds.), *New Perspectives on Encounter Groups.* San Francisco: Jossey-Bass.

Lobsenz, N. M. (1974). "Sex and the senior citizen." *N.Y. Times Magazine,* January 20.

Locke, H. J. (1951). *Predicting Adjustment in Marriage.* New York: Holt, Rinehart and Winston.

Lorion, R. P. (1973). "Socioeconomic status and traditional treatment approaches reconsidered." *Psych. Bull.* **79**:263–270.

Lorion, R. P. (1974). "Patient and therapist variables in the treatment of low-income patients." *Psych. Bull.* **81**:344–354.

Lovaas, O. I., Freitag, G., Gold, V. J., & Kassorka, I. C. (1965). "Experimental studies in childhood schizophrenia: Analysis of self-destructive behavior." *J. of Exp. Child Psychol.* **2**:67–84.

Lovaas, O. I., & Simmons, J. Q. (1969). "Manipulation of self-destruction in three retarded children." *J. Appl. Behav. Anal.* **2**:143–157.

Lowenthal, M. F. (1972). "Some potentialities of a life-cycle approach to the study of retirement." In F. M. Carp (Ed.), *Retirement.* New York: Behavioral Publications.

MacDonald, M., McGuire, C., & Havighurst, R. S. (1949). "Leisure activities and the socioeconomic status of children." *Amer. J. Sociol.* **54**:505–519.

Maher, B. A. (1966). *Principles of Psychopathology.* New York: McGraw-Hill.

Malinowsky, B. (1927). *Sex and Repression in Savage Society.* New York: Harcourt Brace Jovanovich.

Malmo, R. B. (1957). "Anxiety and behavioral arousal." *Psych. Rev.* **64**:276–287.

Mamlet, L. N. (1967). " 'Consciousness limiting' side effects of 'consciousness expanding drugs'." Paper read at American Orthopsychiatric Association, Washington.

Marcson, S. (1953). "Predicting intermarriage." *Sociol. Soc. Res.* **37**:151–156.

Maslow, A. H. (1954). *Motivation and Personality.* New York: Harper & Row.

Maslow, A. H. (1962). *Toward a Psychology of Being.* New York: Van Nostrand Reinhold.

Massarik, F. (1972). "Standards for group leadership." In L. N. Solomon and B. Berzon (Eds.), *New Perspectives on Encounter Groups.* San Francisco: Jossey-Bass.

Masserman, J. H., & Yum, K. S. (1946). "An analysis of the influence of alcohol on experimental neurosis in cats." *Psychosomatic Medicine.* **8**:36–52.

Masters, W. H., & Johnson, V. E. (1966). *Human Sexual Response.* Boston: Little, Brown.

Masters, W. H., & Johnson, V. E. (1968). "Human sexual response: The aging female and the aging male." In B. L. Neugarten (Ed.), *Middle Age and Aging.* Chicago: University of Chicago Press.

Masters, W. H., & Johnson, V. E. (1970). *Human Sexual Inadequacy.* Boston: Little, Brown.

Mathews, L. H. (1964). "Overt fighting in mammals." In J. D. Carthy and F. J. Ebling (Eds.), *The Natural History of Aggression.* New York: Academic Press.

May, M. A. (1943). *A Social Psychology of War and Peace.* New Haven, Conn.: Yale University Press.

Mayo, E., & Lombard, G. F. F. (1944). "Teamwork and labor turnover in the aircraft industry in southern California." In *Publ. Grad. Sch. Bus. Adm. Harvard Univ.*, No. 32.

McCord, W., & McCord, J. (1964). *The Psychopath: An Essay on the Criminal Mind.* New York: Van Nostrand Reinhold.

McDavid, J. W., & Harari, H. (1968). *Social Psychology: Individuals, Groups, Societies.* New York: Harper & Row.

McKinney, F. (1939). "Personality adjustment of college students as related to factors in personal history." *J. Appl. Psychol.* **23**:660–668.

McReynolds, W. T. (1969). *Systematic Desensitization, Insight-Oriented Psychotherapy, and Relaxation Therapy in a Psychiatric Population.* Unpublished doctoral dissertation, University of Texas at Austin.

McReynolds, W. T., & Church, A. (1972). "Self-control, study skills development and counseling approaches to the improvement of study behavior." Unpublished manuscript, University of Missouri, Columbia.

McReynolds, W. T., & Coleman, J. (1972). Token economy: patient and staff changes. *Behavior Research & Therapy.* **10**:29–34.

Mead, G. H. (1934). *Mind, Self and Society.* Chicago: University of Chicago Press.

Mead, M. (1968). "We must learn to see what's really new." *Life.* **23**:30–34.

Meehl, P. E. (1962). "Schizotaxia, schizotypy, schizophrenia." *Amer. Psychol.* **17**:827–838.

Menninger, K. (1938). *Man Against Himself.* New York: Harcourt Brace Jovanovich.

Menninger, W. C. (1949). *Recreation and Mental Health.* Hogg Foundation.

Miller, D. C. (1949). "Economic factors in the morale of college-trained adults." *Amer. J. Sociol.* **47**:139–156.

Miller, D. C., & Form, W. H. (1951). *Industrial Society.* New York: Harper & Brothers.

Miller, S. M., & Riessman, F. (1969). "The working-class subculture: A new view." In A. L. Grey (Ed.), *Class and Personality in Society.* New York: Atherton Press.

Mischel, W. (1970). "Sex typing and socialization." In P. Mussen (Ed.), *Carmichael's Manual of Child Psychology.* New York: Wiley.

Mishler, E. G., & Scotch, N. A. (1970). "Social cultural factors in the epidemiology of schizophrenia." In H. Wechsler, L. Solomon, and B. M. Kramer (Eds.), *Social Psychology and Mental Health.* New York: Holt, Rinehart and Winston.

Moody, H. (1969). "Drugs, the law, and high-minded delusions." *Christianity and Crisis.* **24**:29(20).

Moreno, J. L. (1946). *Psychodrama.* New York: Beacon House.

Moreno, J. L. (1953). *Who Shall Survive?* New York: Beacon House.

Morgan, C. T. (1965). *Physiological Psychology.* New York: McGraw-Hill.

Mowrer, O. H., & Miller, N. E. (1942). "A multi-purpose learning demonstration apparatus." *J. Exp. Psychol.* **31**:163–170.

Mudd, E., Mitchell, H., & Taubin, S. (1965). *Success in Family Living.* New York: Association Press.

Murphy, G. (1945). *Human Nature and Enduring Peace.* Boston: Houghton Mifflin.

Murphy, G. (1947). *Personality: A Biosocial Approach to Origins and Structure.* New York: Harper & Row.

Murphy, L. B. (1962). *Paths Toward Mastery: The Widening World of Childhood.* New York: Basic Books.

Murray, H. A. (1938). *Exploration in Personality.* New York: Oxford University Press.

Mussen, P. H. (1962). "Long-term consequents of masculinity of interests in adolescence." *J. Consult. Psychol.* **26**:435–448.

Mussen, P. H., Conger, J. J., & Kagan, J. (1969). *Child Development and Personality.* New York: Harper & Row.

Naegel, K. D. (1958). "Friends and acquaintances: An exploration of some social distinctions." *Harvard Educ. Rev.* **28**:232–252.

Narrol, H. G. (1967). "Experimental application of reinforcement principles to the analysis and treatment of hospitalized alcoholics." *Quart. J. Stud. Alcohol.* **47**:428–436.

Navran, L. (1967). "Communication and adjustment in marriage." *Family Process.* **6**(2):173–184.

Northway, M. L. (1944). "Outsiders: A study of the personality patterns of children least acceptable to their age mates." *Sociometry.* **7**:10–25.

Nowlis, H. H. (1969). *Drugs on the College Campus.* Garden City, N.Y.: Anchor Books.

Ornstein, R., & Naranjo, C. (1971). *The Psychology of Meditation.* New York: Viking.

Ort, R. L. (1950). "A study of role conflicts as related to happiness in marriage." *J. Abnorm. Soc. Psychol.* **45**:691–699.

Packard, V. (1968). *The Sexual Wilderness.* New York: McKay.

Page, M. L. (1935). "The modification of ascendant behavior in preschool children." *Univ. Iowa Studies in Child Welfare.* **12**:(3).

Partington, J., & Johnson, F. (1969). "Personality types among alcoholics." *Quarterly J. of Studies on Alcohol.* **75**:131–138.

Patterson, C. (1966). *Theories of Counseling and Psychotherapy.* New York: Harper & Row.

Paul, G. L. (1966). *Insight vs. Desensitization in Psychotherapy: An Experiment in Anxiety Reduction.* Stanford, Calif.: Stanford University Press.

Pavlov, I. P. (1929). *Lectures on Conditioned Reflexes.* New York: International Universities Press.

Payne, J. S., Mercer, C. D., Payne, R. A., & Davidson, R. G. (1973). *Headstart: A Tragic-Comedy with Epilogue.* New York: Behavioral Publications.

Pennington, L. A. (1966). "Psychopathic and criminal behavior." In I. A. Berg and L. A. Pennington (Eds.), *An Introduction to Clinical Psychology.* New York: Ronald Press.

Pepinsky, H. B. (1948). "The selection and use of diagnostic categories in clinical counseling." *Amer. Psychol. Monogr.* 15.

Perls, F. S. (1969). *Gestalt Therapy Verbatim.* Lafayette, Calif.: Real People Press.

Phillips, W. S., & Greene, J. E. (1939). "A preliminary study of the relationship of age, hobbies, and civil status to neuroticism among women teachers." *J. Educ. Psychol.* **30**:440–444.

Piaget, J. (1932). *The Moral Judgment of the Child.* New York: Harcourt Brace Jovanovich.

Pineo, P. (1961). "Disenchantment in later years of marriage." *Marr. and Fam. Liv.* **23**:3–11.

Pond, D. A., Ryle, A., & Hamilton, M. (1963). "Social factors and neurosis in a working-class population." *Brit. J. Psychiat.* **109**:587–591.

Powdermaker, F. B., & Frank, J. D. (1953). *Group Psychotherapy.* Cambridge, Mass.: Harvard University Press.

Premack, D. (1965). "Reinforcement theory." In D. Levine (Ed.), *Nebraska Symposium on Motivation.* Lincoln: University of Nebraska Press.

Pressey, S. L. (1946). "Changes from 1923 to 1943 in the attitudes of public school and university students." *J. Psychol.* **21**:173–188.

Provence, S., & Lipton, R. C. (1962). *Infants in Institutions.* New York: International Universities Press.

Raines, G. N., & Kolb, L. C. (1943). "Combat fatigue and war neurosis." *Nav. Med. Bull.* **41**:923–936, 1299–1309.

Ramsey, G. V. (1943). "The sexual development of boys." *Amer. J. Psychol.* **56**:217–223.

Reddy, W. B. (1972). "Screening and selection of participants." In L. N. Solomon and B. Berzon (Eds.), *New Perspectives on Encounter Groups.* San Francisco: Jossey-Bass.

Reisman, J. (1960). "Motivational differences between process and reactive stimuli." *J. Pers.* **28**:12–25.

Roe, A. (1953). *The Making of a Scientist.* New York: Dodd, Mead.

Rogers, C. R. (1951). *Client-Centered Therapy: Its Current Practice, Implications, and Theory.* Boston: Houghton Mifflin.

Rogers, C. R. (1959). "A theory of therapy, personality, and interpersonal relationships, as developed in the client-centered framework." In S. Koch (Ed.), *Psychology: A Study of Science,* Vol. 3. New York: McGraw-Hill.

Rogers, C. R. (1964). "Toward a modern approach to values: The valuing process in the mature person." *J. Abnorm. Soc. Psychol.* **68**:160–167.

Rogers, C. R. (1967). "The process of the basic encounter group." In J. F. T. Bugental (Ed.), *Challenges in Humanistic Psychology.* New York: McGraw-Hill.

Rogers, C. R. (1969). "The group comes of age." *Psychol. Today.* **3**:27–31.

Rogers, E. M., & Havens, A. E. (1960). "Prestige rating and mate selection on a college campus." *Marr. Fam. Liv.* **2**:55–59.

Rosenberg, M. (1962). "The association between self-esteem and anxiety." *J. Psychiat. Res.* **1**:135–152.

Rosenthal, D. (1959). "Some factors associated with concordance and discordance with respect to schizophrenia in monozygotic twins." *J. Nerv. Ment. Dis.* **129**:1–10.

Rosenthal, D., Wender, P. H., Kety, S. S., Schulsinger, F., Welner, J., & Østergaard, L. (1968). "Schizophrenics' offspring reared in adoptive homes." In D. Rosenthal and S. S. Kety (Eds.), *The Transmission of Schizophrenia.* New York: Pergamon Press.

Roth, J., & Peck, R. F. (1951). "Social class and social mobility factors related to marital adjustment." *Amer. Soc. Rev.* **16**:478–487.

Ruch, F. L. (1967). *Psychology and Life.* Glenville, Ill.: Scott, Foresman.

Sameroff, A. J., & Zax, M. (1973). "Perinatal characteristics of the offspring

of schizophrenic women." *J. Nerv. Ment. Dis.* **157**:191–199.
Sanford, F. H., & Wrightsman, L. S., Jr. (1970). *Psychology: A Scientific Study of Man.* Belmont, Calif.: Brooks-Cole.
Sarason, S. B. (1973). *The Creation of Settings: And the Future Societies.* San Francisco: Jossey-Bass.
Savage, C., Savage, E., Fadiman, J., & Harman, W. (1964). "LSD: therapeutic effects of psychedelic experience." *Psychol. Rep.* **14**:111–120.
Schaffer, R. H. (1953). "Satisfaction as related to need satisfaction in work." *Psychol. Monogr.* **67**(14).
Schutz, W. D. (1967). *Joy.* New York: Grove Press.
Sears, P. S. (1940). "The organization of hereditary maze-brightness and maze-dullness." *Genet. Psychol. Monogr.* **39**:279–325.
Sears, R. R. (1936). "Experimental studies of projection: I. Attribution of traits." *J. Soc. Psychol.* **7**:151–163.
Sears, R. R. (1963). "Dependency motivation." In M. R. Jones (Ed.), *Nebraska Symposium on Motivation.* Lincoln: University of Nebraska Press.
Sears, R. R. (1965). "Development of gender role." In F. A. Beach (Ed.), *Sex and Behavior.* New York: Wiley.
Sears, R. R., Maccoby, E. E., & Levin, H. (1957). *Patterns of Child Rearing.* New York: Harper & Row.
Sears, R. R., Whiting, J. W. M., Nowlis, V., & Sears, P. S. (1953). "Some childrearing antecedents of aggression and dependency in young children." *Genet. Psychol. Monogr.* **47**:135–234.
Sechrest, L., & Wallace, J. (1967). *Psychology and Human Problems.* Columbus, Ohio: Merrill.
Segin, C. A. (1950). *Introduction to Psychosomatic Medicine.* New York: International Universities Press.
Shaffer, L. F., & Shoben, E. J., Jr. (1956). *Psychology of Adjustment.* Boston: Houghton Mifflin.
Shanas, E. (1972). "Adjustment to retirement: Substitution or accommodation." In F. M. Carp (Ed.), *Retirement.* New York: Behavioral Publications.
Shannon, J. R. (1940). "A comparison of highly successful teachers, failing teachers, and average teachers at the time of their graduation from Indiana State Teachers College." *Educ. Adm. Superv.* **26**:43–51.
Shannon, J. R., & Kittle, M. A. (1947). "Analysis of 21 groups in one school: Economic discrimination in extracurricular activities." *The Clearing House.* **22**:71–72.
Sherman, M., & Sherman, I. C. (1934). "Psychotic symptoms and social background." In M. Bentley (Ed.), *Problems of Mental Disorder.* New York: McGraw-Hill.
Siegal, S. M. (1956). "The relationship of hostility to authoritarianism." *J. Abnorm. Soc. Psychol.* **52**:368–372.
Silber, E., Hamburg, D. A., Coelho, G. V., Murphy, E. B., & Rosenberg, M. (1961). "Adaptive behavior in competent adolescents." *Arch. Gen. Psychiat.* **5**:354–355.
Skinner, B. F. (1938). *The Behavior of Organisms.* New York: Appleton-Century-Crofts.

Slavson, S. R. (1951). *The Practice of Group Therapy*. New York: International Universities Press.

Smith, H. L., & Hightower, N. C. (1948). "Incidence of functional disease (neurosis) among patients of various occupations." *Occup. Med.* **5**:182–185.

Smith, W. A. (1952). "Rating and dating—A re-study." *Marr. Fam. Liv.* **14**:312–317.

Solomon, R. L., & Wynne, L. C. (1954). "Traumatic avoidance learning: The principles of anxiety conservation and partial irreversibility." *Psychol. Rev.* **61**:353–385.

Sorokin, P. (1927). *Social Mobility*. New York: Harper & Row.

Spielberger, C. D., Parker, J. B., & Becker, J. (1963). "Conformity and achievement in remitted manic-depressive patients." *J. Nerv. Ment. Dis.* **137**:162–172.

Spitz, R. A., & Wolf, K. M. "Anaclitic depression: an inquiry into the genesis of psychiatric conditions in early childhood, II." *Psychoanalytic Study of the Child*, 1946, **2**:313–342.

Srole, L., Langner, T. S., Michael, S. T., Opler, M. K., & Rennie, T. A. C. (1962). *Mental Health in the Metropolis: The Midtown Manhattan Study*. New York: McGraw-Hill.

Stagner, R. (1956). *The Psychology of Industrial Conflict*. New York: Wiley.

Stagner, R. (1965). *Psychology of Personality*. New York: McGraw-Hill.

Stengel, E. (1964). *Suicide and Attempted Suicide*. Baltimore: Penguin.

Stoller, F. H. (1968). "Marathon group therapy." In G. M. Gazda (Ed.), *Innovations to Group Psychotherapy*. Springfield, Ill.: C. C. Thomas.

Strang, R. (1946). *Group Activities in College and Secondary Schools*. New York: Harper & Row.

Stressman, H. D., Thaler, M. B., & Schein, E. H. (1956). "A prisoner of war syndrome: Apathy as a reaction to severe stress." *Amer. J. Psychiat.* **112**:998–1003.

Stroup, A. L. (1953). "Predicting marital success or failure in an urban population." *Amer. Sociol. Rev.* **18**:558–562.

Stroup, A. L. (1966). *Marriage and Family: A Developmental Approach*. New York: Appleton-Century-Crofts.

Sullivan, H. S. (1949). "The theory of anxiety and the nature of psychotherapy." *Psychiat.* **12**:3–13.

Sullivan, H. S. (1953). *The Interpersonal Theory of Psychiatry*. New York: Norton.

Sundberg, N. D., & Tyler, L. E. (1962). *Clinical Psychology*. New York: Appleton-Century-Crofts.

Super, D. E. (1940). *Avocational Interest Patterns: A Study in the Psychology of Avocations*. Stanford: Stanford University Press.

Super, D. E. (1957). *The Psychology of Careers: An Introduction to Vocational Development*. New York: Harper & Row.

Sussman, M. B. (1972). "An analytic model for the sociological study of retirement." In F. M. Carp (Ed.), *Retirement*. New York: Behavioral Publications.

Sutherland, E. H., Schroeder, H. G., & Tordella, C. L. (1950). "Personality traits and the alcoholic: A critique of existing studies." *Quart. J. Stud. Alcohol.* **11**:547–561.

Syme, L. (1957). "Personality characteristics and the alcoholic: A critique of current studies." *Quart. J. Stud. Alcohol.* **18**:288–301.

Symonds, P. M. (1945). "How teachers solve personal problems." *J. Educ. Res.* **38**:641–652.

Symonds, P. M. (1946). *The Dynamics of Human Adjustment.* New York: Appleton-Century-Crofts.

Symonds, P. M. (1951). *The Ego and the Self.* New York: Appleton-Century-Crofts.

Terman, L. M. (1938). *Psychological Factors in Marital Happiness.* New York: McGraw-Hill.

Terman, L. M., & Buttenwieser, P. (1935). "Personality factors in marital compatibility." *J. Soc. Psychol.* **6**:143–171, 267–289.

Terman, L. M., & Miles, C. (1936). *Sex and Personality.* New York: McGraw-Hill.

Tharp, P. (1963). "Psychological patterning in marriage." *Psychol. Bull.* **60**(2): 97–117.

Thomason, B. (1955). "Marital sexual behavior and total marriage adjustment: a research report." In J. Himelhoch and S. L. Fara (Eds.), *Sexual Behavior in American Society.* New York: Norton. Pp. 153–163.

Timmons, W. M. (1944). "Some outcomes of participation in dramatics: II. Likeability and cooperativeness, relationships between outcomes." *J. Soc. Psychol.* **19**:35–51.

Tolman, E. C. (1942). *Drives toward War.* New York: Appleton-Century-Crofts.

Trilling, L. (1963). "The fate of pleasure: Wordsworth to Dostoevsky." In N. Frye (Ed.), *Romanticism Reconsidered.* New York: Columbia University Press.

Truax, C. B., & Carkhuff, R. R. (1965). "The experimental manipulation of therapeutic conditions." *J. Consult. Psychol.* **29**:119–124.

Tuddenham, R. D. (1952). "Studies in reputation: I. Sex and grade differences in school children's evaluations of their peers." *Psychol. Monogr.* **333**:1–39.

Ullmann, L. P., & Krasner, L. (1969). *A Psychological Approach to Abnormal Behavior.* Englewood Cliffs, N.J.: Prentice-Hall.

Ullmann, J. P., Krasner, L., & Edinger, R. L. (1964). "Verbal conditioning of common associations in long term schizophrenic patients." *Behavior Res. and Therapy.* **2**:15–18.

U.S. Bureau of the Census, Census Report of 1964. Washington, D.C.: U.S. Government Printing Office.

Videbeck, R. (1960). "Self conception and the reactions of others." *Sociometry.* **23**:351–359.

Waller, W. (1937). "The rating and dating complex." *Amer. Soc. Rev.* **2**:727–732.

Walters, J., Pearce, D., & Dahms, L. (1957). "Affectional and aggressive behavior of preschool children." *Child Dev.* **28**:15–26.

Watson, J. B., & Rayner, R. (1920). "Conditioned emotional reactions." *J. Exp. Psychol.* **3**:1–14.
Weil, A. T., Zinberg, N. E., & Nelson, J. M. (1968). "Clinical and psychological effects of marijuana in man." *Science.* **162**:1234–1242.
Weiss, J. M. (1968). "Effects of predictable and unpredictable shock on development of gastrointestinal lesions in rats." *Proc. 76th Ann. Conv. APA.* **3**:263–264.
White, R. W. (1959). "Motivation reconsidered: The concept of competence." *Psychol. Rev.* **66**:297–333.
White, R. W. (1966). *Lives in Progress.* New York: Holt, Rinehart and Winston.
Williamson, E. G. (1948). "The group origins of student leaders." *Educ. Psychol. Measmt.* **8**:603–612.
Williamson, R. C. (1952). "Economic factors in marital adjustment." *Marr. Fam. Liv.* **14**:298–301.
Williamson, R. C. (1966). *Marriage and Family Relations.* New York: Wiley.
Winder, A. E., & Hersko, M. A. (1958). "A thematic analysis of an outpatient psychotherapy group." *Int. J. Group Psychother.* **8**:293–300.
Wolf, A. (1951). *The Parent's Manual.* New York: Popular Library.
Wolff, H. G. (1953). "Life stress and bodily disease." In A. Weider (Ed.), *Contributions Toward Medical Psychology.* New York: Ronald Press.
Wolfgang, D. G. (1972). "A Video Tape Microtreatment for Alcoholics." Unpublished doctoral dissertation. University of Missouri, Columbia, Mo.
Wolpe, J. (1958). *Psychotherapy by Reciprocal Inhibition.* Stanford, Calif.: Stanford University Press.
Wrenn, C. G. (1951). *Practical Study Aids.* Stanford, Calif.: Stanford University Press.
Wynne, L. C., Ryckoff, I. M., Day, J., & Hirsch, S. I. (1958). "Pseudomutuality in the family relations of schizophrenics." *Psychiat.* **21**:205–220.
Yablonsky, L. (1965). *The Tunnel Back—Synanon.* New York: Macmillan, Inc.
Zax, M., & Cowen, E. L. (1972). *Abnormal Psychology: Changing Conceptions.* New York: Holt, Rinehart and Winston.
Zax, M., & Stricker, G. (1963). *Patterns of Psychopathology.* New York: Macmillan, Inc.

Glossary

Activity theory. Theory which explains decreased activity and social involvement observed in the elderly as a function of society: withdrawing from the person against his wishes; cf. Disengagement theory.

Adjustment. Behavior that removes an undesirable condition or satisfies an individual's needs.

Affection. Interpersonal need identified by Schutz as reflecting one's desire for emotional closeness with others.

Affective psychosis. Serious psychological disorder marked by psychotic loss of contact with reality expressed by extreme prolonged depression and/or uncontrollable episodes of activity, enthusiasm, and optimism.

Agency. A concept used to describe an individual's sense of assertiveness, responsibility, and control.

Amphetamines. *See* Stimulant drug.

Anal stage. Psychoanalytically hypothesized developmental stage during second and third year of life when attention focuses on toilet training and eliminatory functions. *See* Psychosexual stage.

Analgesic drug. *See* Narcotic drug.

Anxiety. An unpleasant experience producing physiological responses similar to fear. It differs from fear in that there is no objective danger, or the response is disproportionate to the danger.

Apathy. Listless and indifferent behavior to a frustrating or stressful situation accompanied by attitudes of detachment and inattentiveness.

Approach-approach conflict. Conflict in which one is attracted by two desirable but incompatible goals.

Approach-avoidance conflict. Conflict in which one is attracted by a goal that has both attractive and unattractive characteristics.

Autism. Serious psychological disorder observed in very young children marked by massive denial of interpersonal stimuli, withdrawal, and oftentimes, self-punitive behavior.

Autonomy. Eriksonian concept referring to the child's need to feel as if he or she is able to function with some degree of independence and self-direction.

Avoidance-avoidance conflict. Situation in which an individual is forced to respond in an undesirable manner to avoid another even more undesirable situation.

Avoidance conditioning. The acquisition of a response that averts otherwise imminent aversive stimulation; an instrumental conditioning procedure.

Basic trust. Eriksonian concept referring to the infant's developing confidence in the presence, love, and support of his parent, which later generalizes to other close relationships.

Behavior therapy. A therapy approach in which there is a tendency to focus on experimentally established behavior change procedures, usually learning principles, in the modification of problem behavior.

Biogenic needs. Motivational needs that are essentially biologically determined.

Bisexuality. Sexual orientation in which arousal and satisfaction is experienced in either homo- or heterosexual contacts; cf. Homosexuality; Heterosexuality.

Classical conditioning. Acquisition of a new response to a stimulus resulting from the pairing of that stimulus with another stimulus which already elicits the response.

Classical extinction. Repeated presentation of a conditioned stimulus without an unconditioned stimulus, resulting in a decrease in responding.

Client-centered therapy. Therapy in which the client is responsible for exploring his feelings in personality, arriving at insights and making decisions.

Clinical psychologist. A psychologist who has completed an accredited university Ph.D. program plus one year of supervised clinical practice; his professional functions may include psychological testing, psychotherapy, and research.

Cognitive. An aspect of awareness that reflects knowing rather than feeling.

Cognitive dissonance. Conflict in self-awareness in which one discovers an inconsistency between one's own overt behavior and one's covert self-concept.

Commune. Alternative social arrangement in which a number of individuals attempt to achieve greater self-awareness, interpersonal closeness, and personal satisfaction by forming a close-knit, shared, living experience.

Compensation. A defense mechanism that is an impulsive attempt to cover up or balance failure by strenuous effort.

Compromise reactions. One broad arbitrary classification of defense mechanisms, relating behaviors that are somewhat similar and more subtle than withdrawal reactions such as compensation, rationalization, and projection.

Conditioned response (CR). An acquired response to a previously neutral stimulus.

Conditioned stimulus (CS). A previously neutral stimulus which, through the process of learning or conditioning, takes on the property of eliciting a certain (conditioned) response.

Conflict. Motivation that is incompatible with other motivations.

Continuous reinforcement. Reinforcement that follows every correct response.

Control. Interpersonal need identified by Schutz as reflecting one's desire to dominate and manipulate others.

Conversion reaction. Neurotic response to stress by "translating" psychological conflicts into physical symptoms manifested in hysterical psychoneuroses.

Counterconditioning technique. Elimination of unwanted behavior using extinction or punishment while simultaneously replacing it with a more desirable behavior.

Defense mechanism. Pattern of behavior designed to protect the person from the anxiety of facing his own unacceptable feelings.

Deficit motivation. That which usually arises out of a bodily need, such as hunger, thirst.

Delusion. An inaccurate but persistent belief, often characteristic of paranoid ideation; the more common delusions observed include grandiosity (i.e., feelings of being extremely important) and persecution (i.e., feeling that others are "out to get" one).

Denial. A defense mechanism in which the individual attempts to avoid recognition of and dealing with negative feelings.

Dependency. Psychological or physical need to continually secure and ingest a drug; physical dependency develops when continued use results in alterations of normal physiological states; psychological dependency develops when continued use results in anxiety reduction and the onset of a calm, euphoric state.

Depression. Psychological state characterized by feelings of sadness, pessimism, self-defeat, and sluggishness; in its more severe states depression is often marked by serious suicidal potential and loss of contact with reality.

Despair. Eriksonian concept reflecting the mature person's sense of dissatisfaction with his life's accomplishments and his awareness that with death approaching he cannot rectify his failures.

Developmental stage. Period of growth marked by specific physical or psychological characteristics distinct from prior and subsequent levels of development.

Discrimination. Learned differential responses to two stimuli.

Disengagement theory. Theory that explains decreased activity and social involvement observed in the elderly as a function of a mutual process in which society and the aging individual willingly withdraw from each other; cf. Activity theory.

Dissociation. A disunity within the acting organism due to anxiety which may be accompanied by inappropriate response to a situation.

Dissociative reaction. Neurotic response to stress marked by disorders of memory which may be of brief or extended duration and may include unconsciously developing a totally new identity.

Double-bind. Pattern of communication in which two contradictory messages are presented simultaneously; this pattern is believed to be characteristic of the parent-child interactions in a schizophrenic's family history.

Drug abuse. *See* Drug addiction; Dependency.

Drug addiction. State of periodic or chronic physical dependence upon a chemical compound marked by (a) tolerance, i.e., the need to consume increasingly greater amounts of the substance to maintain its physical effect, and (b) the onset of withdrawal symptoms if ingestion of the substance is discontinued. *See* Withdrawal syndrome; Dependency.

Ego. Psychoanalytic concept referring to that segment of personality involved with finding adaptive solutions to the conflicts that arise among the Id, i.e. (libidinal urges), Superego, i.e. (moral reservations), and reality; ego processes are assumed to operate according to the "reality principle" or "secondary process."

Egocentrism. Absence of cognitive differentiation between one's personal experiences and those external to oneself; the term also refers more generally to the inability to appreciate the attitudes and concerns of other individuals.

Ego integrity. Eriksonian concept reflecting a mature person's sense that he has taken care of things and people in his lifetime and has managed to adapt to the various successes and failures that characterize one's life; basically, the term refers to an overall acceptance and satisfaction with one's accomplishments.

Ego strength. Term for one's adaptive potential, including the capacity to cope with the usual and atypical demands of life, to tolerate frustration, and maintain control over anxiety.

Encounter group. Similar to a T-Group in which participants focus primarily on affective reactions to each other in order to achieve a sense of satisfaction in dealing with people.

Epidemiological survey. The study of incidence and spread of mental or physical disease in various segments of the population.

Equal ratio reinforcement. Equal number of responses required per reinforcement (i.e., reinforcement for every *n*th correct response).

Fantasy. Use of imagery to privately satisfy motivation; fantasies may be unrealistic and may depict improbable events.

Feedback. Information returned to the individual by his environment about a behavior he has emitted; the reaction to his behavior.

Fixation. Relatively fixed or attitudinal pattern characteristic of a stage of development earlier than the one in which it is manifested; in the psychoanalytic theory of personality, fixations are a consequence of unresolved conflicts at a particular psychosexual stage.

Fixed interval reinforcement. Reinforcement of a correct response after the passage of a specified amount of time.

Free association. Psychoanalytic treatment technique to overcome a patient's repressive defenses by having him say to the analyst whatever comes to mind.

Frustration. Blocked motivation.

Frustration-aggression hypothesis. Hypothesis stating that aggression is a consequence of frustration.

Generalized reinforcer. Conditioned reinforcer that is prevalent and widespread in our culture, e.g., attention and money.

Genital stage. Psychoanalytically hypothesized developmental stage in which sexuality becomes part of a mature interpersonal relationship following resolution of adolescent conflicts. *See* Psychosexual stage.

Generativity. Eriksonian concept referring to the sense of productiveness and accomplishment experienced by one able to meet successfully the demands of adulthood. *See* Stagnation.

Gestalt therapy. A therapy emphasizing the need to fully experience situations as they are encountered. This involves the expression of feelings previously unexpressed, thus achieving a sense of closure.

Goal-directed behavior. Behavior directed toward an end that will satisfy one's motivation.

Hallucination. Experience of sensations that have no basis in reality, typically involving seeing or hearing things that are not there, although the experience may occur with any sensory modality.

"Head." Slang term referring to one who chronically and dependently uses some drug, e.g., "pot head" for chronic marijuana users and "acid head" for chronic LSD users.

Heterosexuality. Sexual orientation in which arousal and satisfaction are achieved with members of the opposite sex.

Higher-order conditioning. A learning process in which a neutral stimulus when paired with a conditioned stimulus takes on its own properties; the first conditioned stimulus serves as the function of an unconditioned stimulus in the establishment of a new conditioned stimulus.

Homosexuality. Sexual orientation in which arousal and satisfaction are achieved with members of one's own sex.

Hypnotic drug. *See* Sedative drug.

Id. Psychoanalytic concept representing that segment of personality involved with the expression of instinctual (i.e., libidinal) urges; the Id is assumed to operate according to the "pleasure principle" or "primary process."

Ideal self. The self for which the individual strives.

Identification. Psychological process in which an individual assumes as his own aspects those of another person's attitudes, feelings, or behavior patterns.

Identity. An awareness of one's role or roles in life; ability to answer the question "Who am I?"

Inclusion. Interpersonal need identified by Schutz as reflecting one's desire to feel significant in the eyes of others and to receive their concern.

Index of social position. Scale used to determine socioeconomic status in relation to education, occupation, and area of residence.

Industry. Eriksonian concept in which the school-age child seeks to feel that he can successfully accomplish some goal or task.

Inordinate motivation. Motivation that is intense; seemingly insatiable state that lacks the creative aspect of growth motivation, and which rarely achieves the subjective satisfaction sought.

Insight therapy. Therapy in which the focus is on the intrapsychic aspects of the patient, his needs, defenses, and their underlying meanings.

Instrumental conditioning. The acquisition of a response following the positive or negative reinforcement of that response.

Instrumental extinction. Termination of positive or negative reinforcement of a response usually resulting in a decrease in the frequency of that response.

Integrated personality. A personality unified by the association of its various aspects, especially conscious and unconscious processes.

Internalization. Psychological process in which an individual incorporates into his value system the attitudes and moral principles of another.

Intimacy. Eriksonian concept referring to the sense of completeness and personal support characteristic of the young adult able to form a close, meaningful relationship with another; cf. Isolation.

Introjection. Process in which an individual assumes the attitudes and behaviors of an ideal person.

Isolation. Eriksonian concept referring to the sense of loneliness and detachment characteristic of the young adult unable to establish meaningful, intimate personal contacts; cf. Intimacy.

Latency stage. Psychoanalytically hypothesized developmental stage during childhood and preadolescence when it is assumed that libidinal urges are relatively quiescent. *See* Psychosexual stage.

Latent learning. Unintentional learning that may take place without immediately observable changes in behavior.

Learning. A process whereby behavior is changed through interaction of the organism with the environment, when these changes cannot be attributed to maturation or temporary states.

Level of aspiration. Individual estimate of one's anticipated performance on a certain task.

Libido. Psychoanalytic concept referring to the basic psychic energy which is expressed through instinctual urges such as hunger, thirst, sex, etc.

Malevolent transformation. Awareness described by Sullivan that interpersonal relationships can be the cause of pain as well as pleasure.

Marasmus. State of withdrawal, loss of appetite, and affective reaction observed in institutionalized infants without mothering contacts.

Marathon group. Group procedure for facilitating self-awareness and interpersonal skills by providing intense experience concentrated over several days.

Marital schism. Pattern observed in some families of schizophrenics in which each parent is so involved in his or her own problems that neither adopts a complementary role with the other.

Marital skew. Pattern observed in some families of schizophrenics in which one parent is very dominant and the other very submissive.

Masturbation. Self-induced sexual arousal and/or satisfaction involving genital stimulation.

Maturation. Process involving growth or change in which heredity is the main determinant.

Menarche. *See* Puberty.

Menopause. The period between 40 and 50 when women experience the psychological and physiological concomitants of alterations in hormone balance related to sexual reproduction.

Milieu therapy. Treatment approach which aims at modifying negative behaviors and maintaining positive ones by systematically designing the characteristics of the setting and the responsibilities of individuals within the setting in such a way that beneficial effects can result.

Modeling. Change in behavior resulting from the observation of the behavioral patterns in others.

Motivation. A persistent condition that activates and directs the organism until the condition is changed.

Narcissism. Extreme self-centeredness and concern for one's physical appearance and comfort.

Narcotic drug. Chemical substance which when ingested produces marked reductions in the awareness of pain; if ingested in sufficient quantity, narcotic drugs produce a feeling of euphoria (a "high"); continued use results in development of dependency marked by increases in tolerance and presence of withdrawal signs. *See* Dependency; Tolerance; Withdrawal syndrome.

Nature-nurture question. Controversy concerning two determinates of human behavior: the environment or genetic predisposition.

Negative reinforcement. Removal of noxious or aversive stimulus contingent on a response.

Negative reinforcer. A situation or condition not sought or desired by the individual.

Neuropsychiatrist. A physician who practices both neurology and psychiatry.

Nonadjustive behavior. Self-defeating behavior on the part of a frustrated or conflicted individual; by so behaving he obtains relief which results in subsequent difficulties.

Nondeficit motivation. The arousal and direction of behavior which achieves and satisfies tendencies to develop, yet do not relate to specific physiological needs.

Nondirective therapy. A client-centered therapy in which the counselor does not take the major responsibility for directing the session.

Nonintegrative behavior. Behavior that may bring partial or immediate relief, but does not lead to satisfaction of the whole individual.

Observational learning. *See* Modeling.

Operant conditioning. *See* Instrumental conditioning.

Oral stage. *See* Psychosexual stage; psychoanalytically hypothesized developmental stage in which the mouth becomes a central focus of psychological attention and concerns center around incorporation and ingestion during the first year of life.

Paranoia. A character style marked by suspiciousness, distrust of others, grandiosity, and excessive sensitivity to criticism; a serious psychological disorder in which above-mentioned traits are so marked as to impair one's ability for normal functioning.

Parataxic thought. Cognitive pattern described by Sullivan in which causal relationships begin to be perceived between experiences, although, at times, erroneously due to temporal or spatial contiguity.

Partial reinforcement. Noncontinuous reinforcement of a response resulting in increased resistance of the response to extinction.

Peak experience. An experience that stands out in memory as the moment of highest happiness and fulfillment, often accompanied by a feeling of wholeness, aliveness, uniqueness, self-sufficiency, and self-worth.

Perceived self. The self of which the individual is aware.

Personality disorder. Maladaptive behavioral pattern that reflects a lifelong, deeply ingrained style of responding to the normal occupational and interpersonal demands of life.

Phallic stage. Psychoanalytically hypothesized developmental stage during the preschool years when attention focuses on awareness of sexual organs and sensation and conflicts around parental attachments. *See* Psychosexual stage.

Phobia. Psychologically determined fear of an animate or inanimate object or situation in which there is no realistic basis for the presence or intensity of the fear reaction.

Pleasure principle. *See* Id.

Positive reinforcement. Presentation of a desirable or pleasurable stimulus or state of affairs contingent on a response.

Primal therapy. Therapy that sees psychopathology as the result of painful emotions that have been held back. The cure lies in the reexperiencing of these emotions in a therapeutic setting.

Primary process. *See* Id.

Primary reinforcer. Desirable response consequences directly related to primary or biological needs such as thirst and hunger.

Process schizophrenia. Psychotic disorder marked by a long history of emotional disorder and maladjustment.

Projection. A defense mechanism in which the individual protects himself from recognition of an undesirable quality by attributing it to others.

Prototaxic thought. Cognitive pattern described by Sullivan in which experience is processed in an unrelated series of sensation.

Pseudomutuality. Observed characteristic of families of schizophrenics in which there is a strong investment in preserving the impression that close relationships exist between all family members.

Psychiatric nurse. Nurse with specialized education and experience to prepare her/him to care for emotionally disturbed patients.

Psychiatric social worker. A social worker who has completed an M.A. or M.S.W. degree along with an internship in psychiatric setting.

Psychiatrist. A physician who, after completing his M.D. degree, has taken resident training in psychiatry.

Psychodrama. A group therapy situation in which a real anxiety-producing situation to a group member is acted out with others in the group, giving the individual an opportunity for emotional release and catharsis.

Psychogenic drug. Chemical substance which when ingested produces changes in the psychological processes of mood, thinking, and behavior, often evidenced by perceptual distortion, disorientation, and delusion (e.g., LSD, marijuana, mescaline).

Psychoneurosis. Psychological disorder characterized by a variety of maladaptive symptoms or behavior patterns whose aim is to protect the individual against anxiety.

Psychopath. Person displaying signs of psychopathy; Pennington's work with such individuals found psychopaths to be unemotional, socially isolated, and unable to learn from past experiences.

Psychopathy. Personality style characterized by aloofness, solitude, the "absence of conscience," irresponsibility, and exploitative and manipulative interactions with others.

Psychosexual stage. Point of psychological development mediated by a specific erogenous zone of libidinal expression; Freud postulated five such stages including the Oral, Anal, Phallic, Latency, and Genital periods, each of which is marked by specific intrapsychic demands whose resolution determines the ease of transition into subsequent stages.

Psychosis. Psychological disorder characterized by severe disturbances of cognition, affect, and sensation which impairs an individual's ability to continue normal patterns of functioning.

Puberty. Stage of development at which sexual reproduction becomes possible and marked changes in physical appearance and hormonal levels are observable. The stage typically occurs around 12 in females with the onset of menstruation (menarche) and around 14 in males with the appearance of facial hair and structural changes in physical appearance.

Punishment. Presentation of an aversive or withdrawal of a desirable stimulus contingent on a response, usually reducing the frequency of that response.

Rational coping. Synonymous with conscious problem solving; approaching a difficulty by seeking the cause and attempting to manipulate it.

Rational-emotive therapy. Therapy based on the premise that individuals grow by surmounting emotional inhibitions, formed by society; the therapeutic task is to lower defenses sufficiently to release this great store of feelings, following which defenses are unnecessary.

Rationalization. A compromise reaction that involves false explanations for an event which may cause anxiety and loss of self-esteem if honestly faced.

Reaction formation. The defense mechanism in which behavior that is expressed is the opposite of that which is actually felt.

Reactive schizophrenia. Psychotic disorder marked by little prior evidence of instability and history of appropriate, adaptive development.

Readjustment. A program of change to bring about a more adequate satisfaction of motives.

Reality principle. *See* Ego.

Reference group. A group with which an individual interacts, such as the family siblings, or peers, through which self-attitudes develop.

Repression. A defense mechanism; it consists of unconsciously avoiding or denying impulses or memories.

Respondent conditioning. *See* Classical conditioning.

Responses. An activity of the organism, conscious or unconscious.

Response acquisition. Increase in the frequency or probability of a response; cf. Learning.

Response generalization. The "spread" of a conditioned response such that a single conditioned stimulus comes to elicit both a conditioned response and other, related responses.

Role. The function performed by a person in a group, such as role of mother, teacher, secretary, etc.

Role playing. A simpler and less formal form of psychodrama in which an individual's role in a potentially anxious situation is acted out or rehearsed.

Schizophrenia. Psychotic disorder marked by cognitive and affective symptoms including hallucination, dissociation, and inappropriate emotional reactions; this disorder involves an inability to adequately respond to the demands of external reality.

Secondary process. Of "Ego."

Secondary or acquired reinforcer. Desirable response consequences related to but not directly biological in nature.

Sedative drugs. Chemical substance which when ingested results in a noticeable reduction in mood and activity level. These drugs when administered in low doses act as *depressants* and when administered in high doses as hypnotics.

Self actualization. The development of greater fulfillment of one's potential as a person.

Self concept. An individual's enduring consciousness of his own identity as he relates to his environment.

Self control. Therapeutic approach based upon the idea that individuals can exert influence over their own performance and other procedures affecting learning and performance.

Self disclosure. The processes of revealing aspects about oneself to some other person and thereby seeing oneself more clearly and less defensively.

Self esteem. Relative balance of positive and negative feelings a person holds about himself.

Self-ideal discrepancy. An inconsistency between the way one regards himself and what he would like to be.

Self image. How an individual conceptualizes himself both in his eyes and how he thinks others view him; an aspect of his sense of identity.

Set. Psychological expectation of what will occur in a given situation and what behaviors are or are not appropriate.

Shaping. Instrumental reinforcement of successive approximations toward a desired behavior.

Social stratification. Ranking members of a society in vertical series of horizontal layers or strata on the basis of economic-cultural differences between people.

Somatic weakness theory. Hypothesis explaining the form of psychosomatic symptomatology as reflecting the physical or physiological vulnerabilities of individuals.

Specific conflict theory. Hypothesis explaining the forms of psychosomatic symptomatology as resulting from physiological reactions to specific emotional states.

Stagnation. Eriksonian concept referring to the sense of unproductiveness and incompleteness experienced by one unable to successfully confront the demands of adulthood around personal and occupational achievement. *See* Generativity.

Stereotype. Expectations one has about how members of a particular group are supposed to act.

Stimulant drug. Chemical substance which when ingested produces noticeable elevations in mood, increases reductions or delays in fatigue (e.g., benzedrine and the amphetamines).

Stimulus. An event, either within or external to the organism, that is responsible for the response to it.

Stimulus generalization. The "spread" of a conditional stimulus such that stimuli like a conditioned stimulus will elicit the same or similar conditioned response.

Sublimation. A defense mechanism in which there is a substitution of socially accepted means of satisfying impulses that would otherwise be antisocial in nature.

Superego. Psychoanalytic concept referring to that segment of personality involved with restricting the expression of instinctual urges according to rigid, uncompromising moral principles.

Suppression. A conscious and volitional inhibition of unwanted ideas or memories.

Synanon. Organized community of former heroin addicts actively involved in the rehabilitation of drug users.

Syntaxic thought. Cognitive pattern described by Sullivan in which verbal and nonverbal symbols can be processed according to basic principles of logic and reason.

Systematic desensitization. A behavior therapy technique based on operant conditioning paradigm in which relaxation, a fear-inhibiting response, is paired with the fear-arousing stimuli. *See* Counterconditioning technique.

T-group. Group procedure for facilitating interpersonal functioning by having participants openly discuss their perceptions and reactions to each other.

"Taster." Slang term referring to one who irregularly and without dependency experiments with a variety of drugs.

Token economy. Example of a behavior therapy technique utilizing operant reinforcement in the form of a token for retraining to a new desirable behavior. This is usually employed with a given population.

Tolerance. *See* Drug addiction.

Transactional analysis. A therapy used in group situations; a way of examining the communication in which one person does something to another and receives a response from him.

Transference. Psychoanalytic treatment technique whereby remaining detached from and personally unknown by the patient, the analyst becomes a blank screen onto which the patient can project feelings he has toward significant other people in his life.

Unconditioned response. (UCR) Typically expected, automatic, or reflexive response to an unconditioned stimulus.

Unconditioned stimulus (USC). In classical conditioning, a stimulus that elicits a response innately, without training or conditioning.

Unconscious motivation. Behavior influenced by aspects of our personality about which we are minimally, if at all, aware.

Values. Those attitudes that are well established and therefore influence behavior, usually involving one's strong preferences, ethics, and morals.

Variable behavior. Constantly changing behavior aroused by a motivating condition.

Variable interval reinforcement. Reinforcement of the first correct response after a varying interval of time.

Variable responses ratio reinforcement. Variable number of responses required per reinforcement; i.e., reinforcement sometimes after 5 responses, sometimes after 6 responses, etc., defining an *average* ratio of responses per reinforcement.

Waxy flexibility. Symptom of catatonic schizophrenia marked by the tendency to maintain whatever physical position is imposed on one.

Withdrawal reaction. One broad arbitrary classification of defense mechanisms relating behaviors that are somewhat similar; these defense mechanisms allow the individual to deny or withdraw from the situation producing anxiety.

Withdrawal syndrome. Physiological reaction to the cessation of drug use including feelings of nausea, cramps, fever, gastrointestinal disturbances, etc.; the duration and severity of the reaction depend on the specific drug used and the level and duration of its use.

Name Index

Subject Index